COLOR ATLAS OF MICROSURGERY

Sun Lee, MD
Director, San Diego Microsurgical Institute and Training Center at Mercy Hospital; Adjunct Professor of Surgery, University of California at San Diego, School of Medicine; Associate Member, Academic Affairs (Adjunct), Scripps Clinic and Research Foundation, La Jolla, California

Wolff M. Kirsch, MD
Professor of Neurosurgery and Director of Neurological Research, Loma Linda University, School of Medicine

Fu-Chan Wei, MD
Director, Microsurgery and Extremity Reconstruction Center, Department of Plastic Surgery, Chang Gung Memorial Hospital, Taipei, Taiwan

Jonathan Jones, MD
Assistant Clinical Professor of Surgery, University of California at San Diego; Microsurgical Attending Surgeon, Mercy Hospital Medical Center, San Diego, CA; Faculty, San Diego Microsurgical Institute and Training Center at Mercy Hospital

Raphael B. Durfee, MD
Associate Clinical Professor of Reproductive Medicine, University of California San Diego Medical School; Associate Director, San Diego Microsurgical Institute and Training Center at Mercy Hospital

Ishiyaku EuroAmerica, Inc., Publishers
St. Louis · Tokyo

Book Editor: Gregory Hacke, D.C.

Ishiyaku EuroAmerica, Inc.
716 Hanley Industrial Court, St. Louis, Missouri 63144

PHONE ORDERS CALL TOLL FREE 800-MED-1921

Library of Congress Catalogue Number 92-56746

Lee, Sun
COLOR ATLAS OF MICROSURGERY

ISBN 0-912791-64-0

Ishiyaku EuroAmerica, Inc.
St. Louis • Tokyo

Composition by: HiTec Typeset, 101 Orr, Columbia, Missouri 65201
Printed in Japan

Dedicated

To

Mr. and Mrs. Dirk C. Kok, Jr.

NOTICE

CONTRIBUTORS

Zisis Buokuovalas, MD
Research Fellow, Division of Neurosurgery, Loma Linda University School of Medicine, Loma Linda, California

Norman Browse, MD, FACS
Professor of Surgery, United Medical and Dental Schools of Guy and St. Thomas Hospital, University of London, London, England

Robert Chapolini, MD
President, Loma Linda Microsurgical Laboratory, Loma Linda, California

John Chrisler, MD
Director, Loma Linda Microsurgical Laboratory, Loma Linda, California

David Cooley, MD
Resident, Loma Linda University Medical Center, Loma Linda, California

Robert Cushman, MD
President, Cushman Engineering, Albuquerque, New Mexico

Milbhor D'Silva, MD
Instructor, San Diego Microsurgical Institute at Mercy Hospital Medical Center, San Diego, California

Paul J. Formosa, MD
Assistant Professor, Division of Plastic Surgery, University of California Irvine Medical Center, Irvine, California

David Furness, MD
Clinical Professor of Surgery, Chief of Plastic Surgery, University of California Irvine Medical Center, Irvine, California

Robert A. Hardesty, MD
Chief of the Division of Plastic and Reconstructive Surgery, Loma Linda University School of Medicine, Loma Linda, California

Sobhi Hweidi, MD
Instructor, San Diego Microsurgical Institute San Diego, California

David Knierim, MD
Associate Professor and Chairman, Director of Residency Program, Division of Neurosurgery and Pediatric Neurosurgery, Loma Linda University School of Medicine, Loma Linda, California

Edmund LeGrand, DVM, PhD
Pathologist, Ethicon Research Foundation, Somerville, New Jersey

Paul Mann, MD
Associate Professor, School of Pharmacy, University of New Mexico, Albuquerque, New Mexico

Kurt Rohwher, MD
Professor, Neurolisches Zentrum, 3510 Hann Munden, Vogelsang 105, Lower Saxony, West Germany

Derek Rutt, BSc, FRCS
Lecturer in Surgery, United Medical and Dental Schools of Guy and St. Thomas Hospital, University of London, London, England

Winfried R. Schott, MD
Director, Neurologisches Zentrum, 3510 Hann Munden, Vogelsang 105, Lower Saxony, West Germany

David Stoloff, DVM, MS
Section manager, Experimental Surgery, Ethicon Research Foundation, Somerville, New Jersey

Martyn H.C. Webster, MD
Consultant Plastic Surgeon, West of Scotland Regional Plastic and Maxillofacial Surgery Unit, Canniesburn Hospital, Bearsden, Glasgow, Scotland

Nicholas M. Wilson, MD
Lecturer in Surgery, United Medical and Dental Schools of Guy and St. Thomas Hospital, University of London, London, England

Yong Hua Zhu, MD
Assistant Research Professor, Loma Linda University School of Medicine and Jerry L. Pettis Veterans Administration Hospital, Loma Linda, California

CONTENTS

FOREWORD

If the unprecedented and pioneering abilities of Dr. Sun Lee can ever be immortalized in a color atlas, a great cause will have been served. An entire generation of surgeons have looked to his skills for the development of new microsurgical procedures and for personal tutelage on their accomplishment for important surgical research. Sun Lee has avoided the trappings of expensive and cumbersome magnification techniques or elaborate special instruments. With equipment available anywhere in the world, he has demonstrated the length to which microsurgery can be successfully applied in surgical research. We all wish the best success to this atlas documenting his achievements and proselytizing his teachings for the future.

Ruben F. Gittes, MD
Chairman, Department of Surgery,
Urologic Surgeon, Scripps Clinic and
Research Foundation, La Jolla, CA

PREFACE

Over the last several decades, microsurgical techniques that originated and were refined in the laboratory have led to brilliant developments in clinical microvascular, microneural, tubal and vasovasal anastomoses. The application of these microsurgical techniques to tissue and organ transplantation in clinical surgery has produced dramatic results in prolonging life. Those microsurgical techniques have permiated almost every surgical discipline, extending the horizons of clinical reconstructive surgery in general.

In this atlas we have enumerated various microvascular anastomosing techniques, including the conventional, open-loop and the nonsuture silver microclip methods. Pancreaticoduodenal transplantation in the rodent was added to this list by way of symbolizing to the reader the capabilities of this art. The reader can refer to other standard texts for other organ transplantation procedures.

The clinical use of silver clips in microvascular anastomoses is illustrated by Kirsch and Zhu, whereas Wei and Jones elaborate the use of conventional suture techniques in plastic reconstructive surgery. Durfee's illustrations on gynecologic infertility microsurgery are a valuable contribution from the teaching texts at the San Diego Microsurgical Institute and Training Center.

Sun Lee, MD
San Diego Microsurgical Institute
and Training Center at Mercy Hospital
Medical Center, San Diego, California

Section I

Basic
Microsurgical Procedures

Chapter 1

End-To-End Microvascular Anastomosis: Open-Loop Technique

Sun Lee, MD
Milbhor D'Silva, MD
Sobhi A. Hweidi, MD

Employing the open-loop technique, the operator sees each edge he or she should be suturing and there is no blind-needling. Thus, the anastomosis has a lesser possibility of stenosis. Following placement of two stay sutures 180° apart, the anterior edges are loosely sutured using even-distances; then one of the stay sutures is brought under these loose loops by passing a mosquito hemostat through the loops. This stay suture is then retracted gently. Thus, all the loops are put down on one side to avoid entanglement. The first loop is cut close to one stay suture and is tied, avoiding an excessive length for the suture and is tied, avoiding an excessive length for the short tail. This motion is repeated for the remaining loops. As to the continuous technique, each loop is simply pulled consecutively; at the finish it is tied to the stay suture. The posterior edges are treated in the same manner.

A vascular approximator is applied on the vessel, it is divided, flushed with saline, and the adventitia is trimmed.

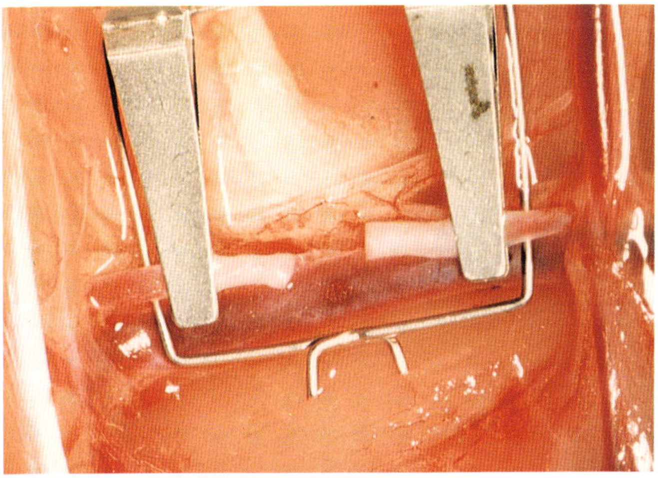

Fig. 1-1

A stay suture is placed on one side.

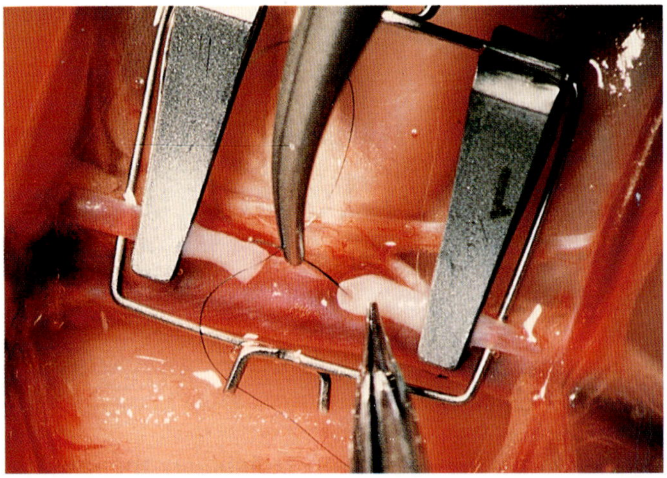

Fig. 1-2

An opposing stay suture is placed 180° apart from the other.

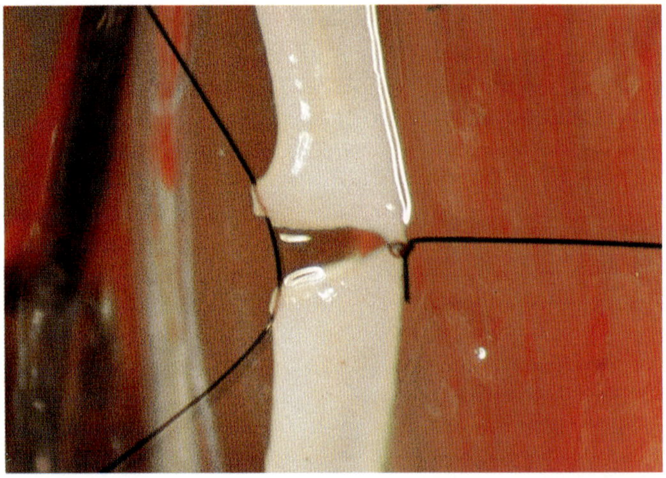

Fig. 1-3

The short tails of the stay sutures are gently retracted.

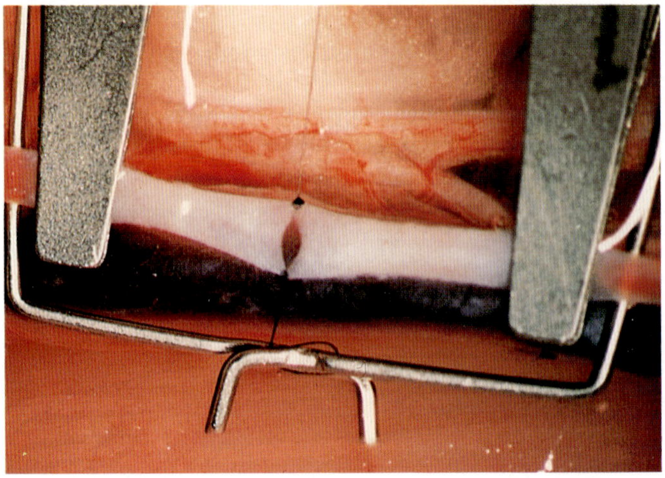

Fig. 1-4

Three open loops have been placed.

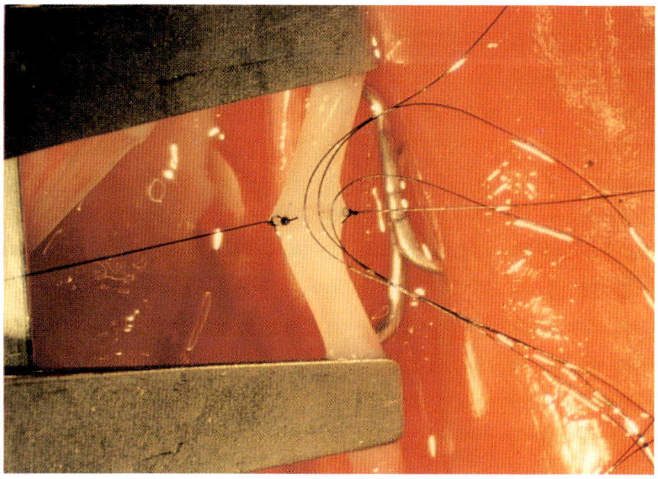

Fig. 1-5

Four equally spaced open loops are visualized between stay sutures (1 mm diameter).

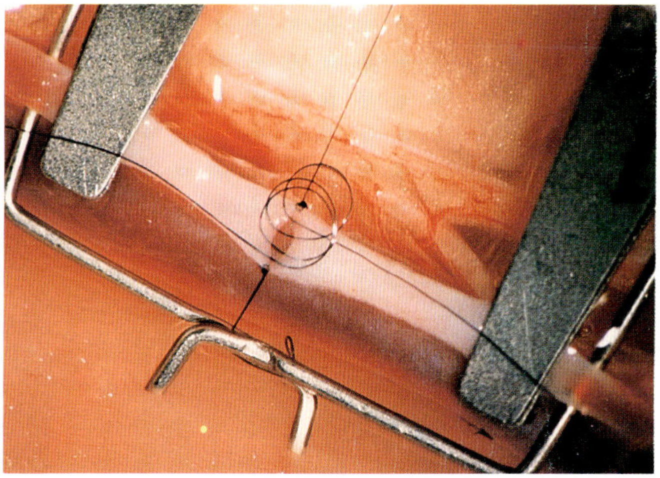

Fig. 1-6

In this higher magnification, the first loop is being cut closely to the stay suture.

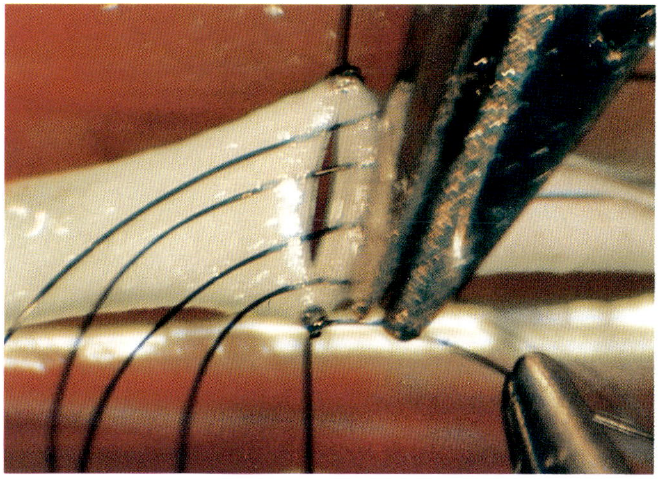

Fig. 1-7

The first loop is gently pulled to bring the suture end near vessel edge for tying.

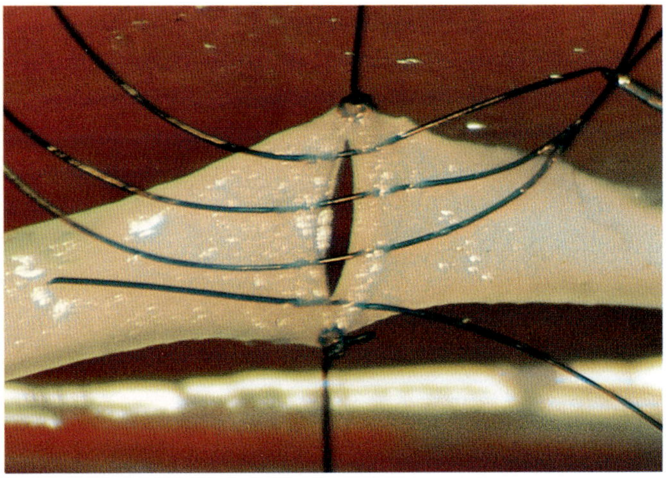

Fig. 1-8

The first knot has been made.

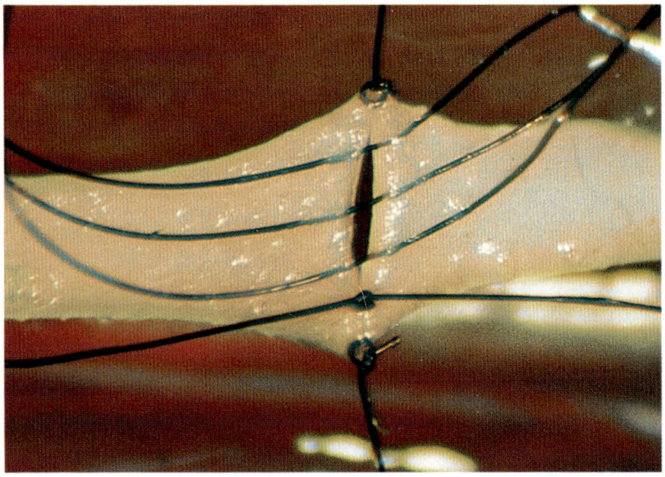

Fig. 1-9

The second knot has been completed.

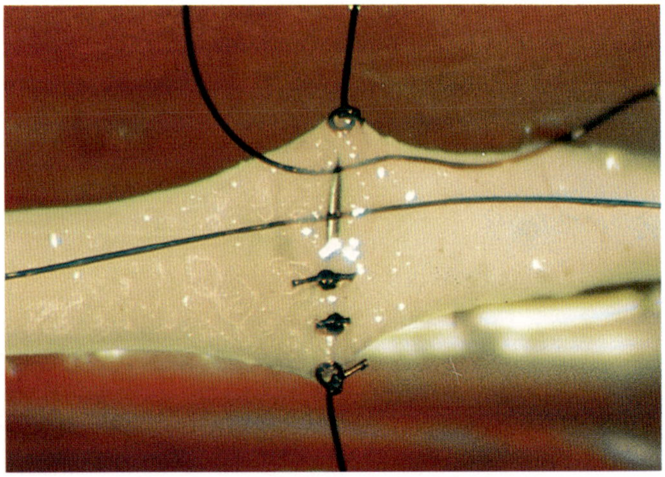

Fig. 1-10

The fourth knot has been completed. A blood vessel of 1 mm in diameter needs four sutures between stay sutures.

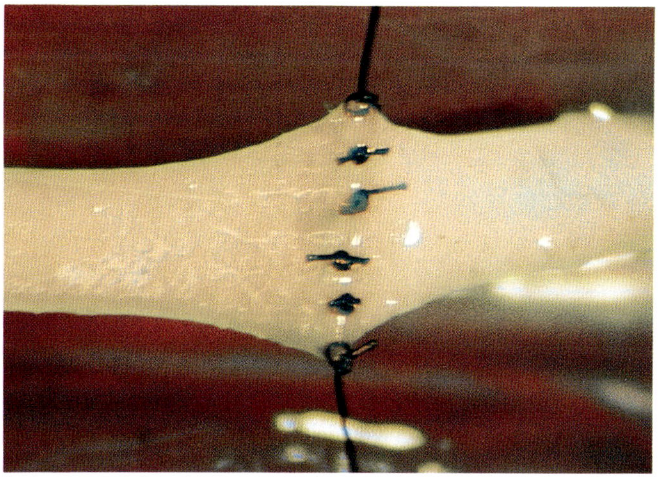

Fig. 1-11

The blood vessel is now flipped and the posterior edges are visualized.

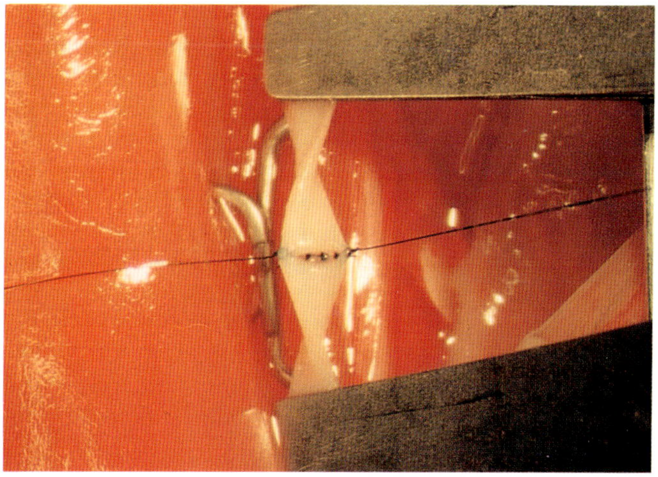

Fig. 1-12

The first suture is placed.

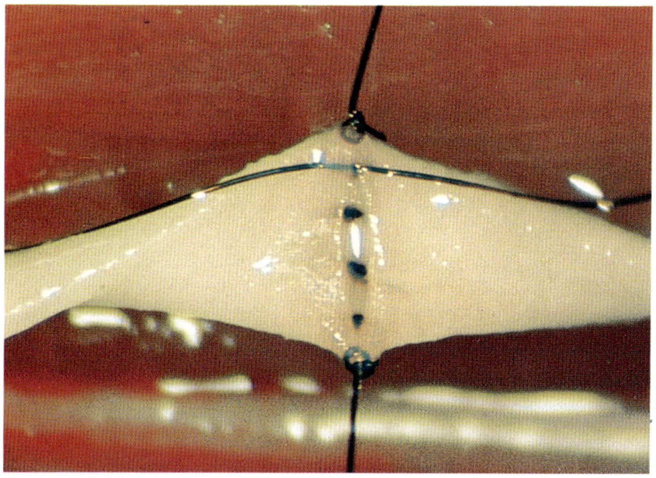

Fig. 1-13

The second loop is being placed.

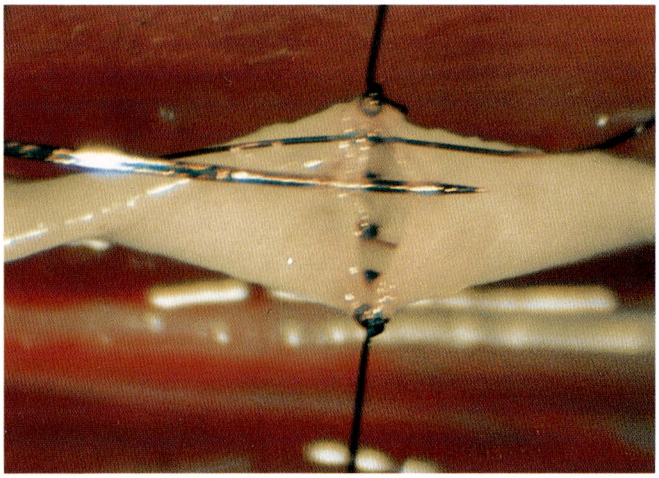

Fig. 1-14

All four loops on the posterior edges have been placed.

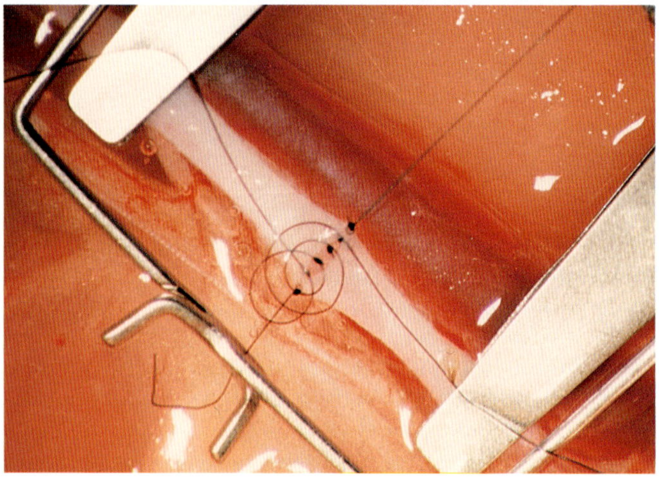

Fig. 1-15

All loops were individualy tied.

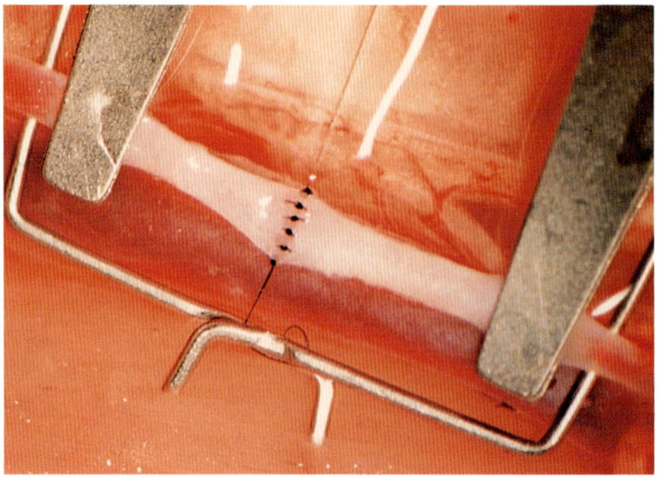

Fig. 1-16

Clamps were released and the circulation has been restored.

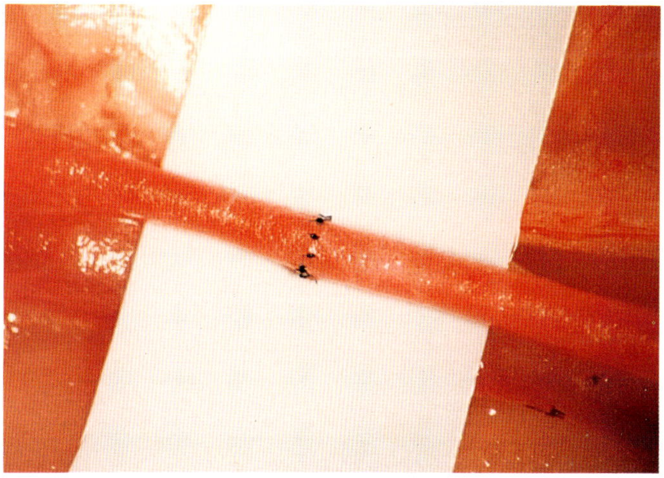

Fig. 1-17

Suggested Reading

Lee S, Hweidi SA, Skivolocki WP. An open-loop technique to facilitate microtubal (microvascular, vasovasal, uterine) anastomoses in the rat. *J Reconstr Microsurg.* 1984;1:45.

Chapter 2

End-To-End Microvascular Anatomosis: Combined Open-Loop and Conventional Techniques

Sun Lee, MD
Milbhor D'Silva, MD
Sobhi A. Hweidi, MD

If the blood vessel segments are not long enough to be turned, it is preferable to start to suture from the posterior edges. With this technique, knots are left outside the vessel. In addition to these interrupted sutures along the posterior lines, the anterior edges may be sutured using the open-loop suture technique to assure that no needle on the anterior edges would have caught the back side.

The blood vessel is cut.

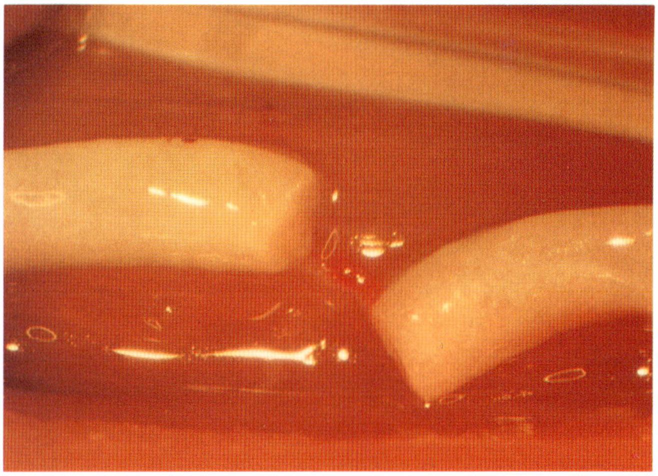

Fig. 2-1

The blood vessel edges are cleaned, including adventitia.

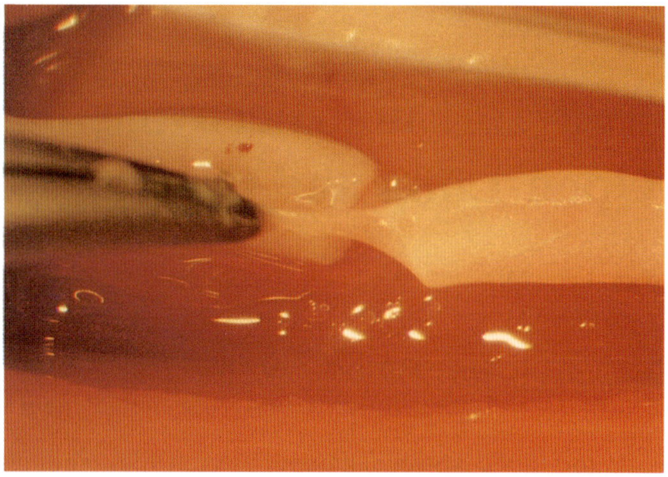

Fig. 2-2

The outside-in suture is placed at the back edge.

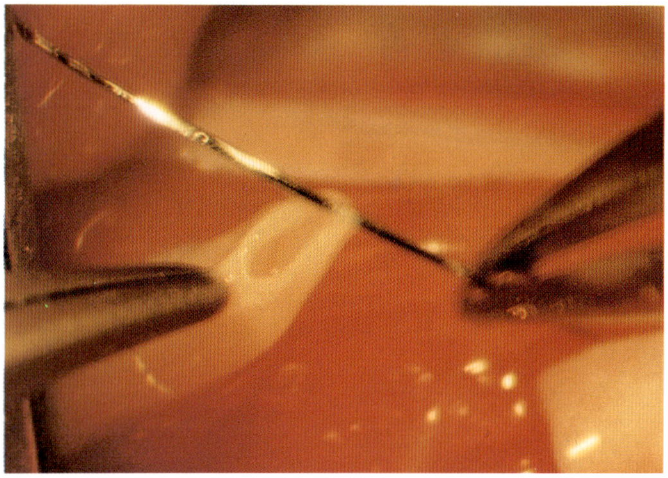

Fig. 2-3

The inside-out suture is placed and tied, leaving the knot in the serosal surface.

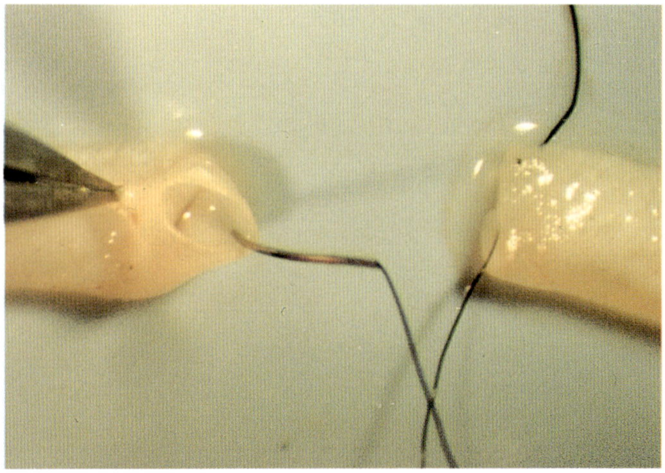

Fig. 2-4

The first suture is tied.

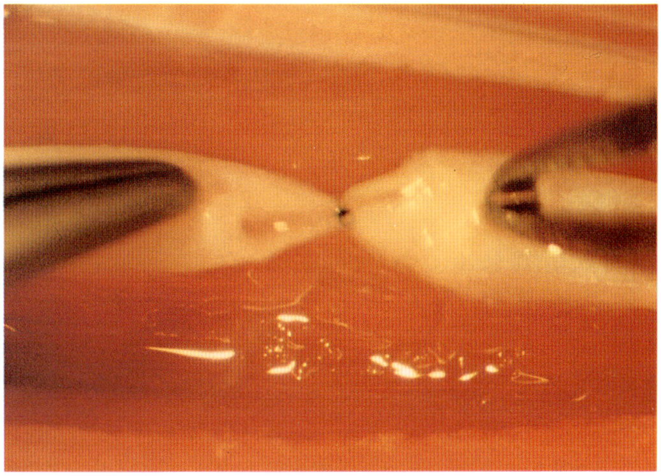

Fig. 2-5

The second interrupted suture is placed next to the first suture and tied.

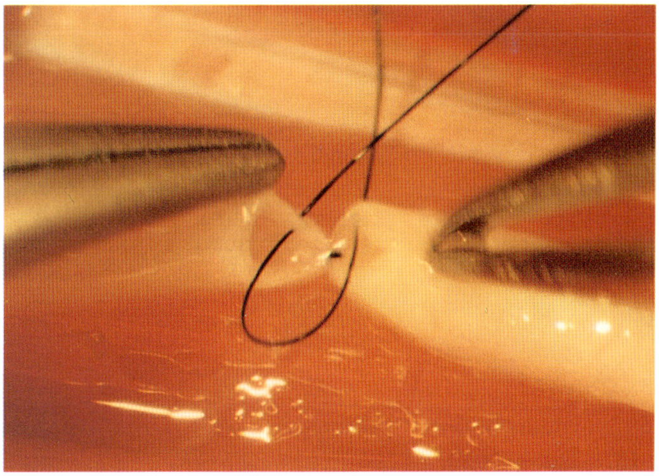

Fig. 2-6

The third suture is placed likewise.

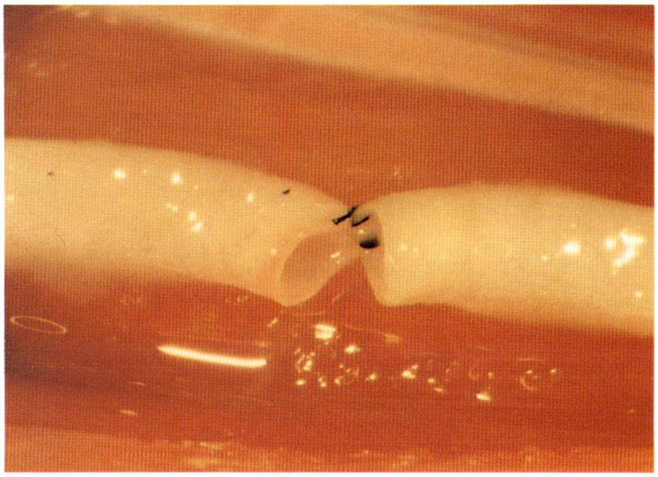

Fig. 2-7

The fifth suture is placed likewise.

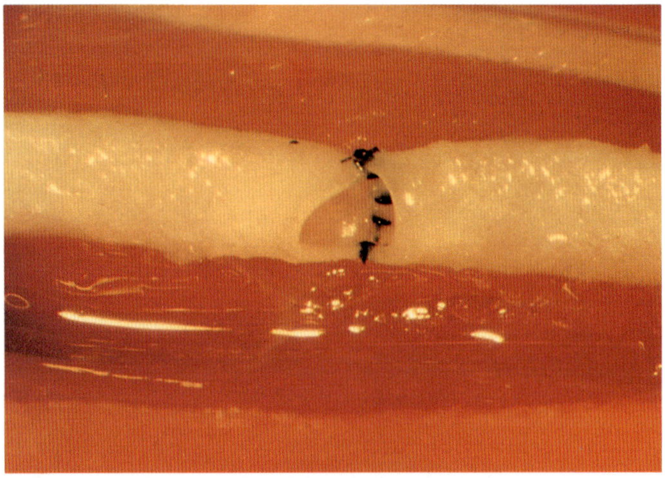

Fig. 2-8

Few open-loop sutures are placed anteriorly.

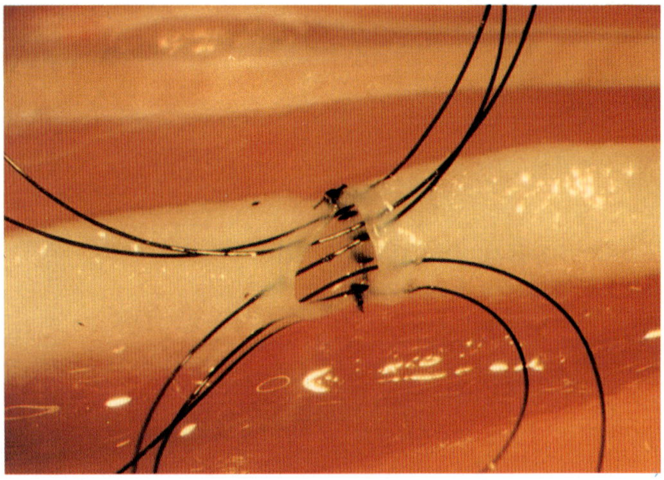

Fig. 2-9

All sutures have been placed.

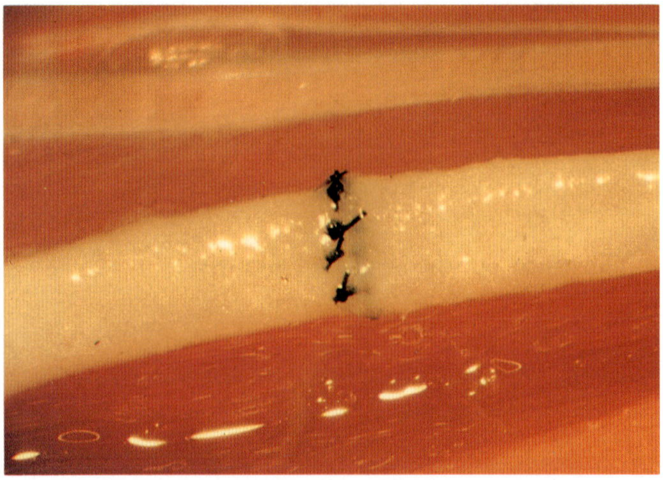

Fig. 2-10

Suggested Reading

Buncke HJ, Schulz WP. Total ear reimplantation in the rabbit utilizing microminiature microvascular anastomoses. *Brit J Plast Surg*. 1966;10:15.

Cobbett JR. Microvascular surgery. *Surg Clin North Am*. 1964;47:679.

Lee S, Hweidi SA, Skivolocki WP. An open-loop technique to facilitate microtubal (microvascular, vasovasal, uterine) anastomoses in the rat. *J Reconstr Microsurg*. 1984;1:45.

Chapter 3
Modified Conventional End-To-End Microvascular Anastomosis

Milbhor D'Silva, MD
Sun Lee, MD
Sobhi A. Hweidi, MD

Even when placing the stay suture either 120° or 180° apart, it is hard to avoid placing the last stitch in the blind manner when the conventional microvascular anastomotic technique is exercised. To avoid such a serious error, this technique has been modified in such a way that at least the last two stitches are left open to see if the needle has caught the back wall of the vessel, after which these sutures are tied.

The blood vessel is severed.

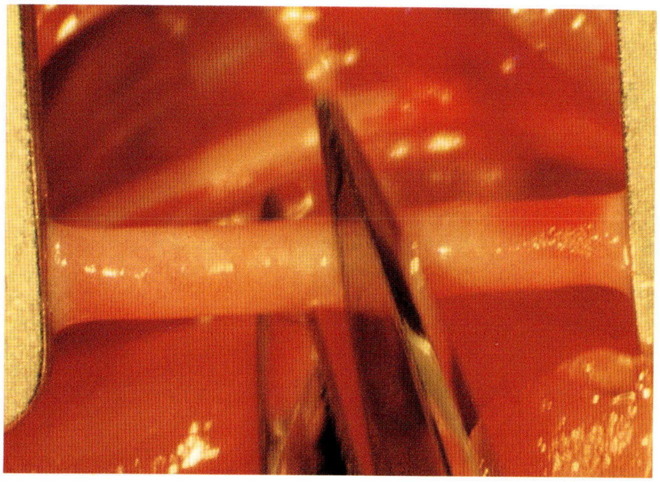

Fig. 3-1

The blood vessel lumens are flushed with saline.

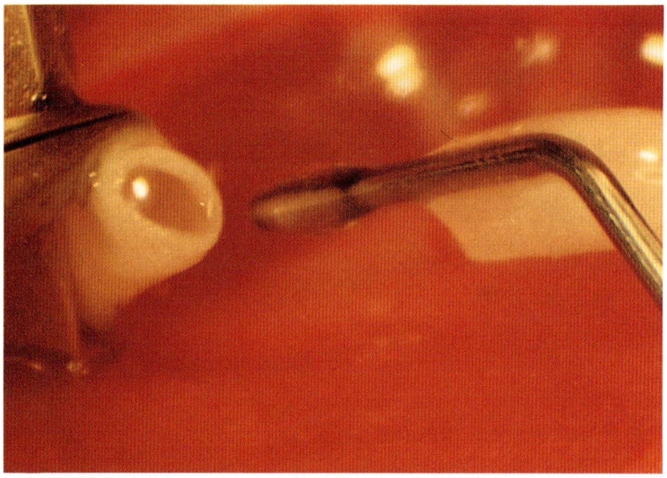

Fig. 3-2

Jeweler's forceps blades are inserted into the vessel lumen to receive the needle.

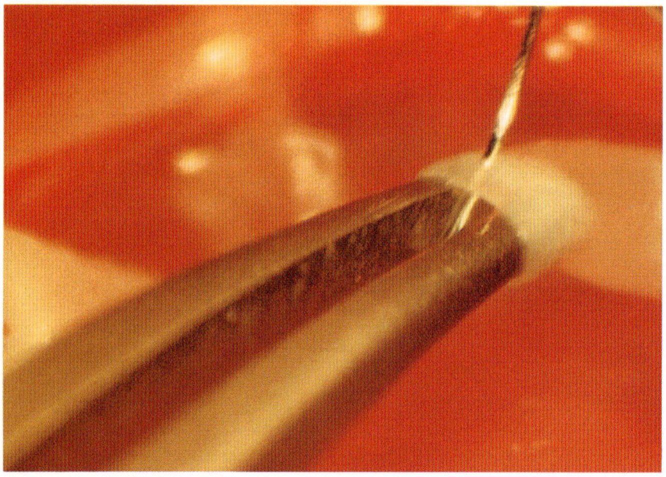

Fig. 3-3

Once the needle has been inserted by an outside-in motion, the needle is employed to pierce the opposite vessel edge by an inside-out motion.

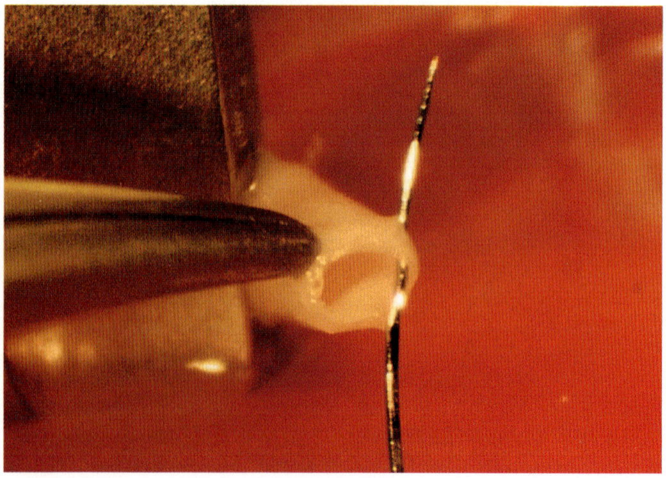

Fig. 3-4

The first stay suture is tied.

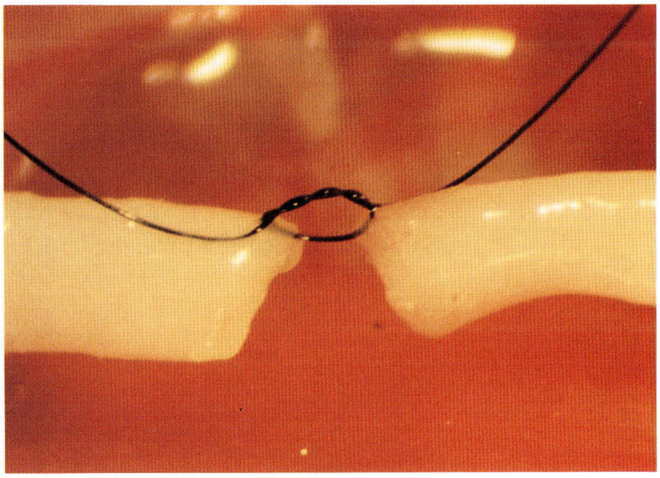

Fig. 3-5

The stay suture is placed either 180° or 120° apart.

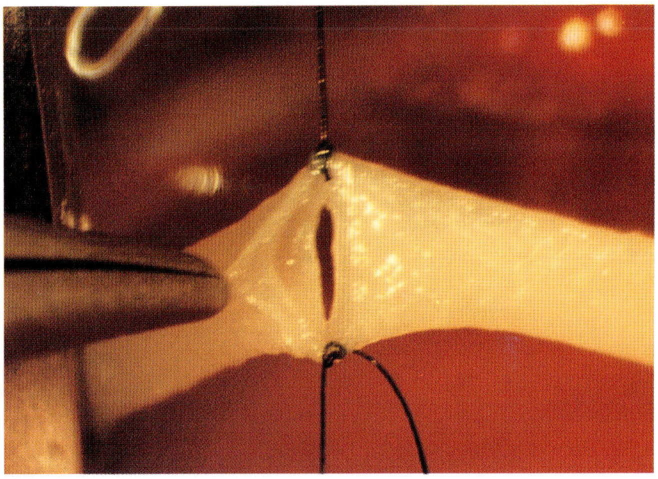

Fig. 3-6

The first interrupted suture is placed next to the stay suture by an outside-in motion.

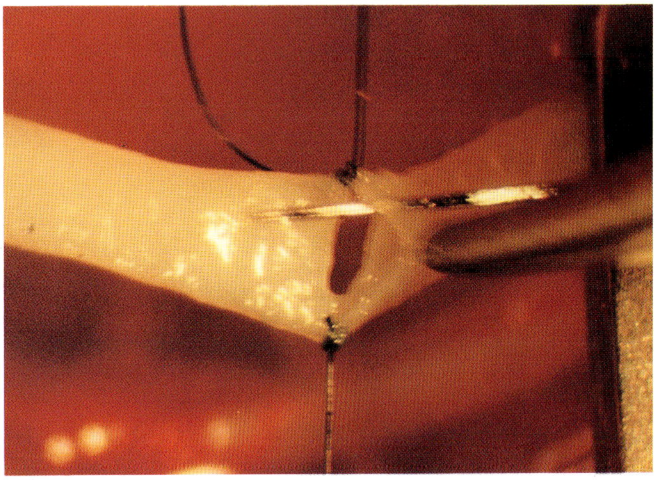

Fig. 3-7

The first interrupted suture is then brought outside of the vessel.

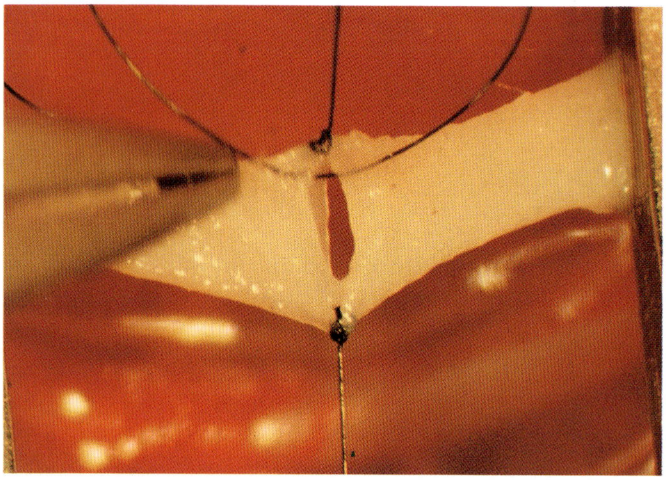

Fig. 3-8

All but two sutures are left open to see if the needle has caught the back edges, after which they are tied.

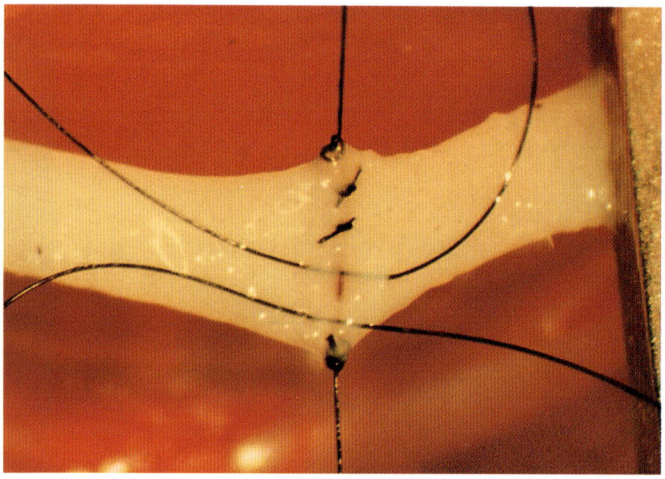

Fig. 3-9

Showing the last tie being placed on anterior edges.

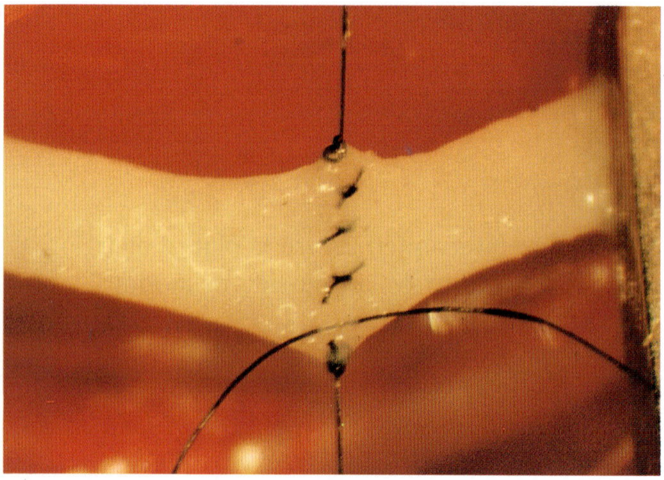

Fig. 3-10

All sutures on the anterior edges are seen.

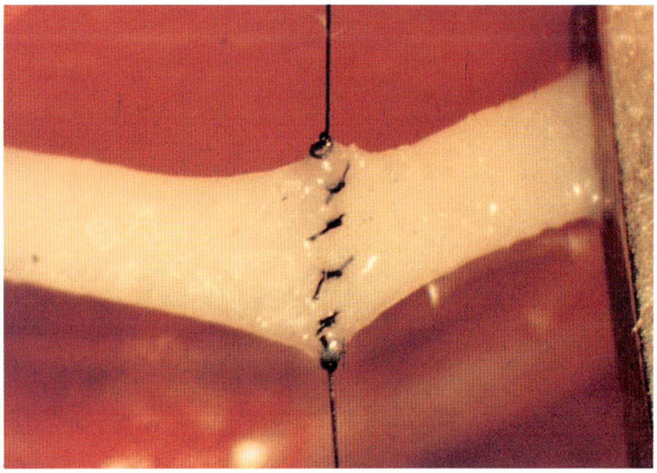

Fig. 3-11

The blood vessel has been reflected and the anterior edge anastomosis is shown through the posterior opening.

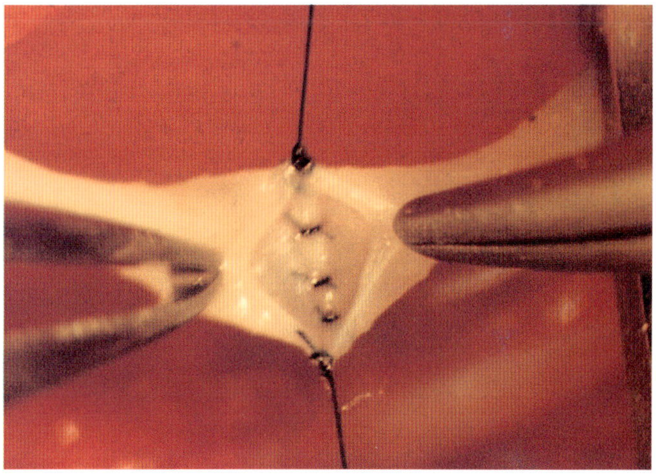

Fig. 3-12

Suggested Reading

Lee S. *Manual of Microsurgery*. Boca Raton, Florida: C.R.C. Press;1985.

Chapter 4

End-To-Side Microvascular Anastomosis

Sun Lee, MD
Milbhor D'Silva, MD

As a typical example, the end-to-side portacaval shunt procedure is described here. The inferior vena cava (IVC) does not need extensive mobilization. The pyloric vein may or may not need ligation and division depending on its proximity to the liver hilum. Clamping the IVC with the Lee Portacaval shunt (PCS) clamp enables the IVC and portal vein (PV) to lie adjacent to each other to make the anastomosis. An eliptical opening is made on the IVC and is flushed with saline. Stay sutures are placed at each end of the opening in the IVC to receive the corresponding edges of the PV, after which the stay suture with the needle is used to pierce the posterior edges of the IVC next to the stay suture in an outside-in fashion. A continuous technique is used to suture the posterior edges. Thereafter, the needle is brought out through the IVC at the lower corner and is tied to the stay suture. Using the open-loop technique, the anterior edges are sutured, usually in continuous manner, after which it is tied to the upper stay suture.

The end vessel (portal vein) is being ligated and clamped proximally and cut.

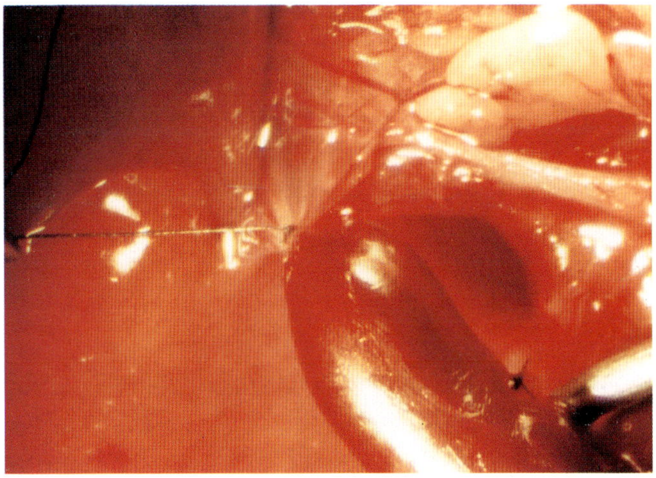

Fig. 4-1

The side vessel is clamped longitudinally and the end of the end vessel is brought closer to the side vessel (vena cava).

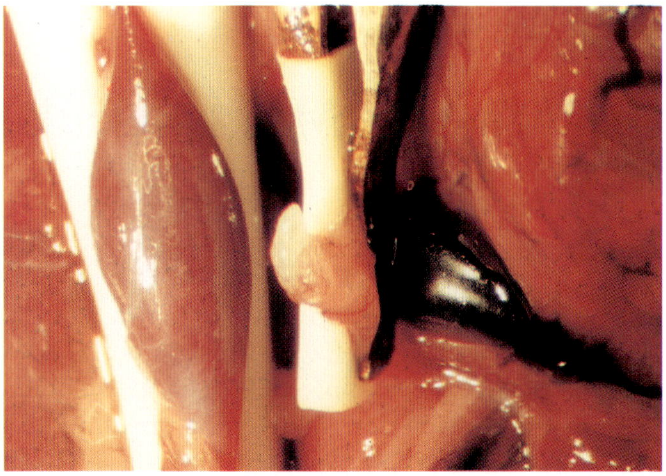

Fig. 4-2

A venotomy is being made using #11 knife blade and flushed with saline.

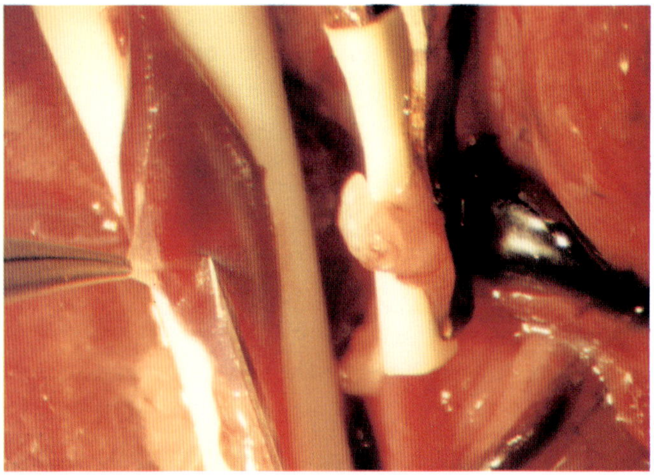

Fig. 4-3

An outside-in suture is placed at the upper corner of the side vessel.

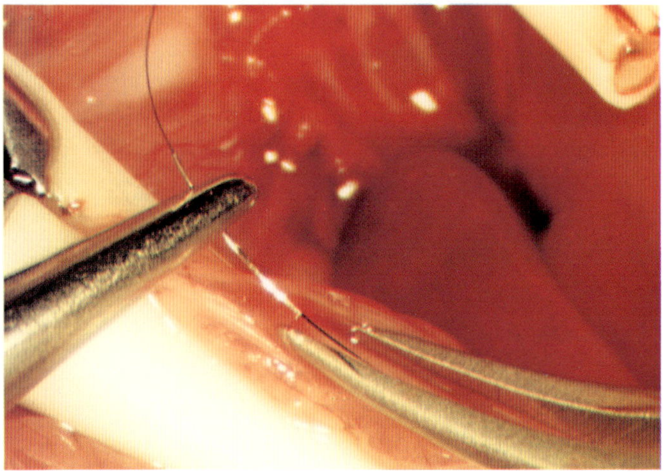

Fig. 4-4

An opening of the side vessel is shown. A lower corner (IVC) suture is placed.

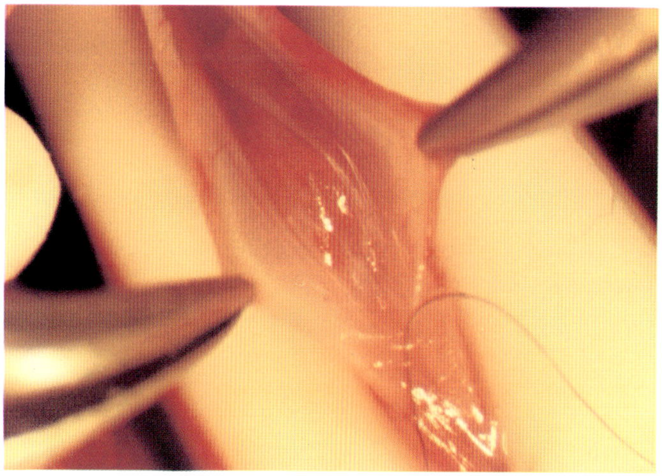

Fig. 4-5

An inside-out suture is placed at the lower corner of the end vessel and tied to bring corners of both vessels together.

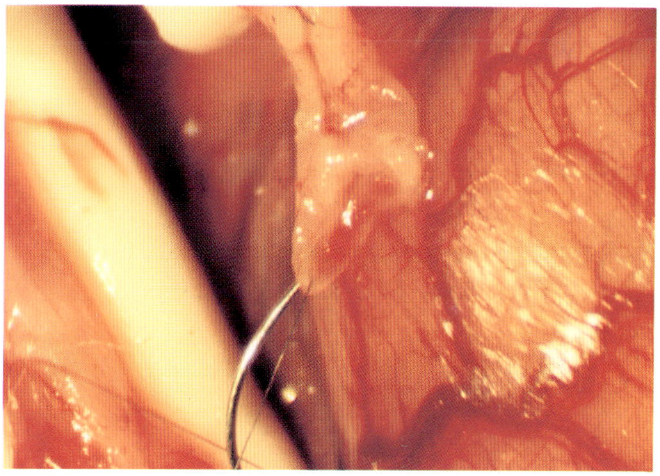

Fig. 4-6

The upper corner suture is placed between two vessels.

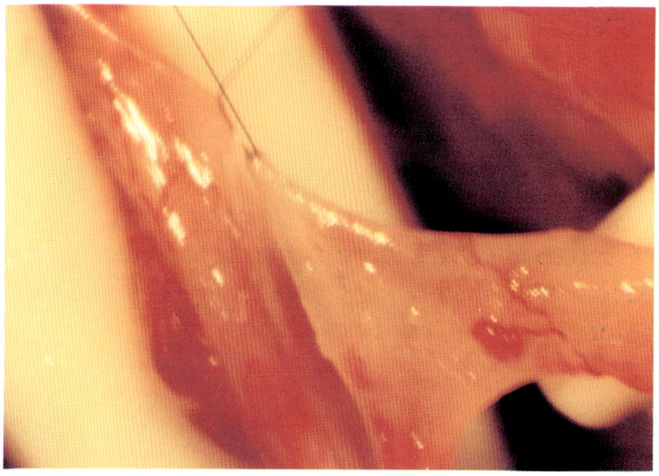

Fig. 4-7

Using the upper suture-needle, the first stitch is entered into the IVC edge.

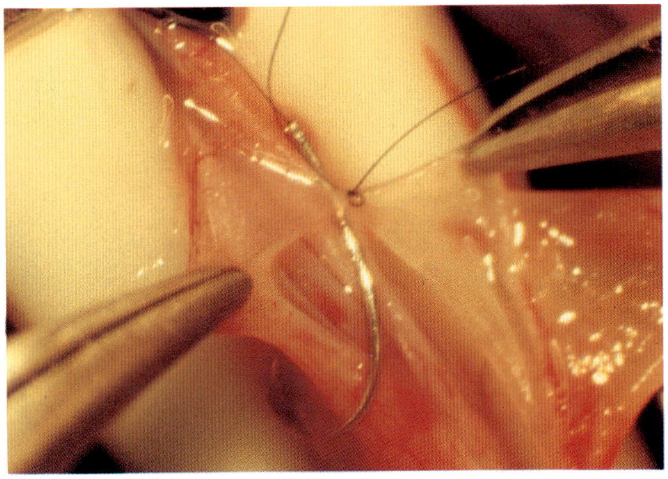

Fig. 4-8

Assisted by the blade of a forceps, the back edge of the portal vein (PV) is pierced. At this time both IVC and PV edges are taken.

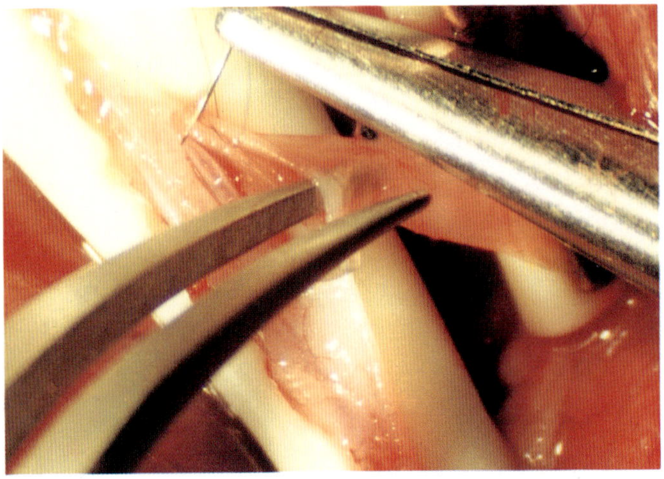

Fig. 4-9

The over-and-over stitching method is used to suture the back edges, after which the needle is brought out through the IVC's anterior wall at the lower corner.

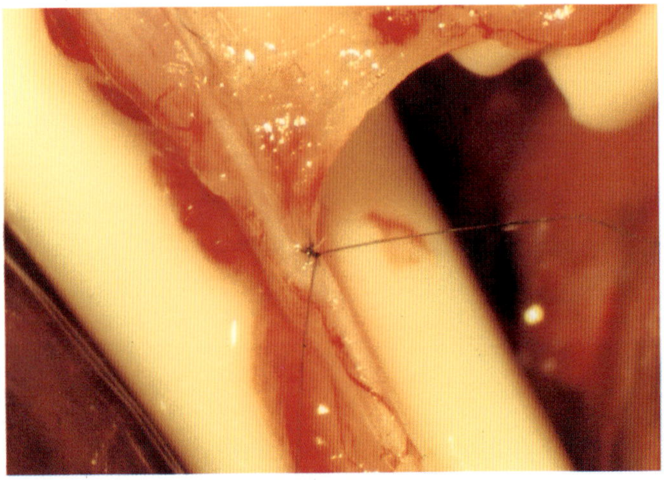

Fig. 4-10

Check to see if any opposite wall has been caught by the needle.

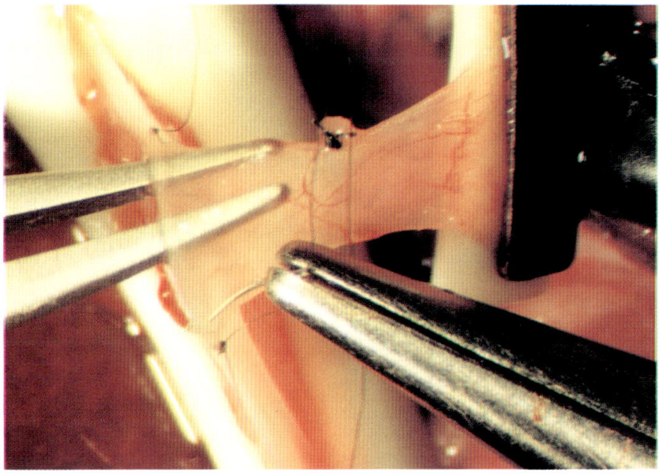

Fig. 4-11

The anterior flaps of both sides are sutured following the one-cell bite concept in continuous fashion.

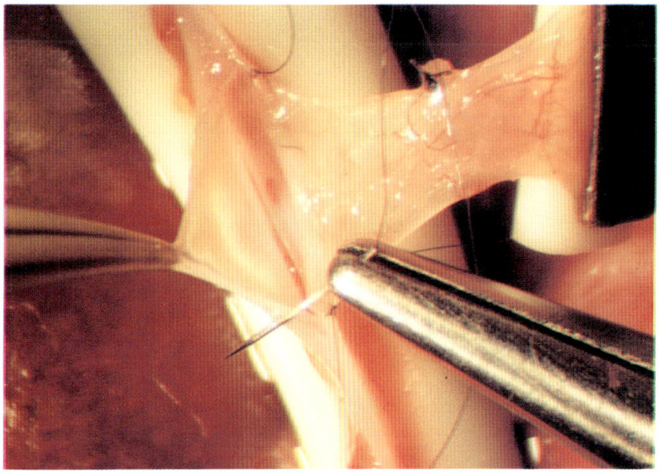

Fig. 4-12

Be careful not to bite the back edges.

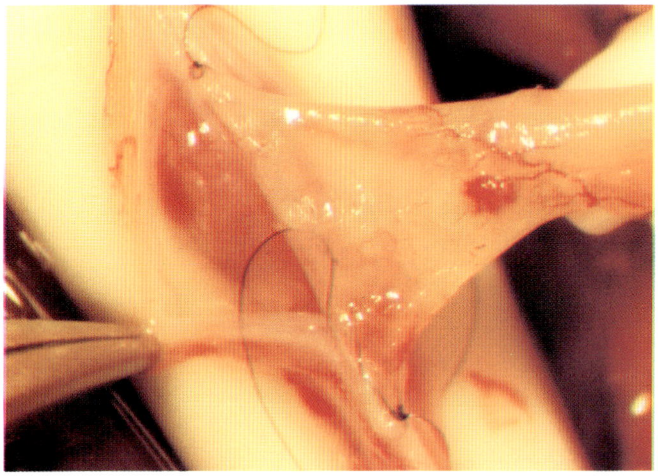

Fig. 4-13

The last two or three stitches are loosely placed to assure that the needle has not caught the back edges.

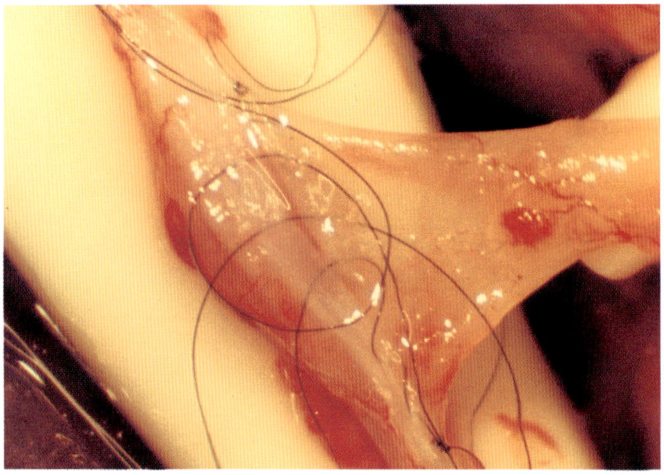

Fig. 4-14

The suture has been pulled gently so as not to cause a purse-string effect, and is tied to the upper short tail.

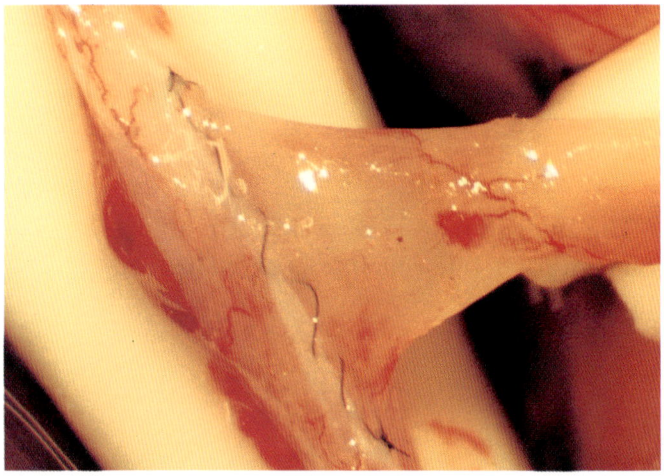

Fig. 4-15

The circulation has been reestablished following clamp release.

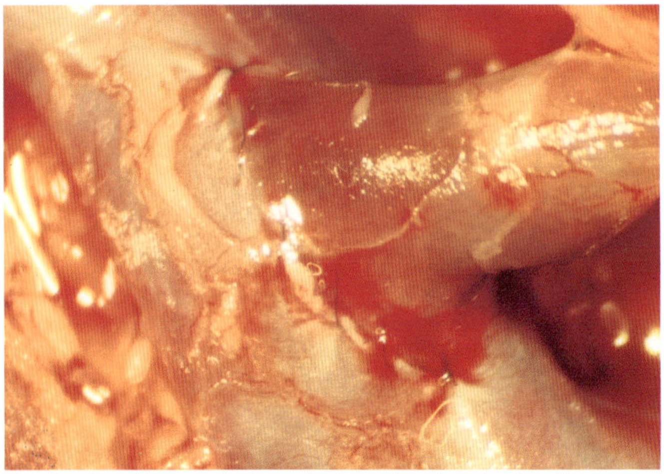

Fig. 4-16

Suggested Reading

Bismuth H, Benhamou JP, Lataste J. L'anastomose porto-cave experimentale chez le rat normal: Technique et resultats preliminaire. *Presse Med.* 1963;25:1858.

Lee S, Fisher B. Portacaval shunt in the rat. *Surgery.* 1961;50:668.

Chapter 5

End-To-Side Microvascular Anastomosis: Large to Small Caliber

Milbhor D'Silva, MD

Sun Lee, MD

Whereas the portacaval shunt deals with a small caliber end vessel that is sutured to the side of a larger vein, the cavalportal shunt involves a larger caliber end vessel that is sutured to the side of a smaller vessel. The IVC between the right renal vein and the lower margin of the liver is completely freed from its surrounding attachments, clamped at the right renal vein entrance level and is tied at the lower margin of the liver, following which it is cut and flushed with saline. The portal vein is clamped longitudinally with the Lee PCS clamp. An appropriately sized venotomy is made (elliptical excision will cause narrowing of the lumen) to receive the IVC. The anastomosis is conducted in a similar manner as for the portacaval shunt.

A large caliber end vessel (IVC) is being prepared in such a way that the cardiac end is ligated; it is clamped at the splenic vein entrance.

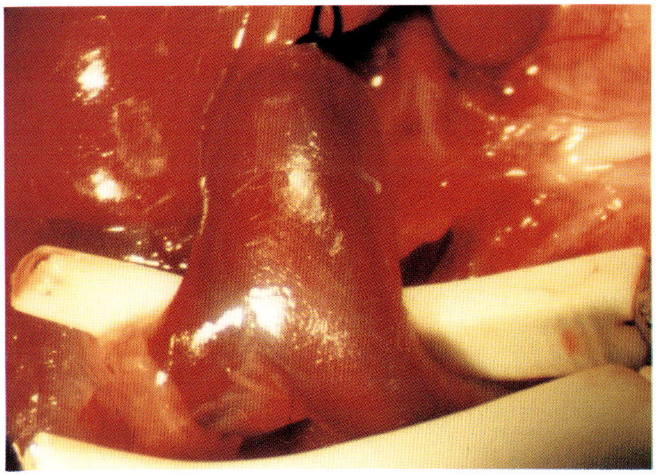

Fig. 5-1

The IVC is cut at the tie.

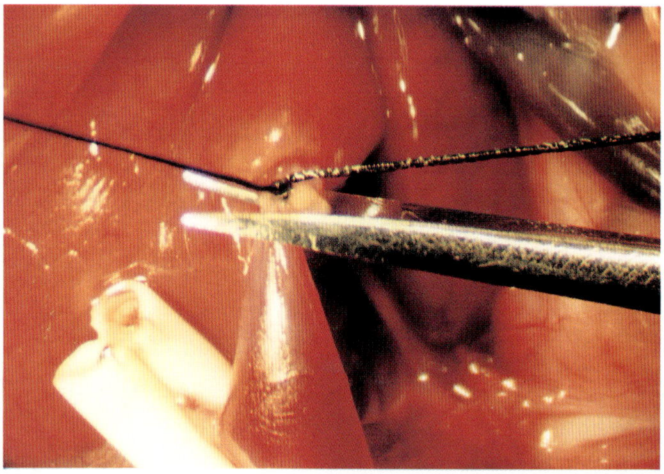

Fig. 5-2

The IVC stump is irrigated and the size estimated in order to make an incision on the side vessel (portal vein).

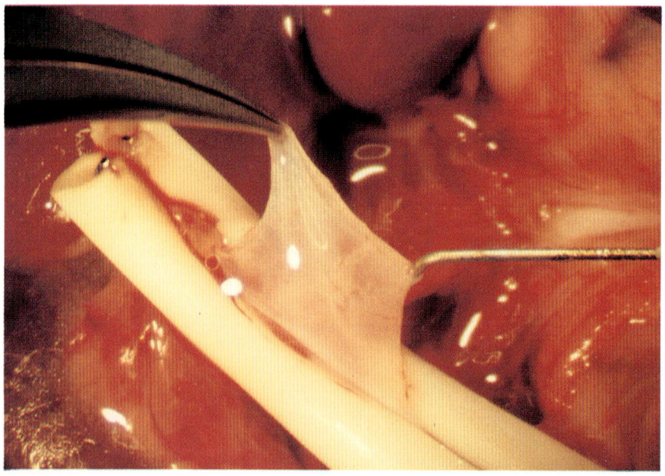

Fig. 5-3

The side vessel (PV) is clamped longitudinally.

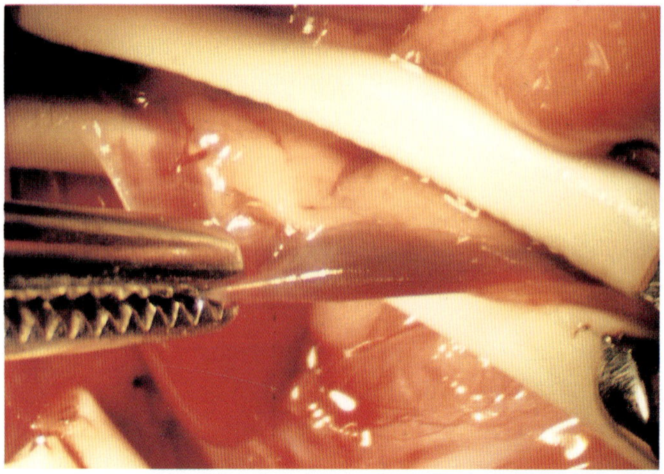

Fig. 5-4

A longitudinal opening is made with a #11 knife blade.

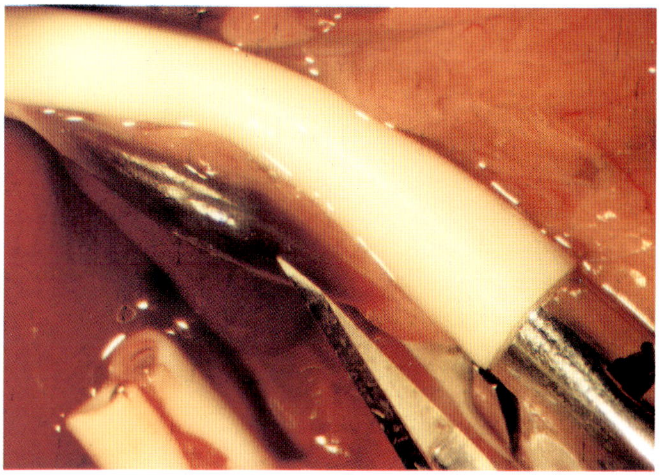

Fig. 5-5

An opening is enlarged to accommodate the IVC.

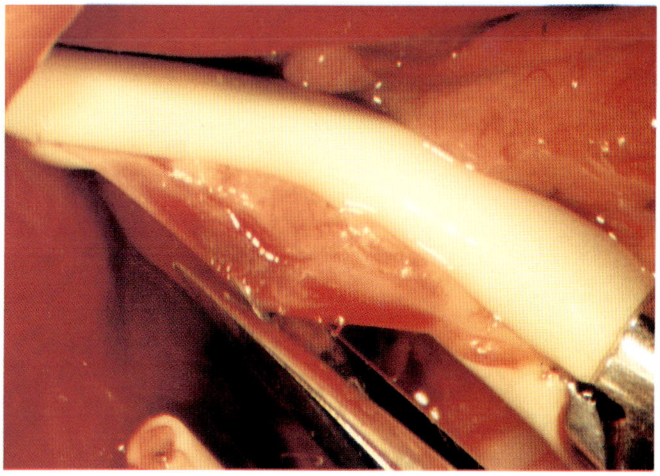

Fig. 5-6

A lower corner stitch is made between IVC and PV.

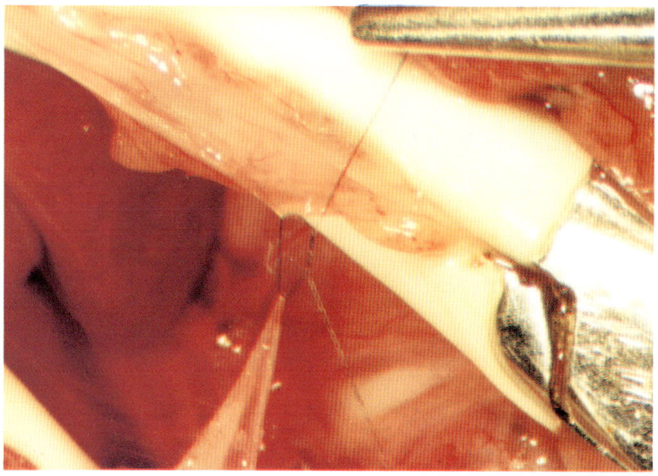

Fig. 5-7

An upper corner stitch is placed between IVC and PV.

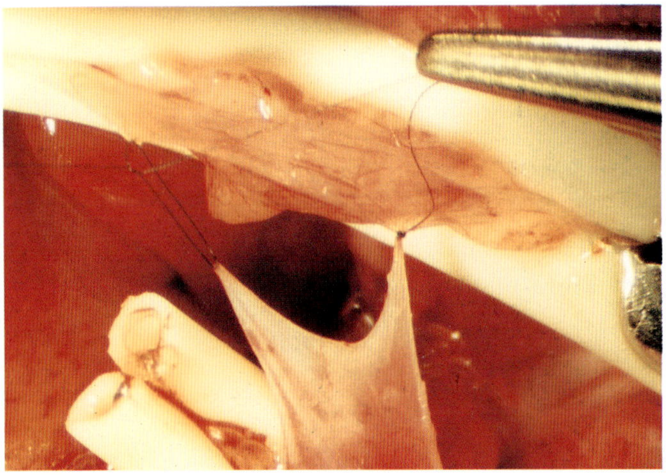

Fig. 5-8

The upper corner stay suture needle is used to enter the IVC's back edge.

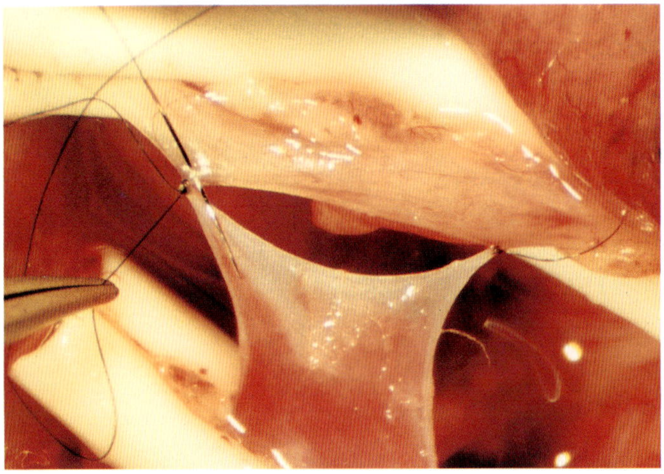

Fig. 5-9

The posterior edges are then sutured in continuous fashion.

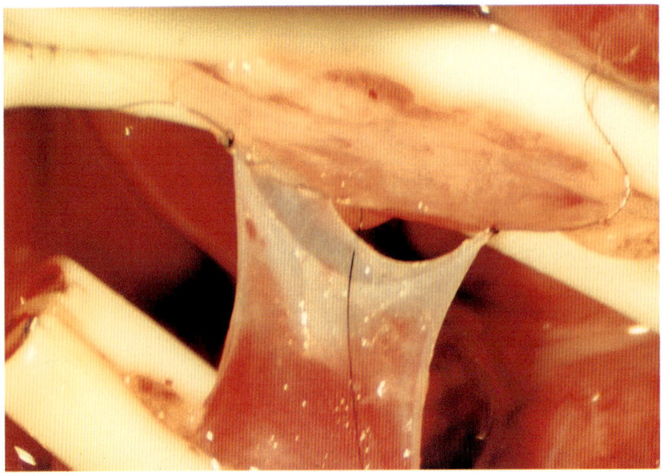

Fig. 5-10

If one wishes to use the open-loop suture technique, do so.

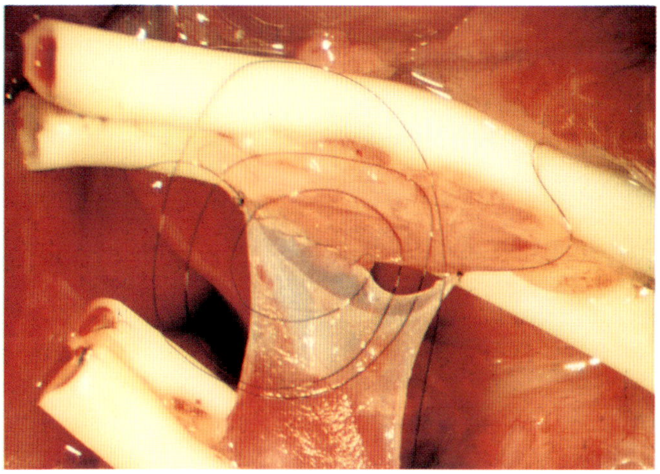

Fig. 5-11

When the suture reaches to the lower corner, the needle is brought out of the IVC and tied to the stay suture to prevent the purse-string effect.

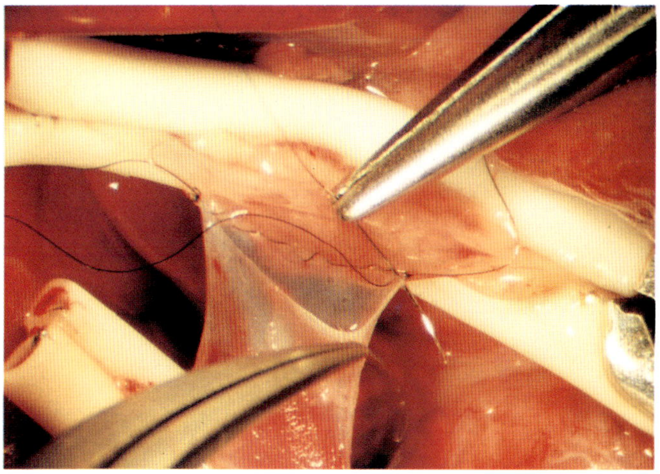

Fig. 5-12

Using the same needle, the anterior edges are sutured.

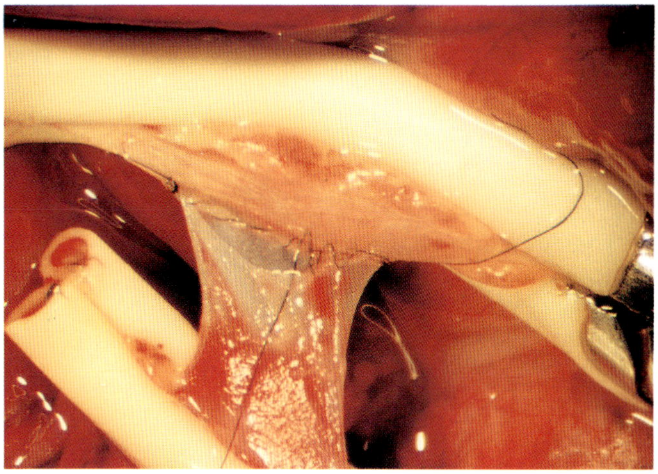

Fig. 5-13

The last two or three stitches are loosely placed in an open-loop fashion, after which each loop is pulled and tied to the upper stay suture.

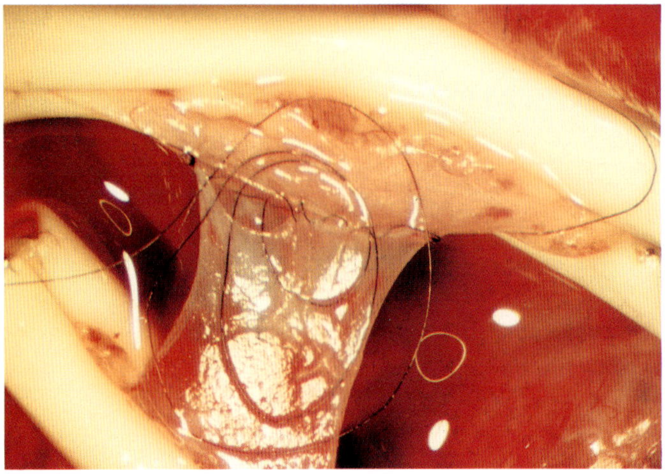

Fig. 5-14

The anastomosis has been completed.

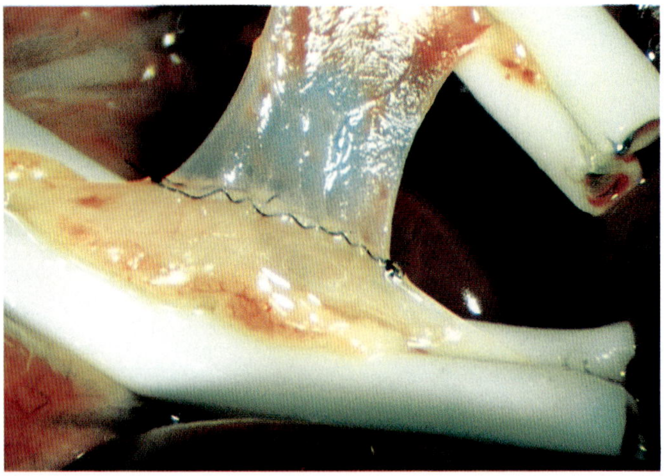

Fig. 5-15

The circulation has been restored following the clamp release.

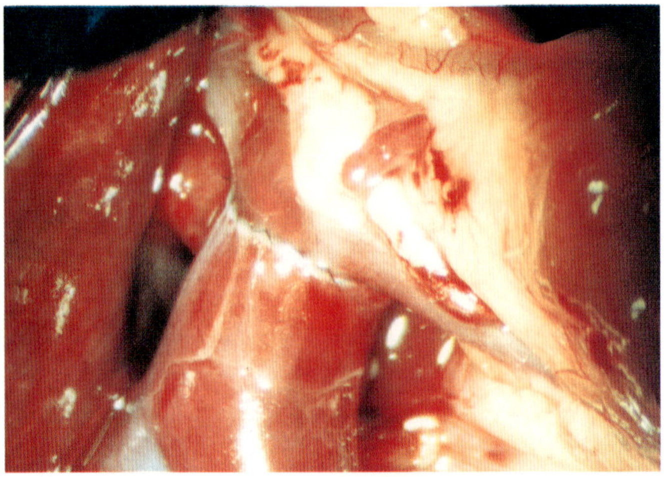

Fig. 5-16

Suggested Reading

McCullough D, Gittes RF, Lee S, Judd HL. Testicular-caval-portal venous shunt in the rat: effects on testosterone, FSH, LH and prolactin. Presented at the 57th Endocrine Soc., St. Louis, 1975.

Chapter 6

Vasovasostomy

Sun Lee, MD

Milbhor D'Silva, MD

Deferential vessels are doubly ligated using 9-0 suture and the vas is divided. Two seromuscular stay sutures are placed 180° apart. These sutures traverse at least two thirds of the wall thickness between the luminal margin and serosal surface. They are retracted without tying. Four equally spaced sutures are placed in a fashion identical to that previously described for the stay sutures, using an open-loop technique. These are then tied. The vasal anastomotic area is inverted by flipping the stay sutures. The posterior face of the anastomosis now visible should make the identification and alignment of both vasal luminal surfaces possible. Proper symmetrical alignment is mandatory for a successful outcome. Clear visualization of the luminal surfaces is greatly aided by periodic flushing of the area with physiological saline. The posterior face is treated similarly as the anterior. Lastly, the stay sutures are tied.

The vas deferens is exposed.

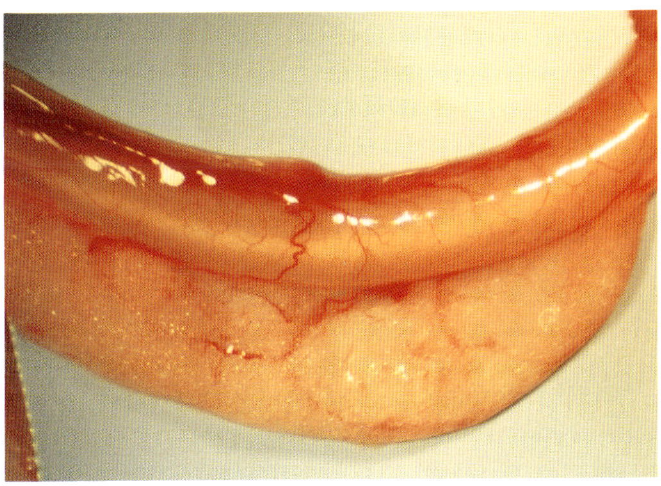

Fig. 6-1

Using 9-0 microsuture-ligature, the vasal vessels are doubly ligated.

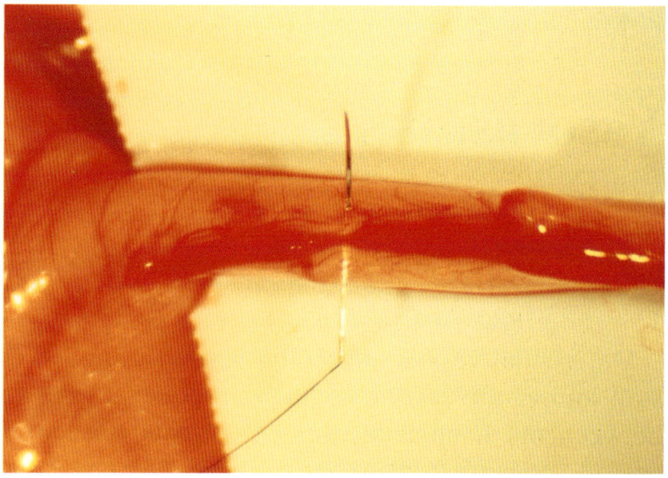

Fig. 6-2

The vas is sharply divided between these ties.

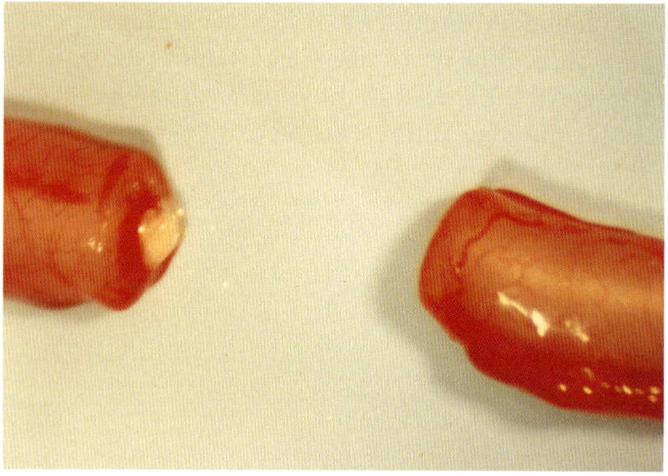

Fig. 6-3

The first seromuscular stay suture is placed outside-in fashion, making the suture traverse two thirds of the wall thickness.

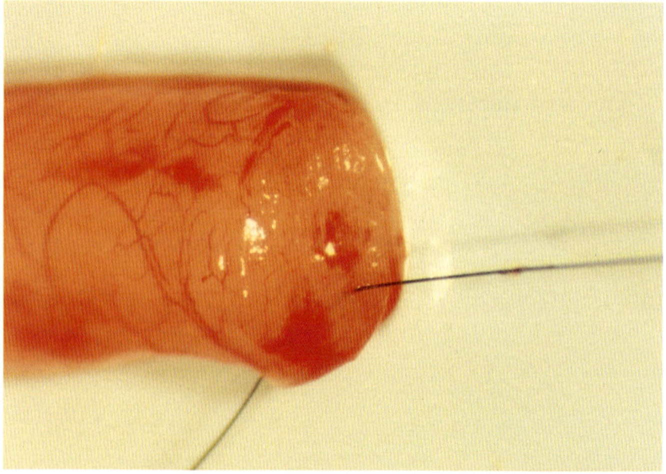

Fig. 6-4

A similar method is used to traverse the needle through the opposite vessel wall by the inside-out manner.

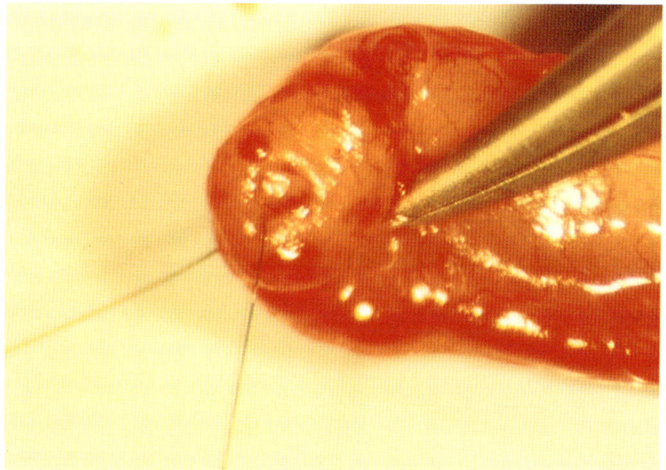

Fig. 6-5

The stay suture is retracted without tying.

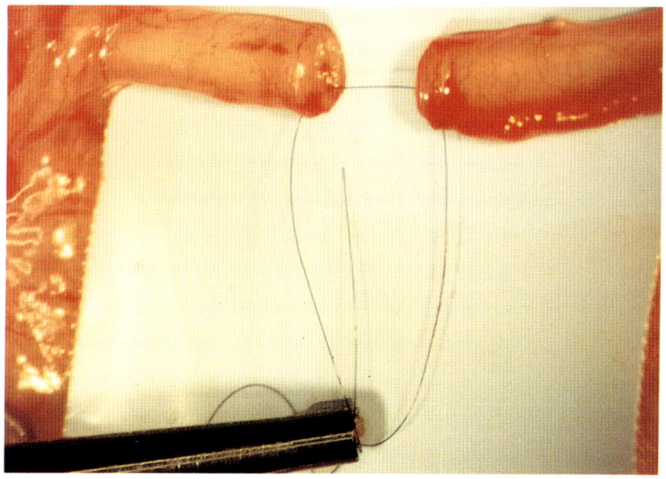

Fig. 6-6

The second stay suture is similarly placed 180° apart from the first one, and retracted without tying.

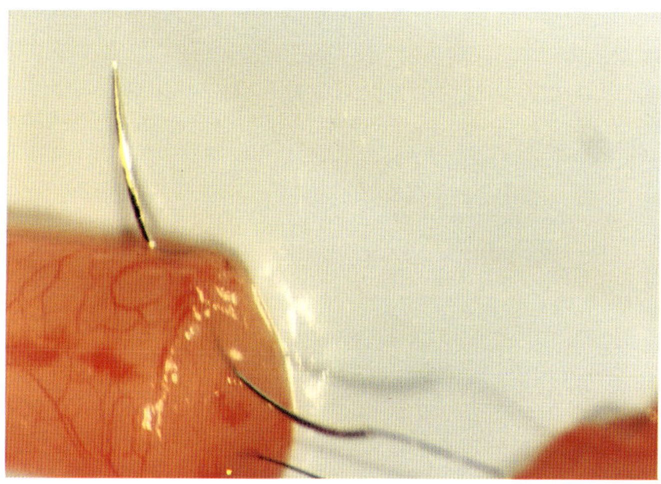

Fig. 6-7

These stay sutures are gently retracted.

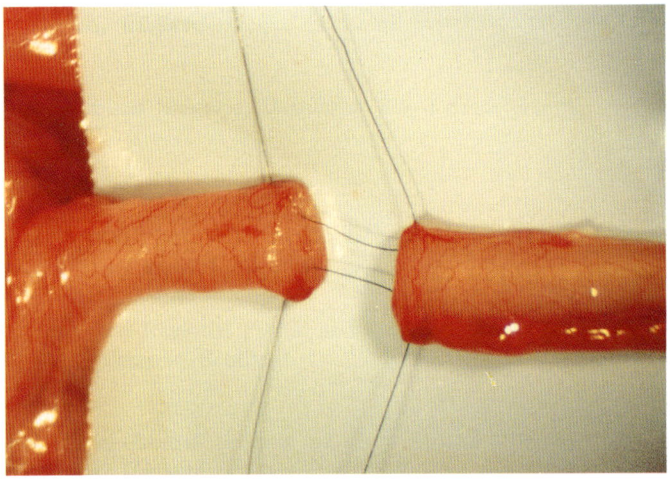

Fig. 6-8

Using a separate suture, a seromusculo-submucosal stitch is made between the two segments of the vas deferens and left untied.

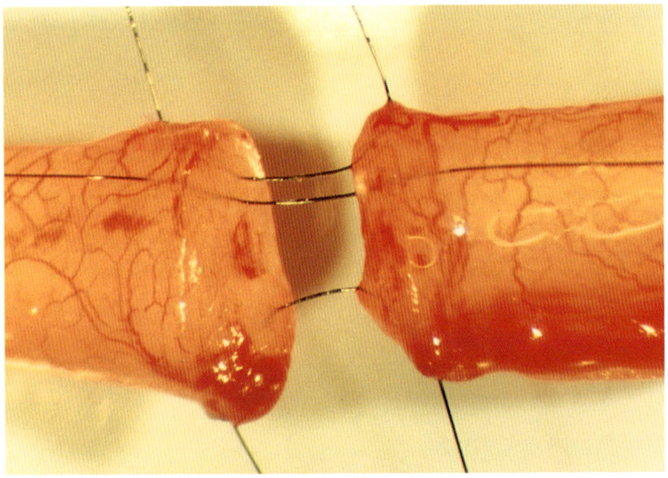

Fig. 6-9

The second open loop suture is placed and untied.

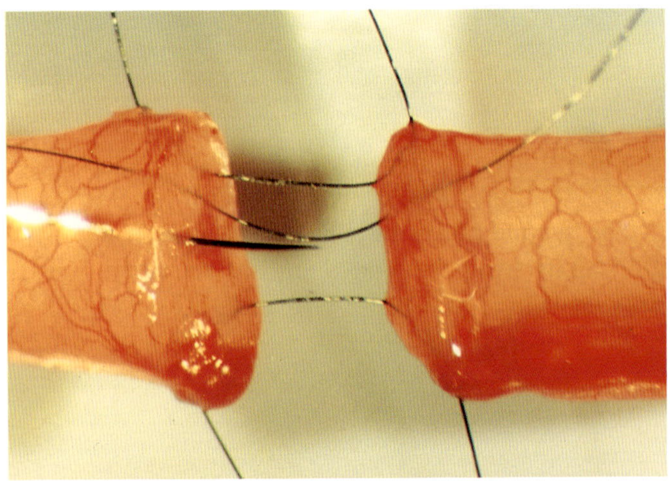

Fig. 6-10

The third open loop suture is placed.

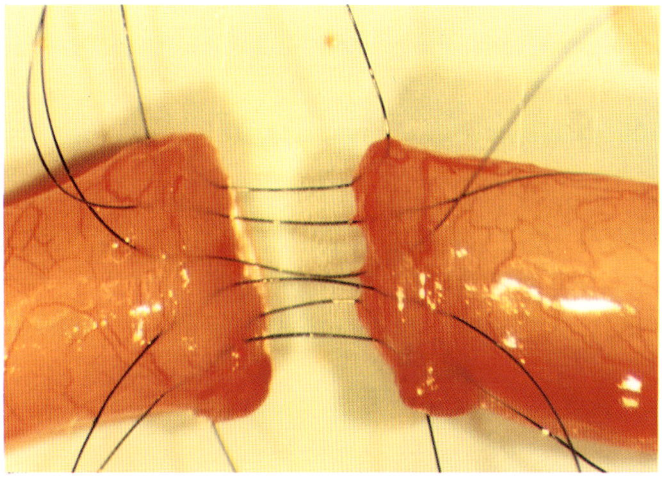

Fig. 6-11

The first suture is tied.

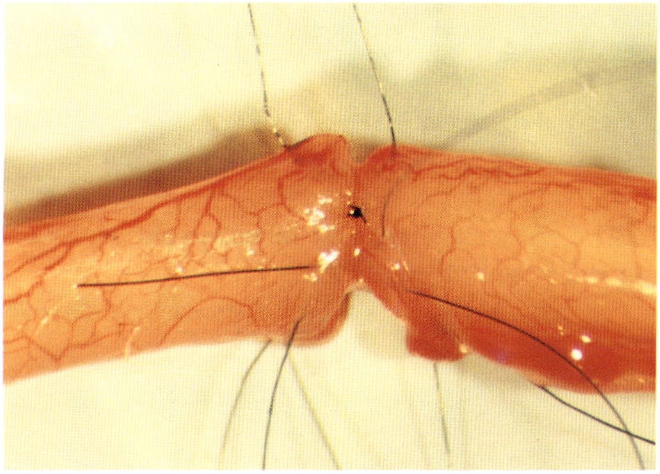

Fig. 6-12

The second suture is tied.

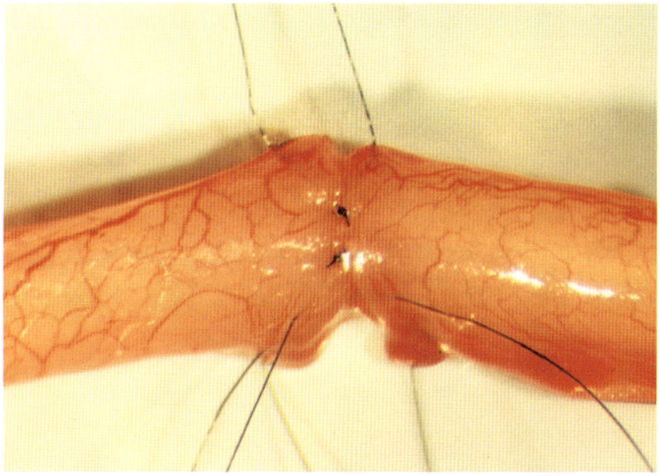

Fig. 6-13

The third suture is tied. Stay sutures are not tied and the vas is flipped.

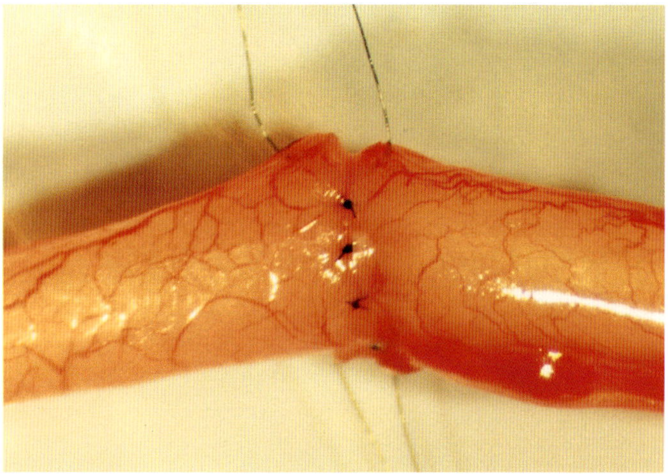

Fig. 6-14

Three more interrupted sutures are placed on the posterior edges.

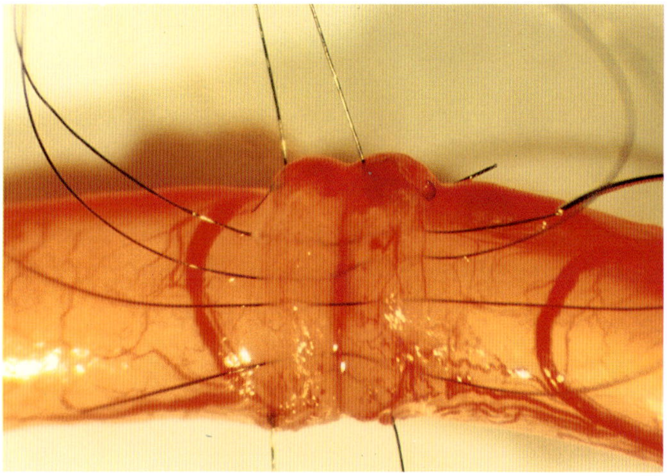

Fig. 6-15

All sutures are tied, including stay sutures.

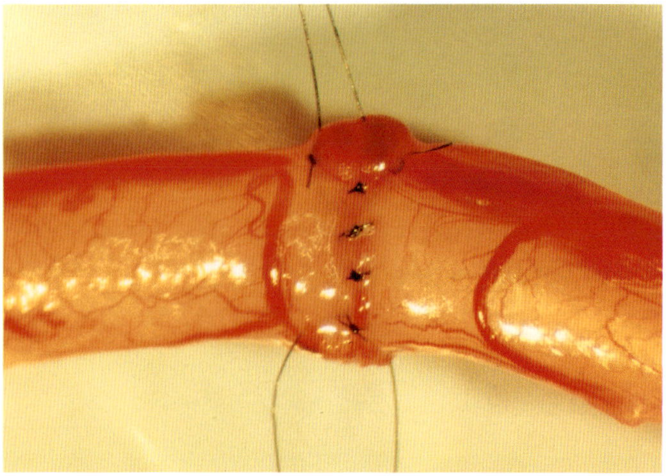

Fig. 6-16

Suggested Reading

Lee S, Han K, Li SJ, Wolf P, Orloff MJ. Vasovasostomy in the rat. *Urol.* 1982;22:418.

Chapter 7

Tubal Reconstruction

Milbhor D'Silva, MD

Sun Lee, MD

The mesosalpinx is devascularized by cauterizing it for about 1 cm, and then the devascularized uterine segment is removed. Two stay sutures (one at the mesosalpingeal border, the other at the anti-mesosalpingeal end), positioned 180° apart, are placed such that the needle traverses the serosubmucosal layers. They are then tied and retracted. Using the open-loop technique, six or seven interrupted sutures are placed in a manner similar to that described for the stay sutures. The posterior face of the anastomotic region is treated likewise. The stay sutures are then cut closely to the knot.

Mesosalpingeal vessels and a segment of the rat uterus are seen.

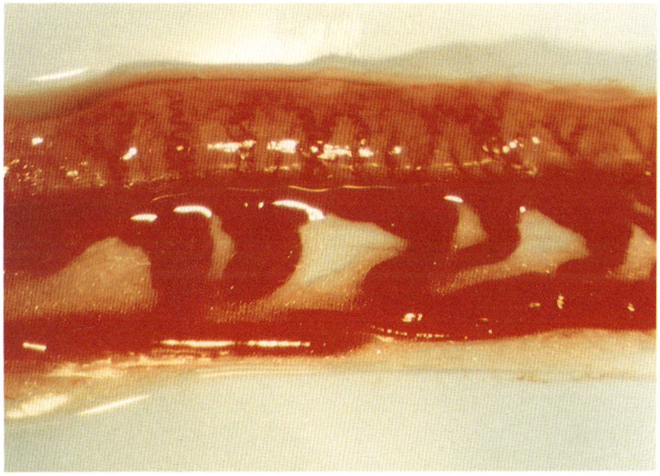

Fig. 7-1

Few salpingeal vessels are cauterized.

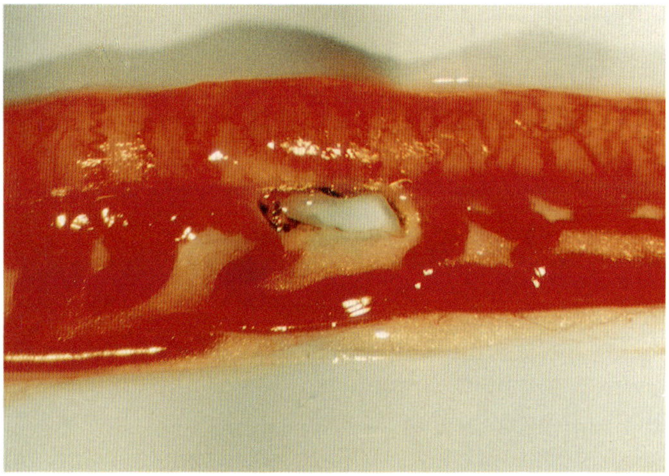

Fig. 7-2

A segment of uterus is resected.

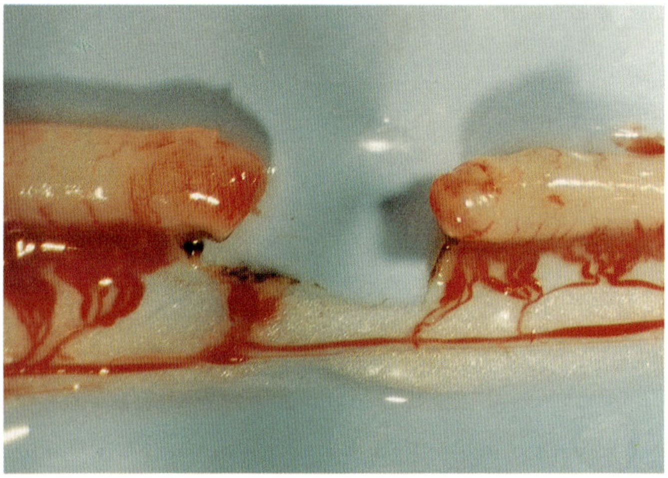

Fig. 7-3

An outside-in stitch is placed through the seromusculo-submucosal layers.

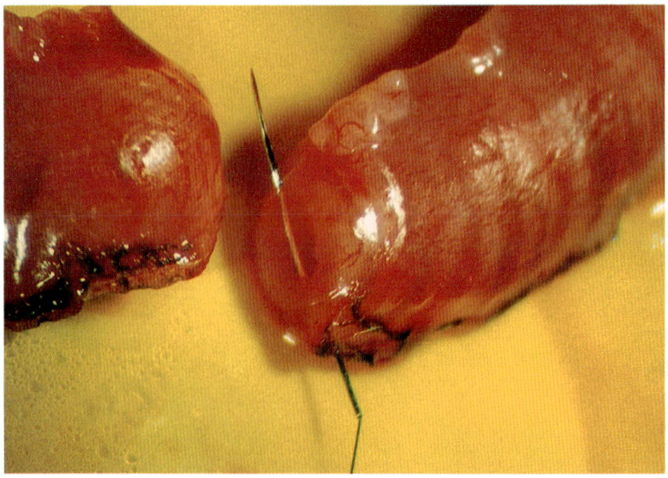

Fig. 7-4

An inside-out stitch is placed through the submucosal-musculoserosal layers and tied.

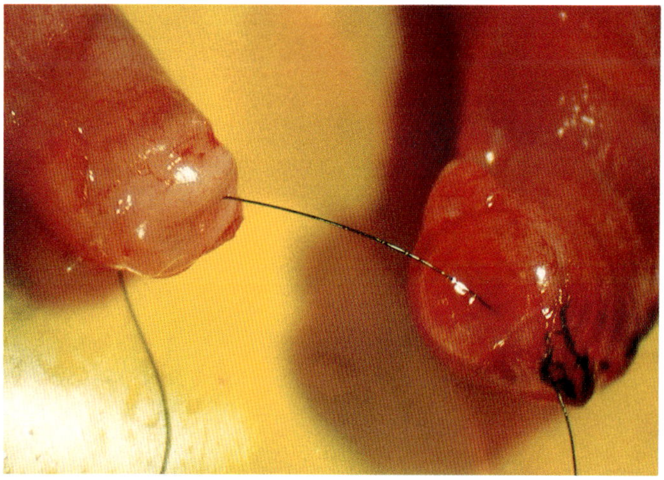

Fig. 7-5

An opposing stay suture is placed likewise 180° apart and retracted gently.

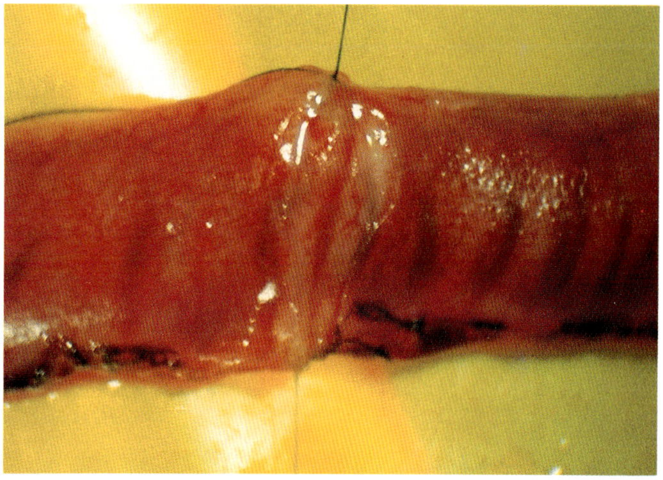

Fig. 7-6

A similar maneuver is employed to pierce the seromusculo-submucosal layer of one segment of the uterus.

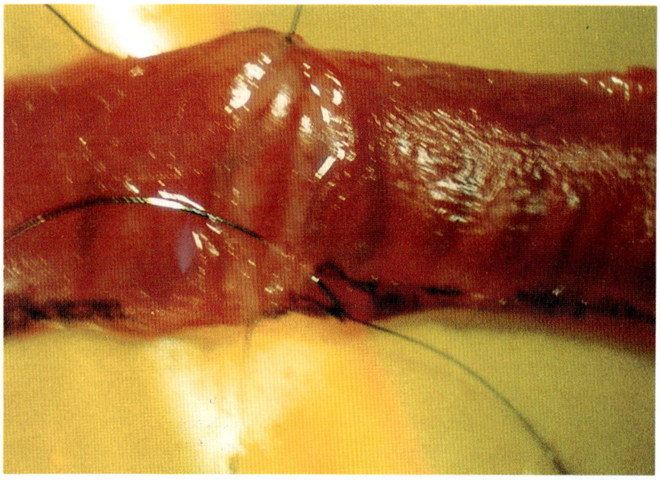

Fig. 7-7

The needle is then brought out through the opposite flap of the uterine wall in similar manner.

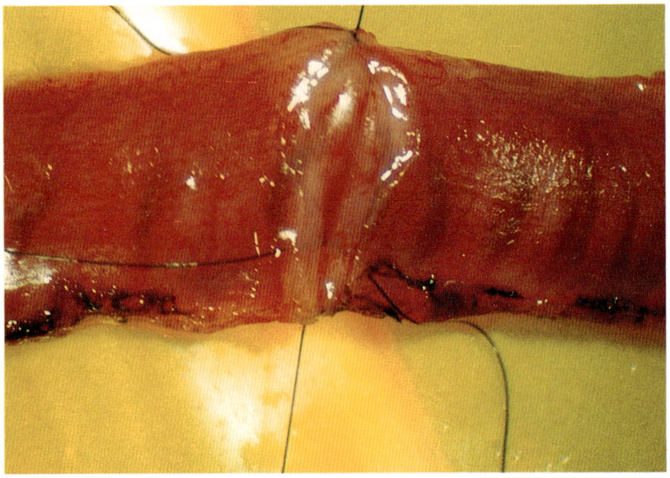

Fig. 7-8

An open-loop suture technique is exercised to assure that the needle has not caught the back edges, after which each loop is cut and tied.

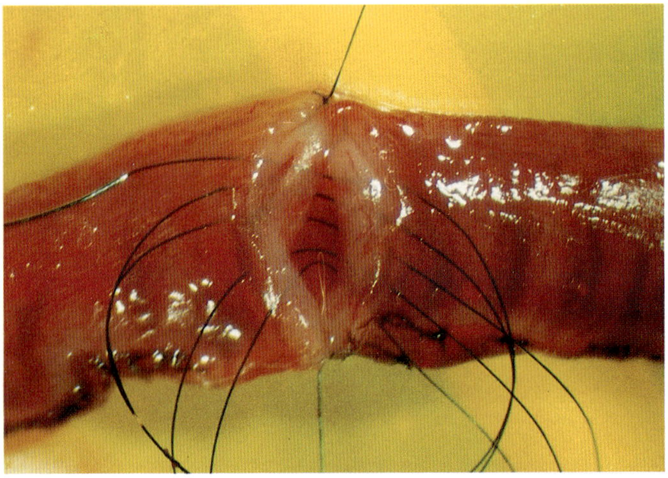

Fig. 7-9

All anterior sutures have been tied.

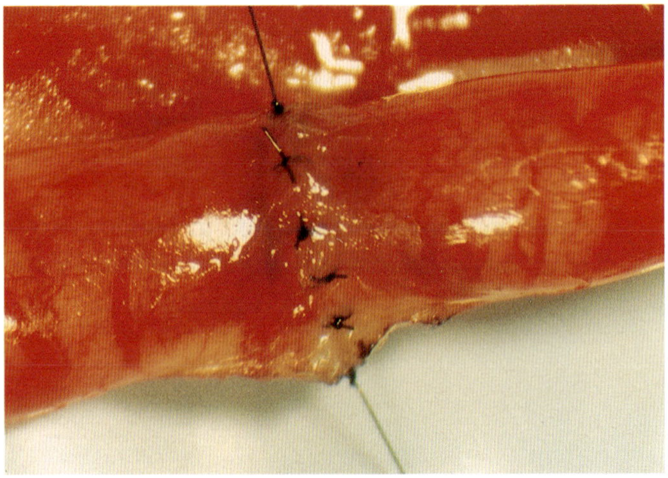

Fig. 7-10

The uterine segment is flipped and the suture-line is examined.

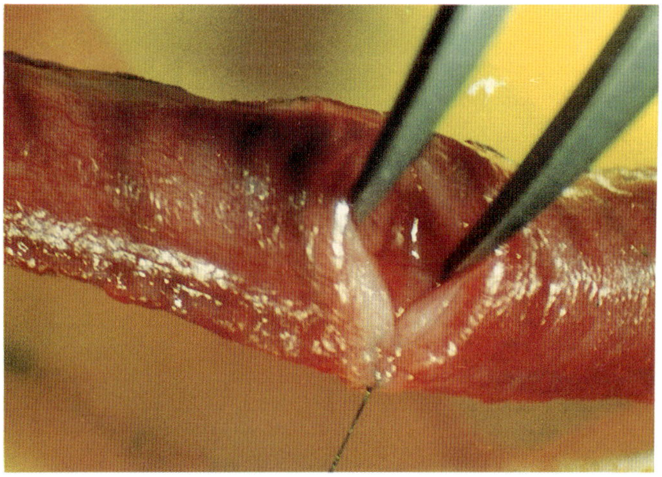

Fig. 7-11

Several open-loop sutures are placed.

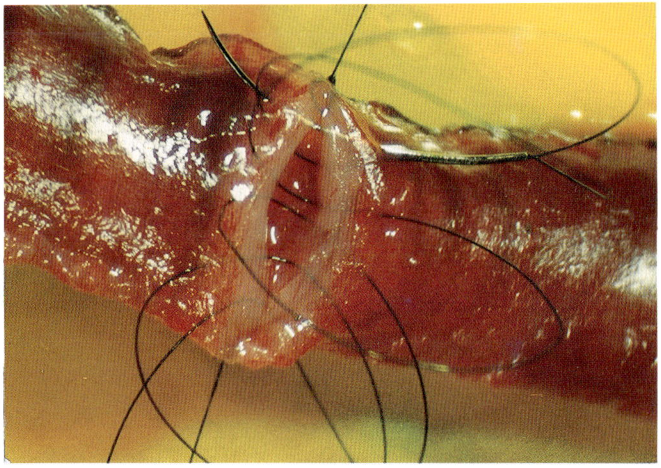

Fig. 7-12

The open-loop stitches are individually tied.

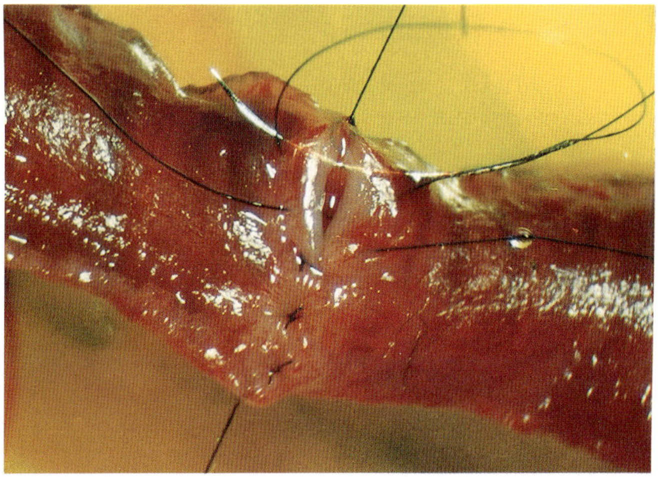

Fig. 7-13

The anastomosis has been completed.

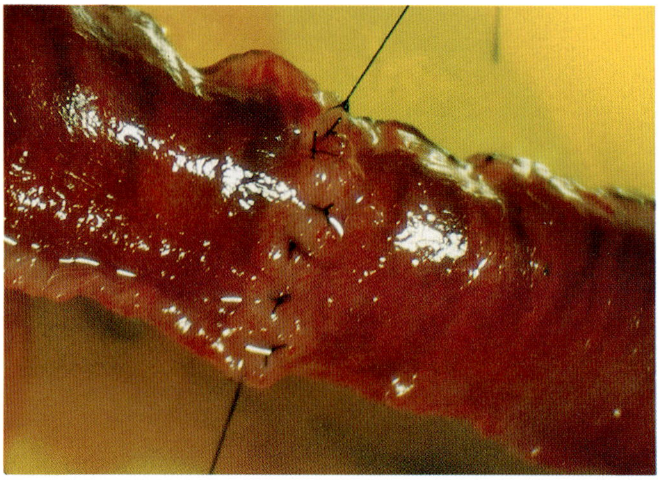

Fig. 7-14

The uterus is cut longitudinally to show that the lumen is free of suture materials.

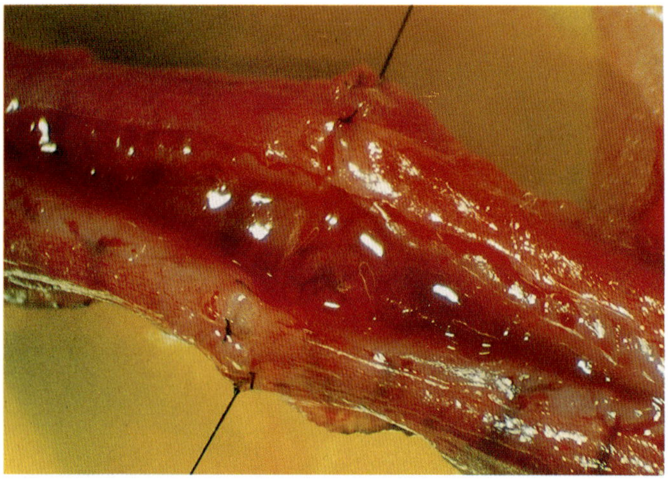

Fig. 7-15

Suggested Reading

D'Silva M, Durfee R, Wolf P, Lee S. A comparative study of Dexon and Nylon microsutures in rat uterine anastomoses. *Microsurg.* 1989;10:183.

Chapter 8

Organ Transplant Microsurgery: Pancreatic Transplant in Rats

Sun Lee, MD
Milbhor D'Silva, MD

Donor Preparation

Upon entering the abdomen, the right abdominal flap is retracted to the left and the intestines are retracted to the right of the operator. The Ligament of Treitz is cut and the aorta, celiac, superior mesenteric (SMA) and right renal arteries are dissected; the right renal artery is doubly ligated and cut between the ties. The duodenum is gently retracted to the left of the operator and the right colic vessels are doubly ligated and cut. A splenectomy is performed by ligating the pedicle vessels, and the left gastric vessels are ligated and cut at this time. The pancreas is gently freed from the greater omentum by serial ligation of its vessels, and the right gastroepiploic vessels are ligated close to the pyloric ring. The gastroduodenal artery and pyloric vein are doubly ligated and cut. The superior mesenteric vein (SMV-PV) is ligated at the lower margin of the pancreaticoduodenum (PD) and the pylorus is ligated and cut above the ligature. A loose ligature is placed on the aorta below the SMA and a right angle clamp is placed on the aorta about 1 cm above the celiac artery, after which about 2 to 3 ml of cold saline (7° C) is used to perfuse the PD via the aorta at the level of about 0.5 cm below the SMA. As the perfusate enters the organ, the loose ligature is tied over the needle and is tightened on removal of the needle. The aortic segment, which includes the SMA and celiac artery, is obtained by cutting the aorta below the tie and below the clamp. The portal vein is cut at the liver hilum, leaving a small piece of the liver on the right hilar portal vein. The duodenum is cut at the demarcation line and the SMV is cut distal to the tie. The PD graft is stored in cold saline.

Recipient Preparation and Transplantation

The right abdominal flap is retracted to the left and the intestines are retracted to the right of the operator. The aorta and IVC below the left renal vein are dissected free from each other, but are not completely mobilized from their posterior attachments. The IVC and aorta are clamped together using the Lee PCS clamp and a venotomy is made in the anterior aspect of the IVC, after which an elliptical excision or aortotomy (depending on the aortic size) is made to accommodate the end of the donor aorta. Using 9-0 or 10-0 microsutures (according to the size of vessels), an end-to-side aorto-aortic anastomosis is performed. The PV-IVC end-to-side anastomosis follows thereafter. At this time, the right hilar portal vein margin is positioned lower to prevent venous kinking. Thus, a piece of liver can prove useful as a position marker. Since the venous outlet of the transplant needs to be wide so as to promote unimpeded egress of venous flow, the right and left hilar portal veins are obliquely cut open proximally. An end-to-side duodeno-duodenostomy is made according to Connell, using 7-0 silk suture.

A band between pancreas and duodenum is freed. At this time Treitz ligament is also cut.

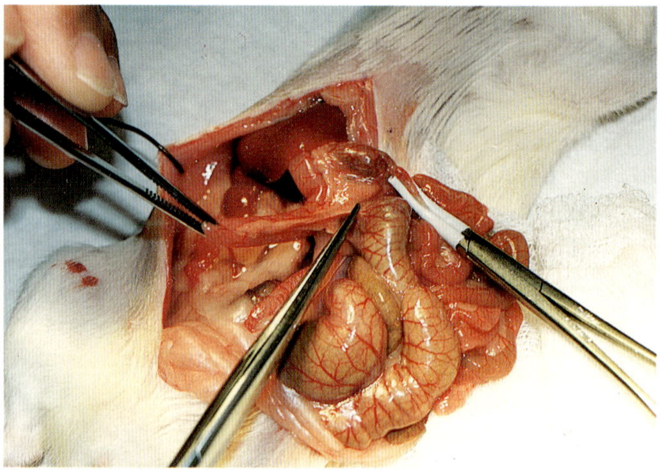

Fig. 8-1

A gentle dissection of the pancreas from the duodenum exposes the superior mesenteric and portal veins.

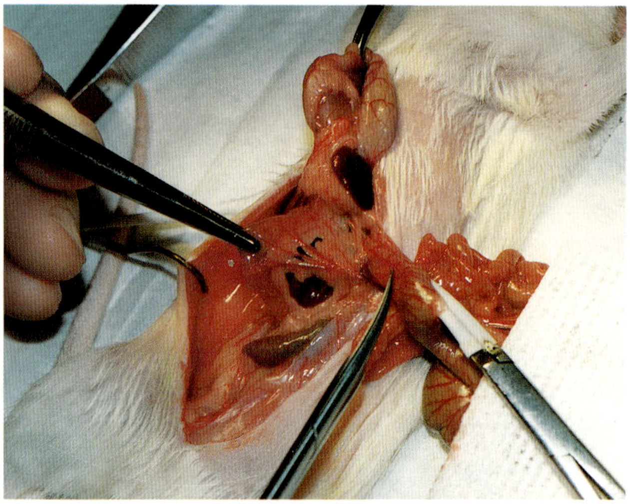

Fig. 8-2

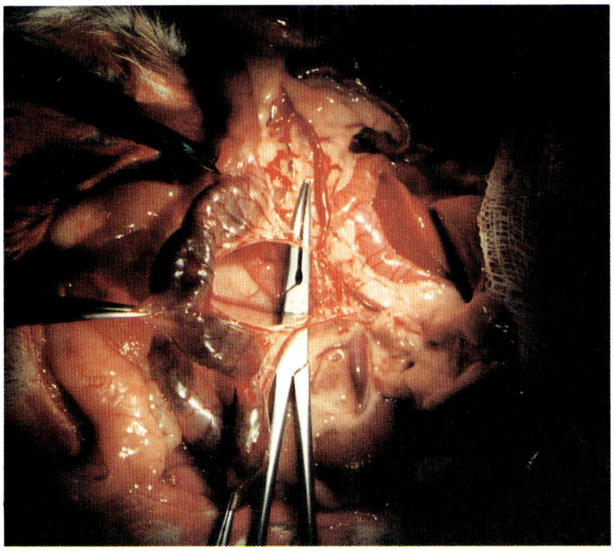

Fig. 8-3

The right and midcolic vessels are identified.

Those colic vessels are doubly ligated and divided.

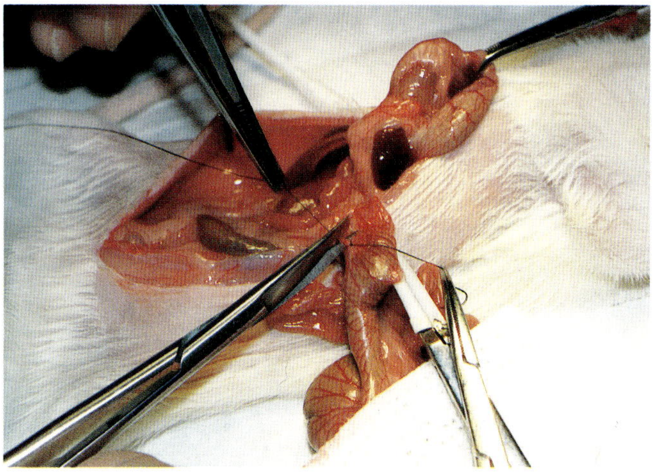

Fig. 8-4

A splenectomy is performed.

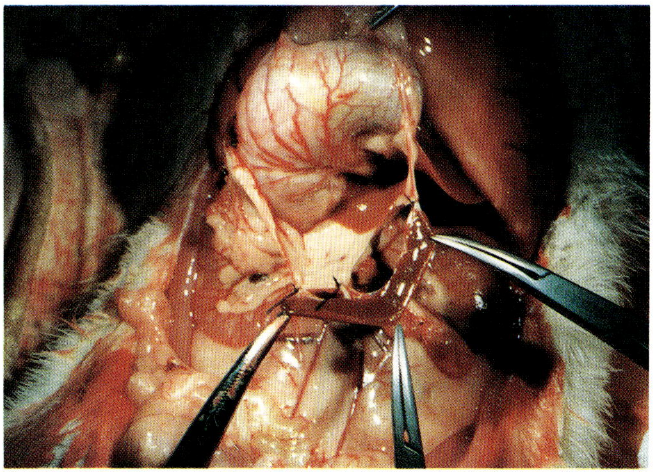

Fig. 8-5

The pancreatic element is being freed from the greater omentum.

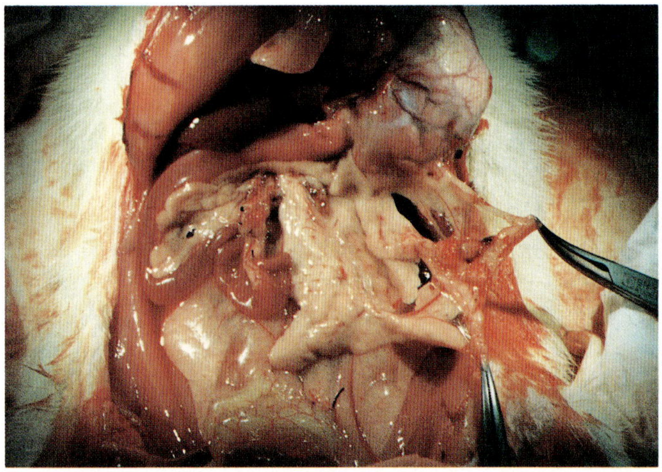

Fig. 8-6

The left gastric and splenic vessels are tied together and cut distally.

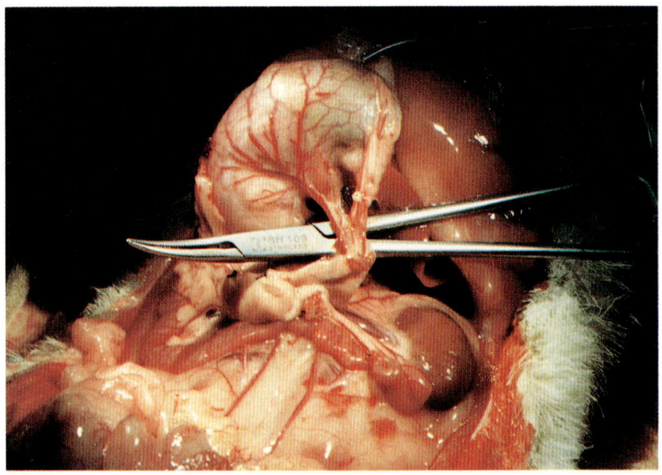

Fig. 8-7

The right gastroepiploic vessels are ligated and the pylorus is freed from minute vessels.

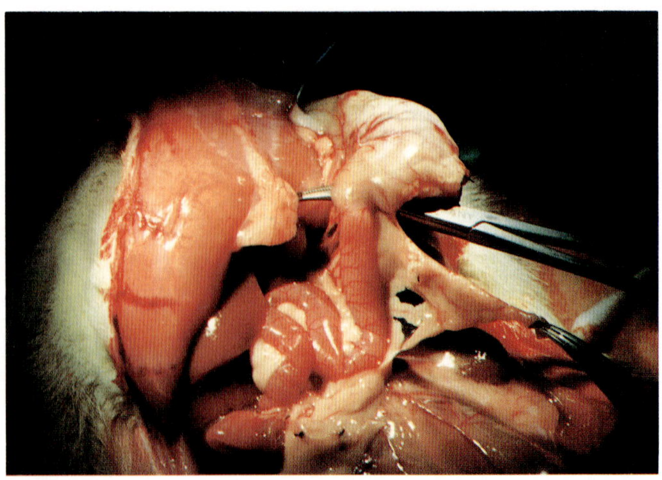

Fig. 8-8

The pylorus is tied.

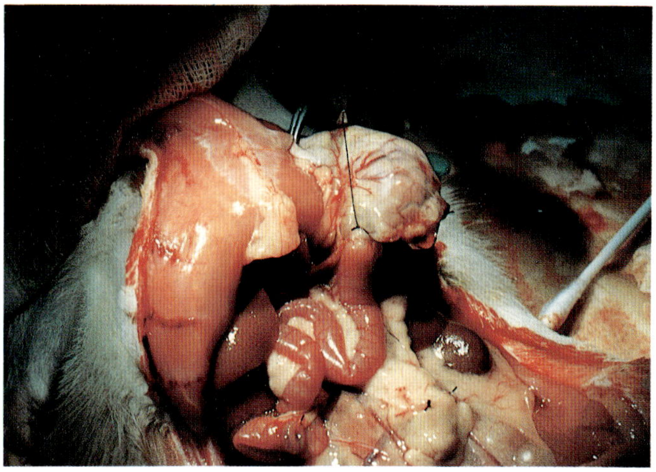

Fig. 8-9

The duodenum is severed from the stomach above the pyloric ligation.

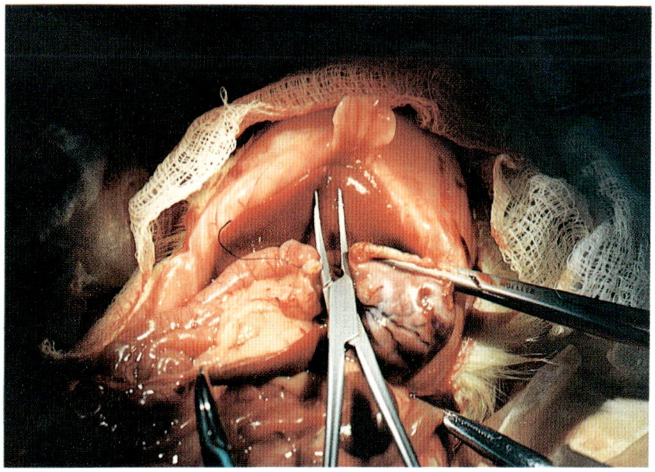

Fig. 8-10

The portal vein is being freed from the hepatic artery and bile duct and these are ligated together and cut.

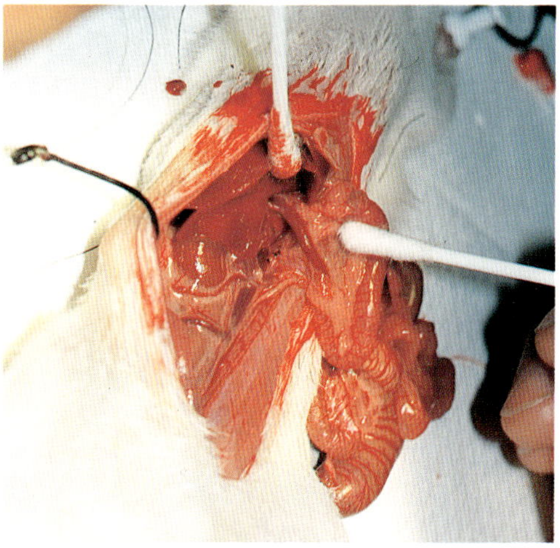

Fig. 8-11

The celiac and superior mesenteric arteries are freed from surrounding structures.

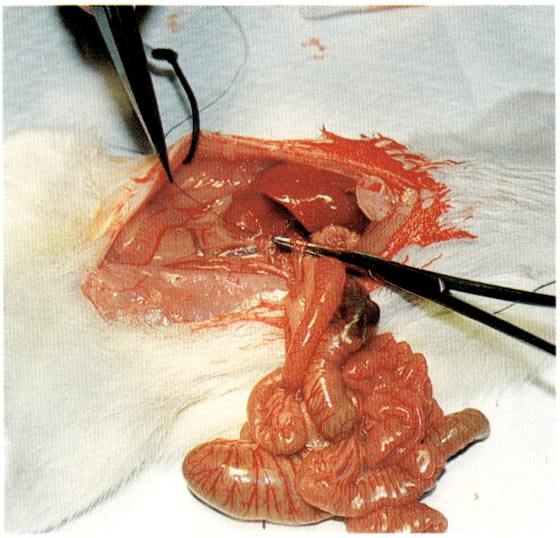

Fig. 8-12

The superior mesenteric vein is dissected at the lower margin of the pancreas.

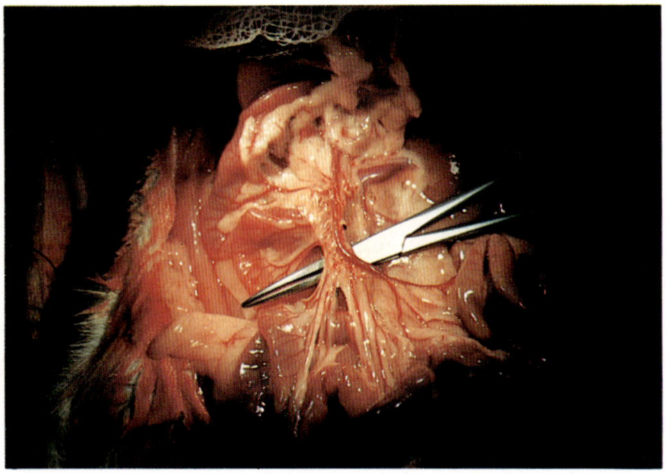

Fig. 8-13

The superior mesenteric vein is ligated at the lower margin of the pancreas.

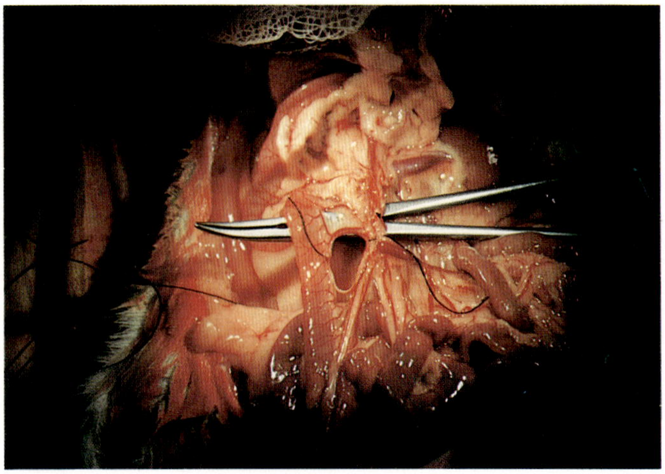

Fig. 8-14

Lumbar branches of the aorta at the celiac and mesenteric arteries are ligated and cut.

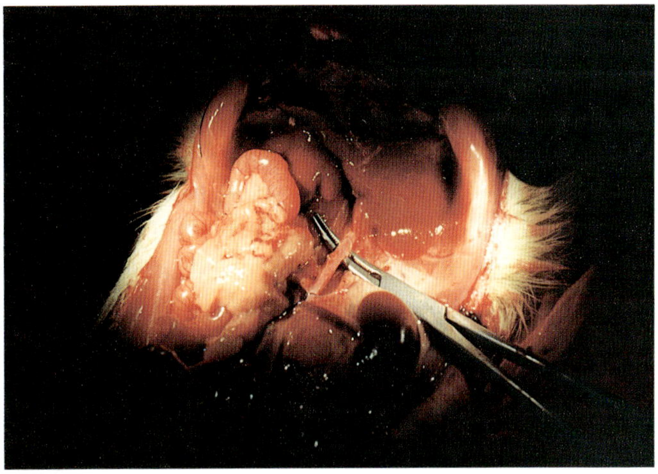

Fig. 8-15

The pancreaticoduodenum (PD) is perfused via the aorta using 3 to 4 ml of cold saline (7° C); the aorta is ligated below the superior mesenteric artery level.

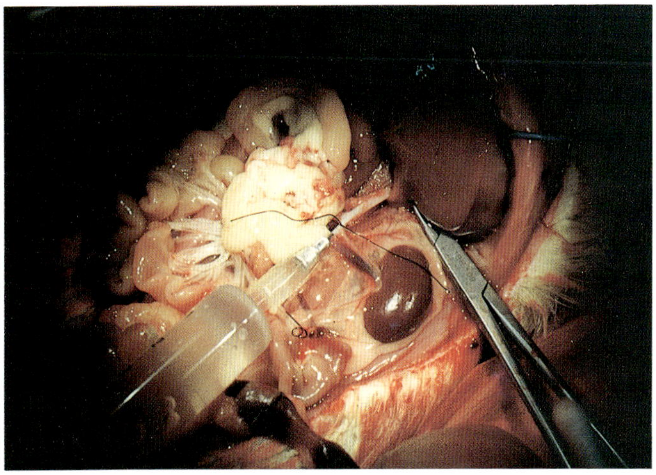

Fig. 8-16

The portal vein is cut at the liver hilum, leaving a small portion of the liver on the right end of the portal vein.

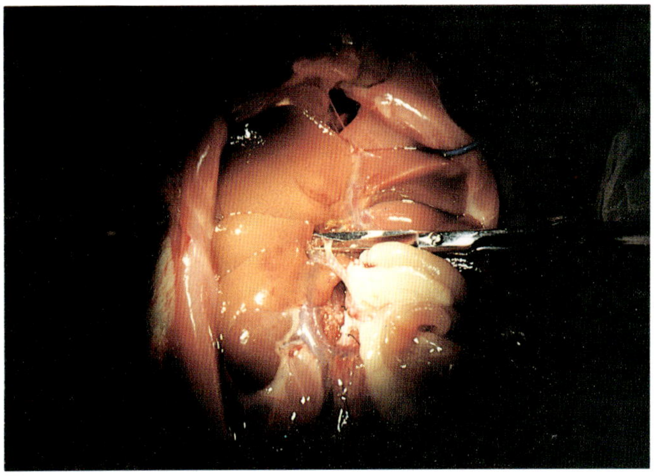

Fig. 8-17

The pancreaticoduodenum is removed by cutting the aorta below the tie and above the celiac artery, and cutting the duodenum at the demarcation line. The superior mesenteric vein is cut below the tie.

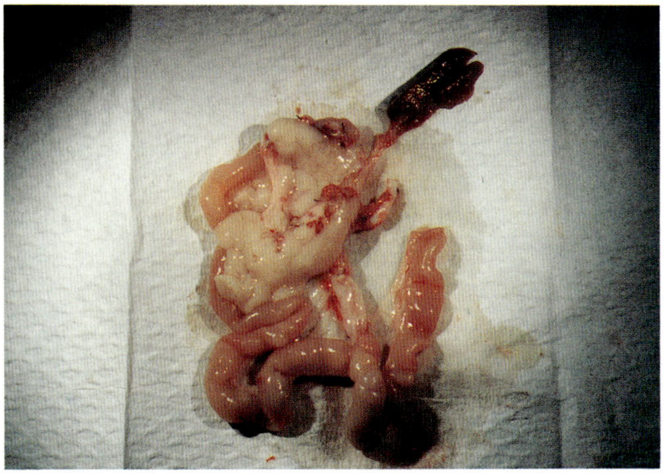

Fig. 8-18

Following the application of a clamp on both the aorta and IVC of the recipient, an aorto-aortic end-to-side anastomosis is made. The anterior edges have been approximated.

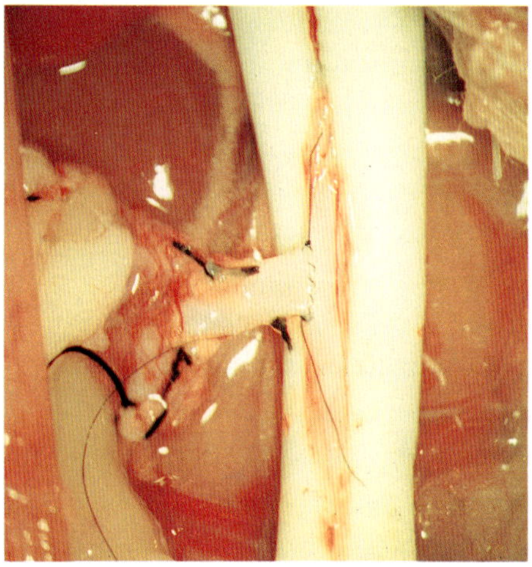

Fig. 8-19

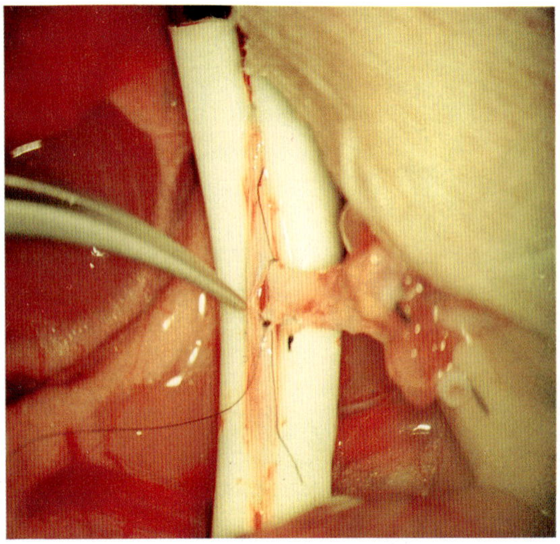

Fig. 8-20

The posterior edges of the aortas have been sutured.

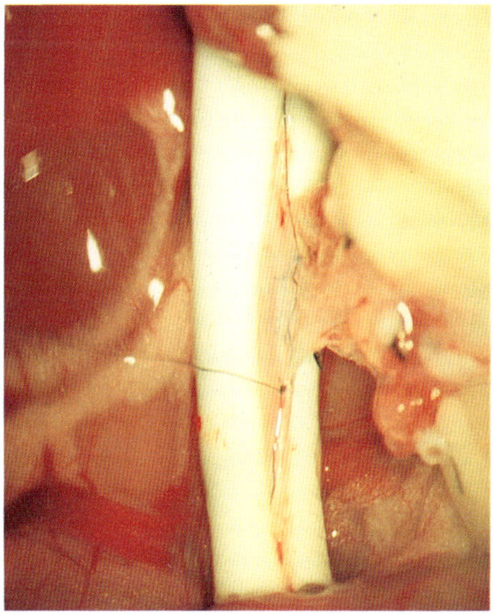

Fig. 8-21

The end of the portal vein is being anastomosed in an end-to-side fashion to the IVC. The anterior edges have been sutured.

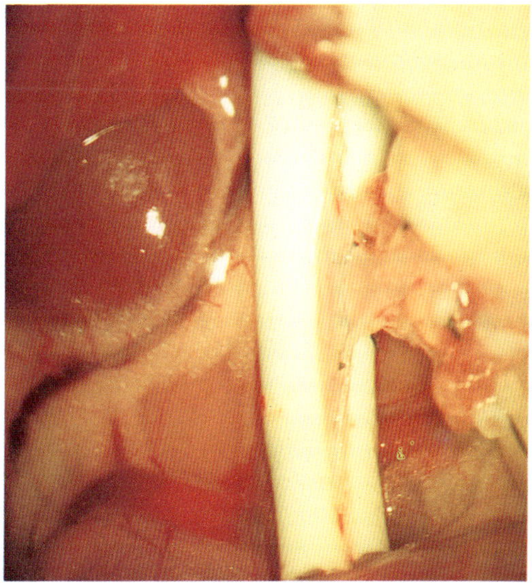

Fig. 8-22

The posterior edges of those veins have been sutured using a continuous suture technique.

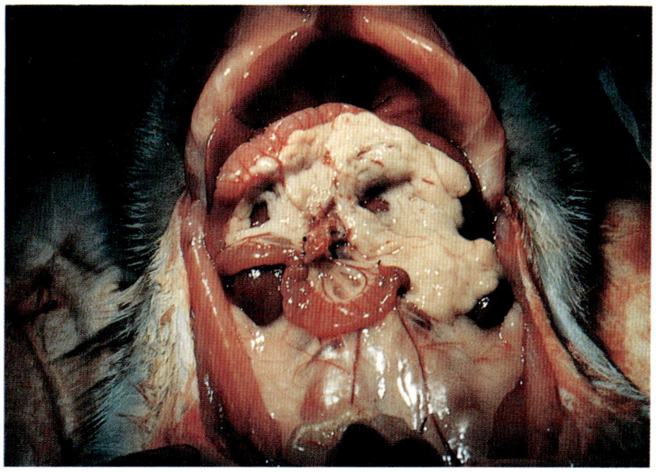

Fig. 8-23

The circulation of the pancreatico-duodenum has been restored upon release of the clamp.

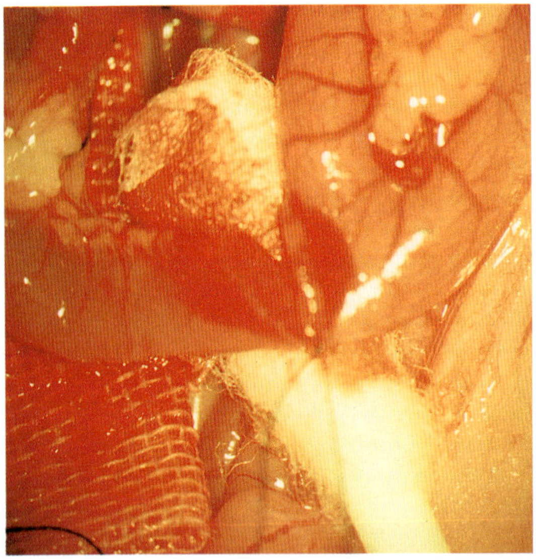

Fig. 8-24

An end-to-side duodeno-duodenostomy is being performed.

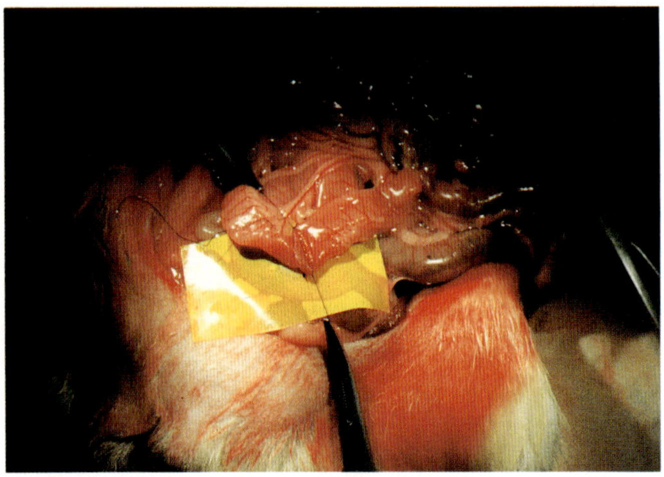

Fig. 8-25

Two opposing stay sutures have been placed 180° apart.

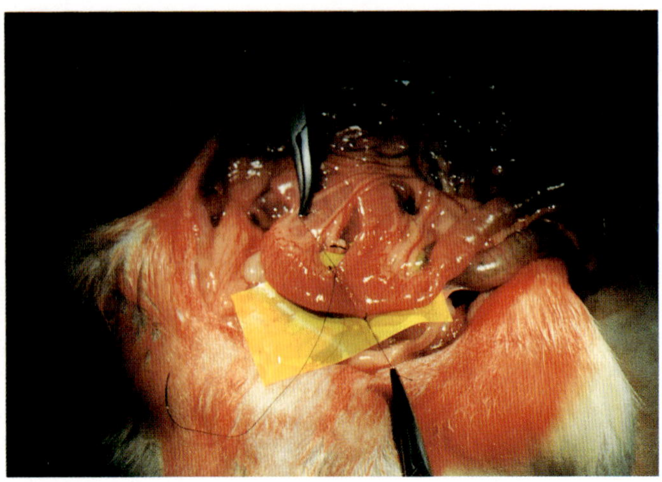

Fig. 8-26

A continuous Connel suture technique has been applied to invert the intestinal edges. One row needs three or four such stitches.

The high magnification shows the suture site immediately following anastomosis.

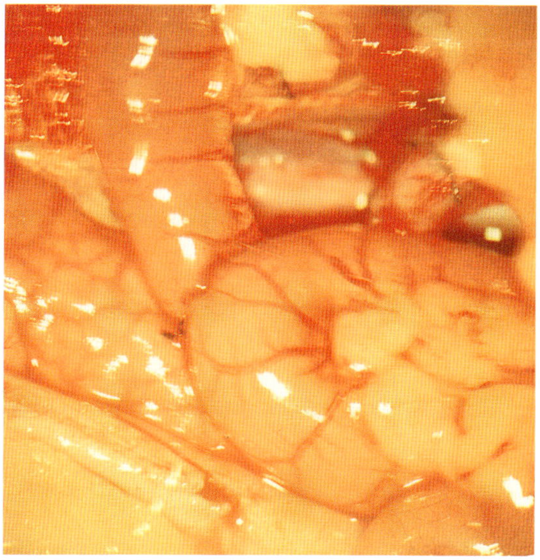

Fig. 8-27

The pancreatico-duodenal graft is shown well vascularized (arrow) immediately following transplantation.

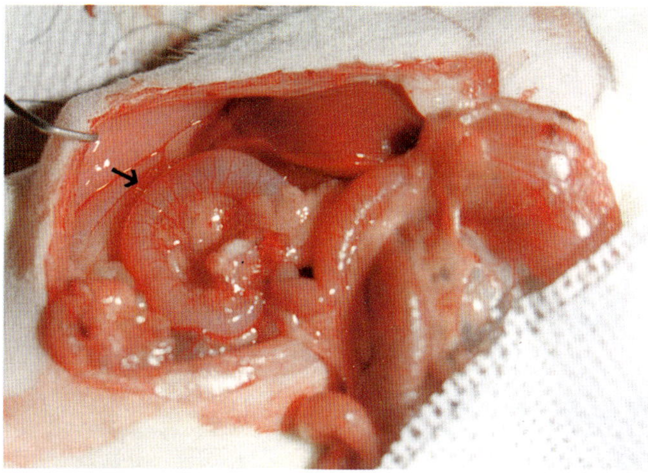

Fig. 8-28

Suggested Reading

Lee S, Tung KSK, Koopmans H, Chandler JG, Orloff MJ. Pancreaticoduodenal transplantation in the rat. *Transplantation*. 1972;13:421-425.

Nozawa M, Weil R, McIntosh R, Reemtsma K. Vascularized transplantation of the rat pancreas without duodenum. *Transplantation*. 1974;17:137-140.

Section II

Kirsch Microsurgical Clips And Their Clinical Application

Chapter 9

Instrumentation for Tissue Reconstruction With Nonpenetrating Clips

W.M. Kirsch, MD

Y.H. Zhu, MD

Z. Boukouvalas, MD

R. Cushman

R.A. Hardesty, MD

The recognized difficulties attending contemporary microvascular reconstructions, especially venous anastomoses, warrant ongoing testing of alternative nonsuture methods. These trials have included fixed rings, cuffs, pins, glues and adhesives, laser energy and penetrating staples.[1-6] Needle and suture continue to be used in microsurgery because alternative methods are so far either impractical or inferior. This chapter describes the instruments that enable the construction of a nonpenetrating, clipped and flanged microvascular anastomosis with intima-to-intima contact. Nonpenetrating microclips are applied in an interrupted fashion to create end-to-end, end-to-side, or vessel diameter mismatch anastomoses, with either normal or diseased arteries, autogenous grafts, or vascular prostheses. The elastomeric flange formed by clips has unique biological and physical properties that will be discussed in other chapters.[7]

The first generation microclips were fabricated from ultrathin silver by computer assisted, wire electrocorrosion technology. "H"-shaped clips (700 microns long, 100 microns thick) were applied with a suction adapted microneedle holder and special everting forceps. The latter are jeweler's forceps with blunt, angled tips. Microclip loading and application is now expedited by development of a modified clip and applier. The clip is incorporated on a detachable tang with an enlarged head, enabling unambiguous loading into a recessed slot on the applier. The loaded applier functions as a dissecting microfork, embracing everted vessel walls and interposed intima prior to firing.

The clip proper consists of a pair of curved arms, interconnected by a bridge attached to a frangible tang. The two arms terminate at rounded tips that focally squeeze but do not penetrate the flanged vessel walls when set to close as "zero gap." The shoulders of the clip engage the jaws of the applier, with the centered bridge connected by a neck to a tang designed to break at a predetermined tension. The breaking strength of the tang neck is designed to exceed the tension required to deform by bending the bridge portion of the clip. Microclips, fabricated from pure silver, have the following dimensions: 2.3 mm long tang, 0.4 mm long clip, 150 microns thick, tip radius of curvature 17.5 microns with a gap between the open clip tips of 0.3 mm. Clip closure is generated by tension applied to the tang by a pinch pressure between thumb and forefinger on the forward wings of the clip applier, a desirable maneuver for any microinstrument. This enables fine motor control of the instrument. The clip shoulders are supported by the stationary jaw faces on

the applier, with the relationship of jaw faces and the clip shoulders designed so that the points of engagement are remote from the neck. The bending movement for this geometric configuration is defined:
Tension (T) on the tang produces a bending moment $(M) = \frac{(T)(X)}{2}$ at the center of the bridge, with X the distance from tang axis to either symmetrical shoulder contact point. During the course of actuation, X becomes progressively smaller as the symmetrical shoulder contact points advance medially, until the bending moment is zero. The neck is designed with sufficient tensile strength to permit a bending moment large enough to deform the bridge portion. As bending deformation proceeds, contact points move closer to the neck until increasing tang tension generates no further bending moment, but instead is directed to reproducibly separating the tang neck. The advantage of this design is that bridge deformation is precisely determined by clip/jaw face geometry and is independent of the surgeon's manipulating force. Actuation provided by the surgeon's forefinger and thumb is translated into a reproducible pincer movement measured in microns. Precise and reproducible manipulation parameters now approach the limits of optical resolution. Changes in jaw face/clip shoulder-geometry will produce any desired degree of clip closure. An angulation allowing for "zero gap" closure of pure silver microclip tips has worked very well in all surgical situations thus far evaluated, both at micro and macro level. Though set for "zero gap," the clip tips in actual practice compress the two everted vascular walls at a discrete point but do not penetrate intima. The tissue above the tips forms the flange. As silver or titanium clips are fired they remodel into a curved configuration without sharp projections.

The applier jaw is supported on a body that terminates at a forward end, with the stationary jaw face straddling the slot to engage the shoulders of the loaded clip. For silver clips, jaw faces are planar at an obtuse angle of 120° with clip shoulders at 150° to produce "zero gap" closure. Tension on the clip is produced by a cam-actuated response to a squeezing pressure from the surgeon's thumb and forefinger on the distal wings. Clip loading requires actuating the proximal wings (cams) on the applier to expose the slot. The same maneuver after clip firing allows for ejection of the expended tang. Microclips require magnification for loading; mini, mezzo and macroclips are easily loaded without optical aid. Tang extraction is accomplished with a jeweler's forceps. Malapplied clips are removed by squeezing the bridge of the clip with a modified, sharp pointed, microneedle holder. This maneuver opens the arms and separates the tips. Since clips are nonpenetrating, no intimal damage is incurred after removal.

Instrument design remains in evolution with conservation of the basic principle of forming a nonpenetrated, elastometric flange with clips. Though silver has a long history as an acceptable material for surgical closure and suture, it may not be ideal since recent studies suggest slight tissue reactivity.[8] Silver combines with proteins to form stable soluble complexes that decompose into black silver sulfite. This discoloration is associated with a low-grade inflammatory reaction in surrounding tissues. Though no clinical reports of surgical complications attributable to silver clips have been described, silver may be slightly toxic to nervous tissue. Titanium clips are now available. Titanium is far less reactive, has no known neurotoxicity, is not paramagnetic and thus does not interfere with MRI studies. Further instrument improvement is anticipated with development of a bioabsorbable clip, and endoscopic utilization. The ideal anastomotic nonsuture device may be a repetively fired bioabsorbable microclip. This instrument could permit the rapid construction of the flanged microanastomoses without the need of removing any instrument from the operating field, leaving no traces after resorption and vessel wall remodeling.

Anastomosis of a rat femoral artery (1 mm O.D.) with the first generation microclips. Note the apparent fusing of intima that masks the actual anastomotic line, ears on the clips, and the relative size of the clips to arterial wall thickness. The clip is 700μ long, 100μ thick. The artery has been opened and the intimal surface is inferior. (Immediate post-operative period.)

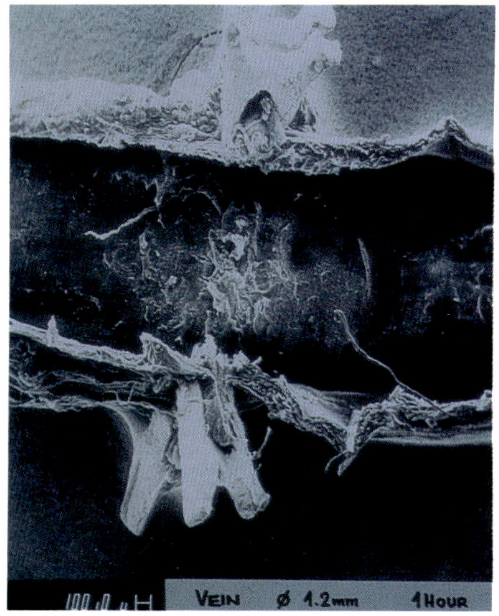

Fig. 9-1

The tips of jeweler's forceps are modified and angled to form a pincer that enables mobilization of the adventitia and formation of the flange. Varying angles are sometimes necessary for forming the flange at the heel-and-toe of the end-to-side anastomoses.

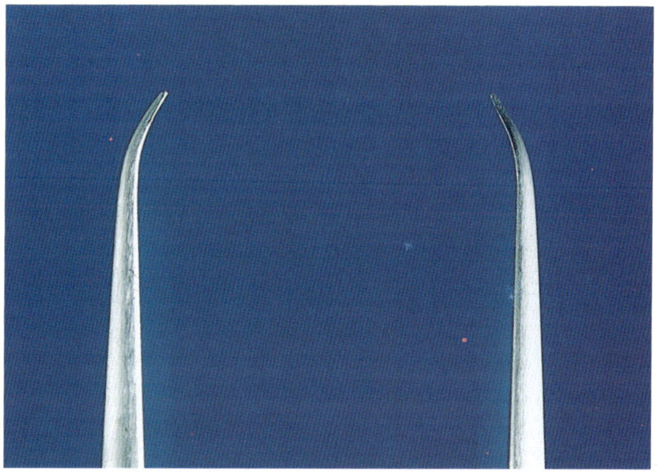

Fig. 9-2

The principle of the nonpenetrating clip and applier. Note the differential angulation of clip and jaw shoulders with **A** the initial contact point, **B** the rounded clip tips, **C** the frangible tang, and **D** the enlarged clip head that fits into the puller slot.

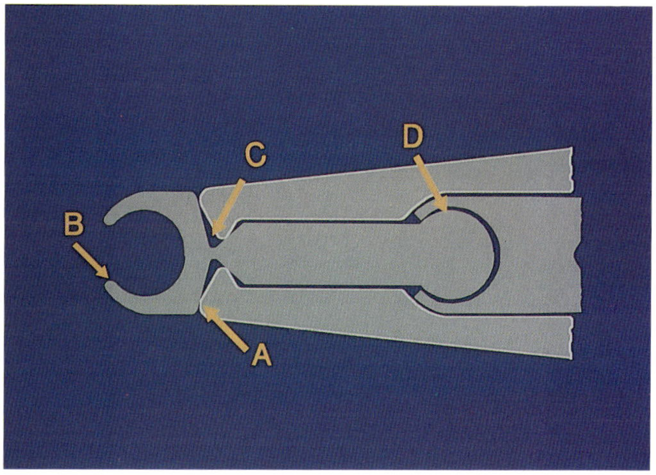

Fig. 9-3

Activation of the nonpenetrating clip; **A** is the clip jaw contact point that has been moved centrally towards the detachable tang with remodeling of the clip; **B** is the "zero gap" at the tips resulting from the bending movement; **C** is the smooth break from the clip bridge; and **D** the clip head being withdrawn by the puller.

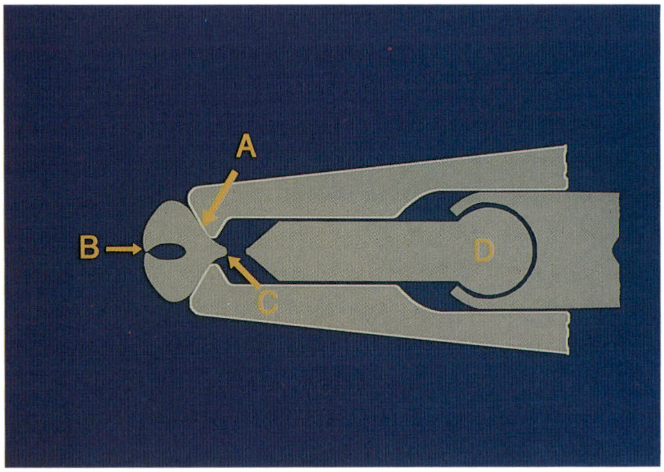

Fig. 9-4

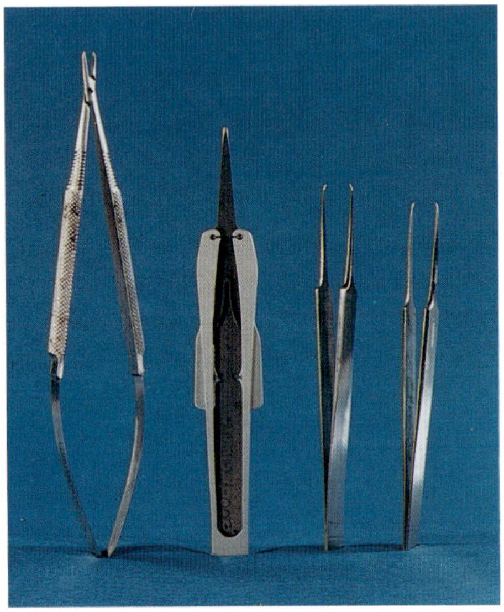

Fig. 9-5

Instruments necessary for microclip application and removal. From the left: clip remover consisting of a modified Castroviejo needle holder; clip applier, the distal wings are the actuators for clip firing, the proximal wings extend the tip to accommodate clip loading or tang removal. Two everting forceps with different angles at their tips.

The four currently utilized clips and their dimensions. Microclips and miniclips require separate appliers; mezzoclips and macroclips use the same applier. These sizes cover all experimental and clinical tissue approximations so far encountered to include human dural closure and severely atherosclerotic human arteries.

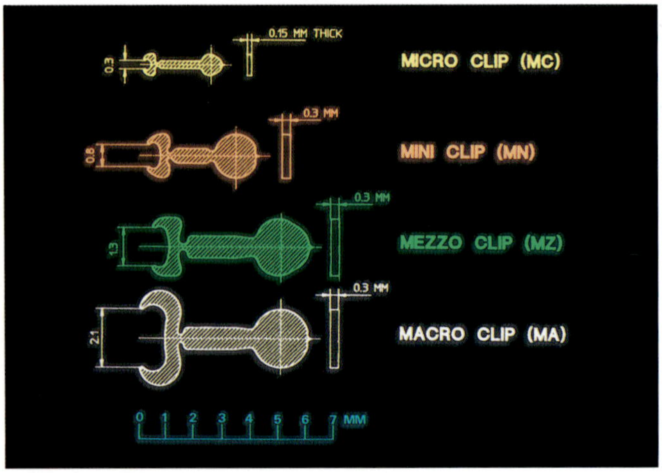

Fig. 9-6

The applier tip prior to actuation of the proximal cam for clip loading. Note the jaw angulation.

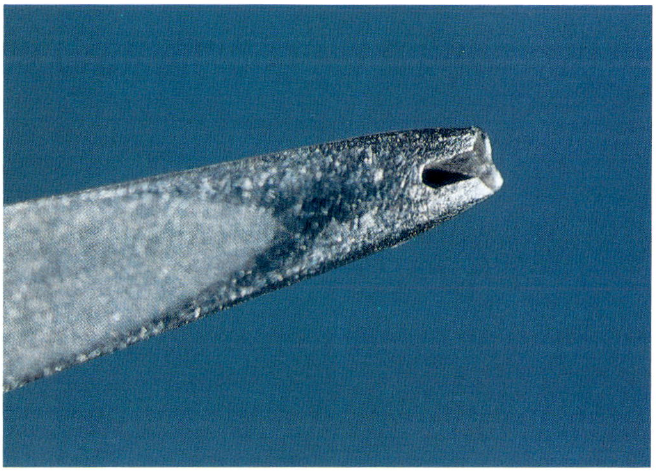

Fig. 9-7

Actuation of the applier's proximal wings extends the applier tip, exposing the slot to receive the microclip. This identical maneuver exposes the expended tang after clip application.

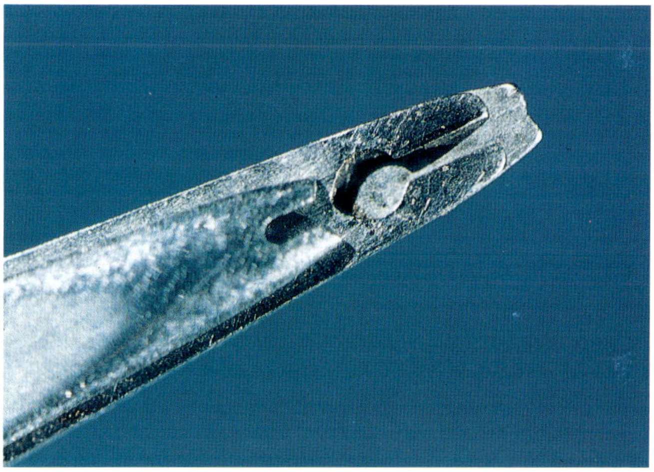

Fig. 9-8

A microclip has been loaded in the applier. Note the configuration of the clip head. Microclips are easily loaded with a fine curved forceps and magnification. Pressure on the proximal wings maintains this configuration of the applier, relaxation of pressure readies thc applicr for firing.

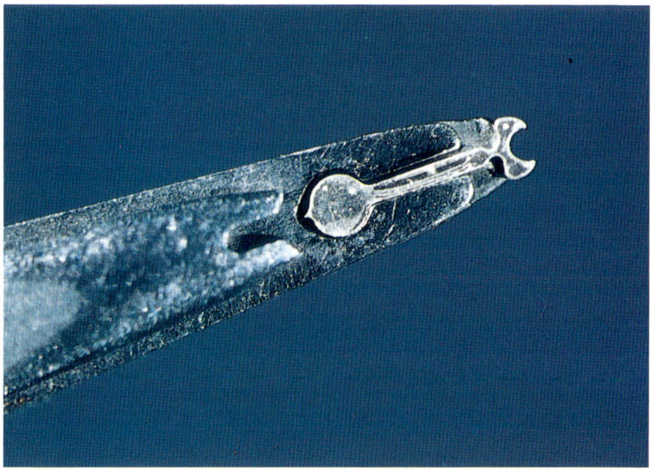

Fig. 9-9

The clip has been loaded, the proximal wings relaxed, and the clip is now ready to be fired. Notice the relationship of the clip shoulders to the jaw angulation. Clip firing is instantaneous with a squeezing motion between thumb and forefinger. Tactile feedback is associated with neck detachment.

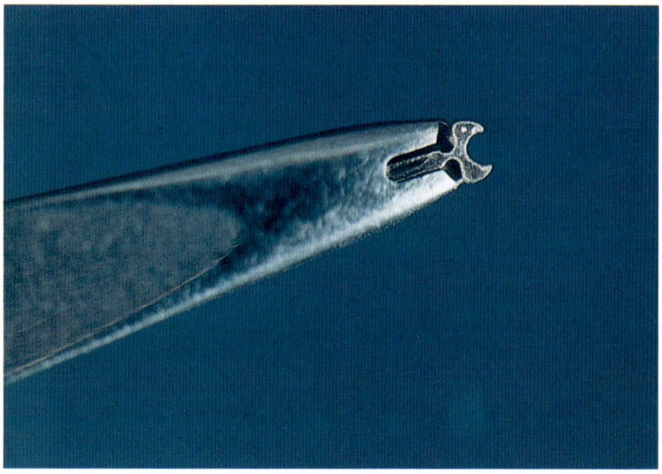

Fig. 9-10

This series of illustrations reviews the procedure for microclip loading and application.

The clip is held with a fine curved forceps by its tang in order to be placed unambiguously into the slotted receiver.

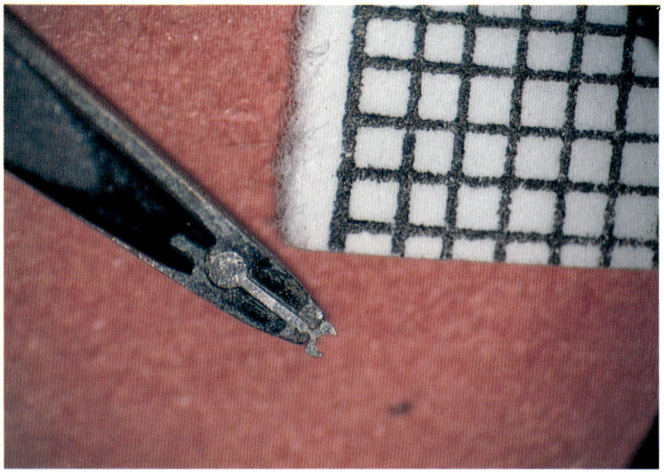

Fig. 9-11

The proximal actuator is squeezed, causing the jaws to be withdrawn, exposing the clip slot.

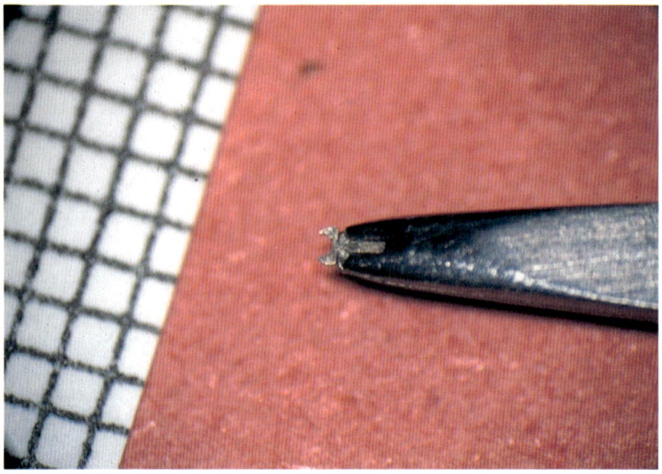

Fig. 9-12

The clip is loaded, the priximal actuator relaxed, and is now ready for application.

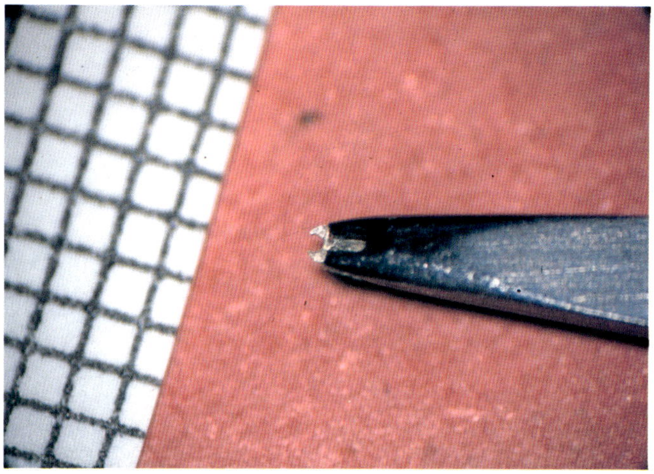

Fig. 9-13

The process of clip firing. Pressure on the distal actuator causes the jaws to make contact at the lateral shoulders of the clip resulting in clip closure.

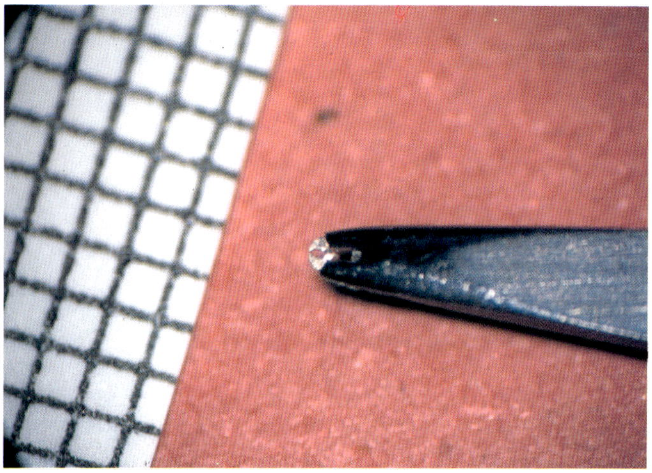

Fig. 9-14

As actuation continues and after the clip closes, the clip separates from its tang at a predetermined point.

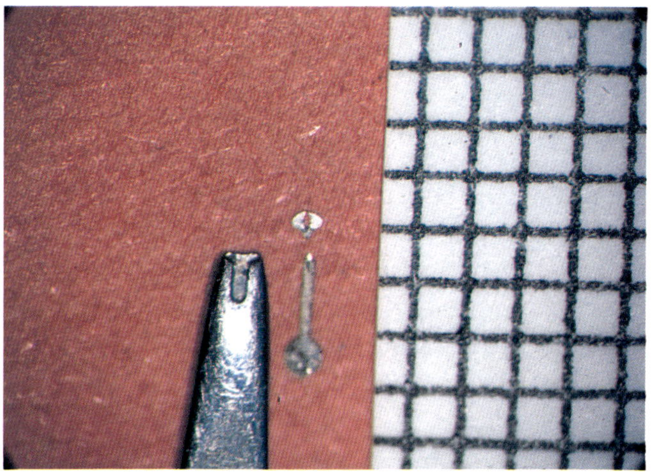

Fig. 9-15

The expended tang is easily removed by reexposing the slot and grasping the tang with fine forceps. Scale 1mm.

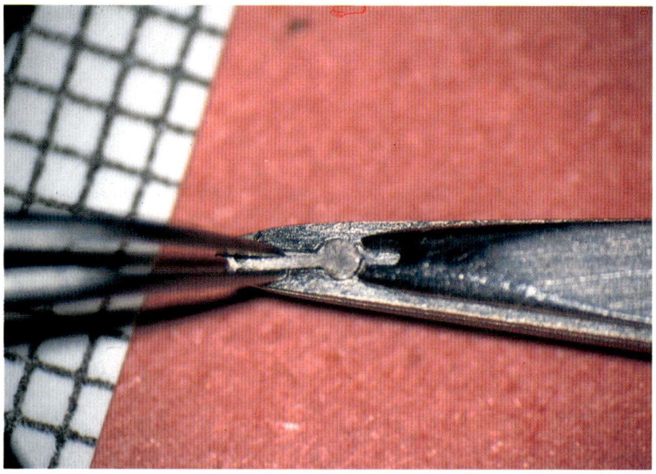

Fig. 9-16

Clip remover. The jaws of the Castroviejo needle holder have been reduced to a fine point. Squeezing the applied clip neck with the jaw points opens the clip and permits easy clip removal without intimal damage.

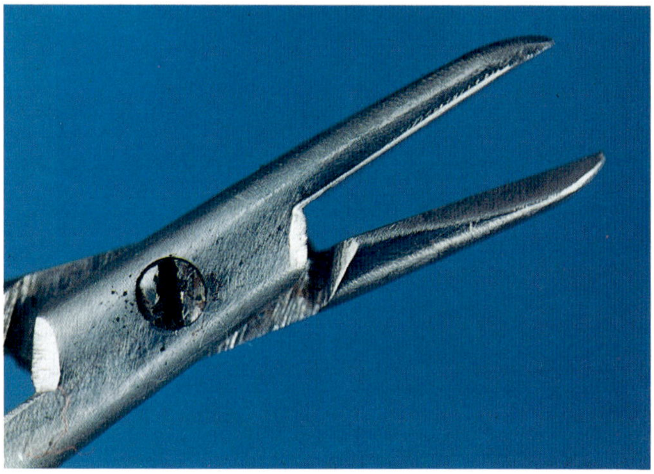

Fig. 9-17

Procedure for clip removal. **A.** A microclip applied to a sheet of plastic contrast material. **B.** The clip remover squeezing the bridge of the clip. **C.** Clip removal without tearing or damage to contrast material as a consequence of the nonpenetrating feature of the clip.

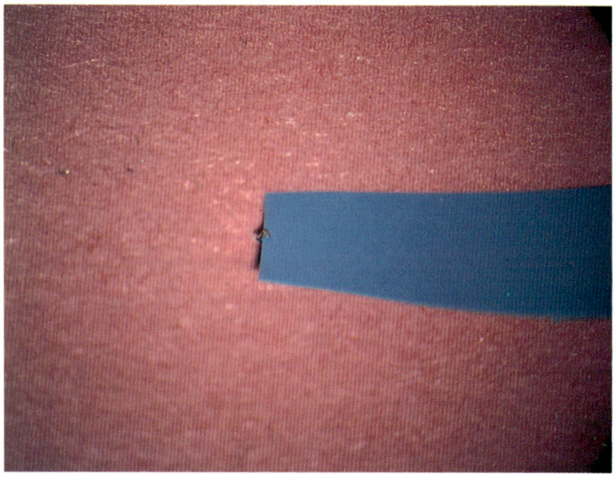

Fig. 9-18 A

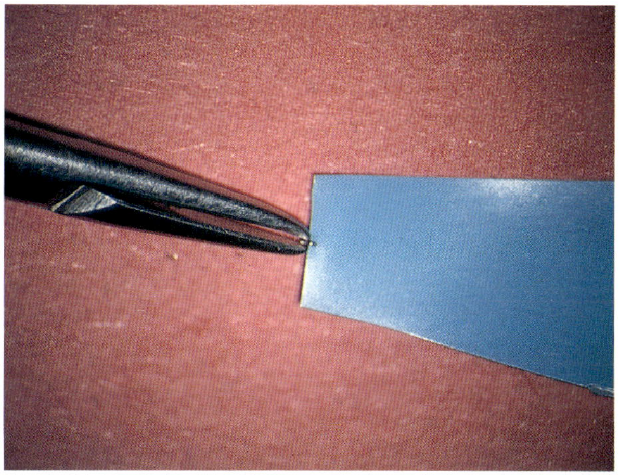

Fig. 9-18 B

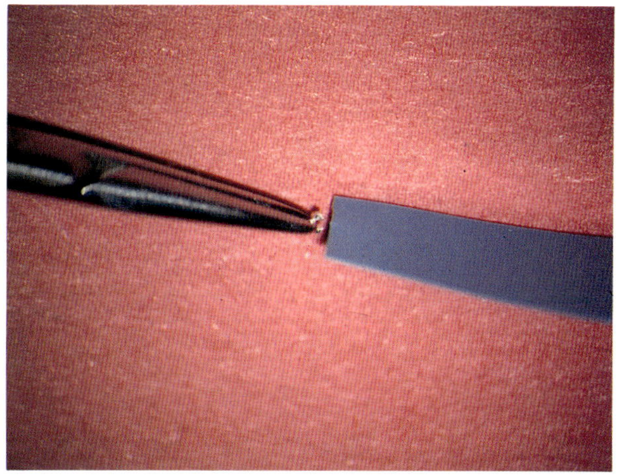

Fig. 9-18 C

References

1. Ostrup LT, Berggren A. The Uni-link instrument system for fast and safe microvascular anastomosis. *Ann Plast Surg*. 1980;17:521.
2. Nakayama K, Tamiya T, Yamamoto K, Akimoto S. A simple new apparatus for small vessel anastomosis (free autograft of the sigmoid included). *Surgery*. 1952;52:913.
3. Gottlob R, Blumel G. Anastomoses of small arteries and veins by means of bushings and adhesive. *J Cardiovasc Surg*. 1968;9:337.
4. Daniel RK, Olding M. An absorbable anastomotic device for microvascular surgery: experimental studies. *Plast Reconstr Surg*. 1984;74:329.
5. Obora Y, Tamaki N, Matsumoto S. Nonsuture microvascular anastomosis using magnetic rings: preliminary report. *Surg Neurol*. 1978;9:117.
6. Gang Z, Yi CL, Qun Q. Experience using microvascular anastomotic rings for the transplantation of 20 free flaps. *Plast Reconstr Surg*. 1989;84:822.
7. Zhu YH, Kirsch WM, Cushman R. Comparison of suture and clip for microvascular anastomosis. *Surg Forum*. 1985;36:492.
8. von Holst H, Collins P, Steiner L. Titanium, silver, and tantalum clip in brain tissue. *Acta Neurosurg*. 1956;56:239.

Chapter 10

Microvascular Anastomoses: Surgical Technique

W.M. Kirsch, MD

Y.H. Zhu, MD

Z. Boukouvalas, MD

R.A. Hardesty, MD

Dr. Lee's book *Experimental Microsurgery* provides the necessary technical background information for the construction of a sutured microvascular anastomosis. These details will enable the reader to place the clip technique into proper perspective. This amply illustrated volume reviews the development of techniques for microvascular anastomoses, discusses alternative nonsuture methods, and provides a practical guide for the design of microsurgical experiments. Special attention is directed to experimental microsurgical organ transplantation. There are basic surgical principles of arterial and venous exposure that are common to all anastomotic techniques, as well as precautions to minimize pitfalls. These details are important, and not generally published. The microsurgeon expert with needle and suture is in a better position to perceive the technical and biological advantages offered by the microclip.

The basic instruments necessary for performance of a clipped microvascular anastomosis have been described in the preceding chapter. The minimum requirements are two pairs of everting forceps, the clip applier, microclips, and clip remover. A stent is not necessary. The availability of more than one applier expedites the procedure. Figure 10-1 diagrams the technique and Figures 10-2 through 10-10 illustrate an end-to-end, microclipped anastomosis of a 0.8 mm rat femoral artery. Shuttling two appliers enables this procedure to be routinely performed in five to six minutes, about one third of the time required for microsuturing. Since vein walls are predominantly adventitia, the flanged microvenous anastomosis is actually easier than the arterial procedure. Microclips are applied sequentially, using about the same number of clips as microsutures for an appropriate sized vessel. The clipped anastomoses are usually "blood-tight," but in the event of leakage at a single point of the anastomotic sight, it is unnecessary to reapply temporary occluding clips. Reapplication of occluding clips to a previously ischemic segment is a threat to anastomotic patency. Any bleeding point at the clipped anastomotic site is easily sealed by grasping with the tips of the everting forceps and placing another microclip. Anastomotic bleeding from a microvascular anastomosis requiring control by either pressure or application of hemostatic agents is a serious threat to patency.

The end-to-side anastomosis requires the use of two everting forceps in order to form the flange for clip application. The heel is molded and clipped first, manipulating two everting forceps with both hands to shape the flange. The acute angulation at the "heel" restricts flange molding and application of the clip to the everted edges, therefore, the "heel" *must* be constructed first. Once the "heel" is secured, the "toe" is formed into a flange and clipped. After "heel" and "toe" are constructed, clipping proceeds rapidly along both walls to construct a "blood-tight" anastomosis. Formation of a well flanged "heel" is critical for success of the procedure. The "zero gap" microclip can accommodate different wall thicknesses and consistency, (vein, artery, prosthesis) at the flange.

The learning curve for the microclip anastomotic technique is very rapid. Excellent patency rates and "blood-tight" anastomoses are quickly achieved. Inexperienced surgeons can be taught within hours to successfully anastomose 1 mm rat femoral veins. Improved instrumentation and clip loading systems may permit even speedier construction of microvascular anastomoses. Clip application is a highly reproducible maneuver and consistent procedure, well tolerated by the microvasculature. In a laboratory demonstration of the clip, a rat femoral artery (0.8 mm O.D.) was serially reanastomosed at the same site within a two-hour time frame. Clips were applied, removed, and reapplied eight times, resulting in persistent patency of the artery.[2]

As with any surgical procedure, there are pitfalls to be mindful of. Silver microclips are fragile, soft, and easily bent. A bent clip has the precise geometric relation of shoulders to the jaw angles distorted and may scissor, or worse yet, not detach from the tang after closure. The clip should be inspected after loading into the applier to assure its alignment. There is a definite tactile feedback of the tang breaking. If the neck does not break after the clip is applied, pulling back on the applier will tear the vessel wall. This event is signalled by the absence of tactile feedback associated with the clip detaching. In the exceptional event of the tang not breaking, the clip is easily detached by the clip remover squeezing the tang neck. Microclips, appliers, everting forceps, and removers are precision instruments and will malfunction if caked with blood, not lubricated, or not treated with an ultrasonic cleaner between applications. Currently used appliers are remarkably durable, but the fine-tip everting forceps can be bent or broken if mishandled. Precautions are necessary in the handling and sterilizing of clips to avoid bending.

The principle of microclip application for vessel anastomosis. The loaded applier functions as a microfork after the flange has been shaped with everting forceps. Clips are applied at a 90° angle to the vessel axis. About the same number of clips as interrupted sutures are required for a blood-tight anastomosis.

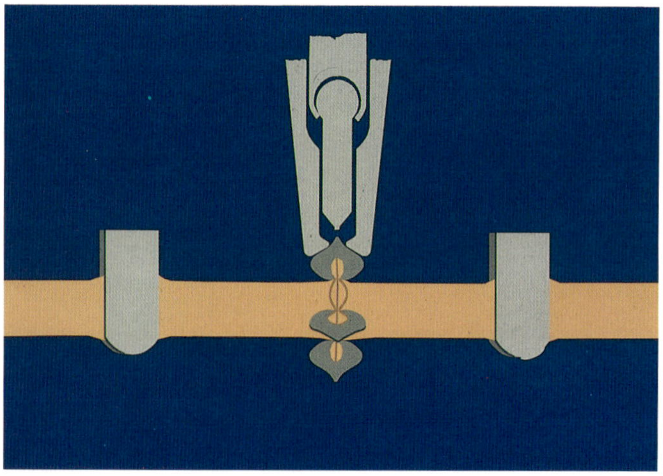

Fig. 10-1

A 0.8 mm O.D. rat femoral artery is prepared for anastomosis. The artery has been sectioned sharply. A mm rule demonstrates the size of the vessel and the size of microclips to be used for the anastomosis. Note that the adventitia is not extensively stripped.

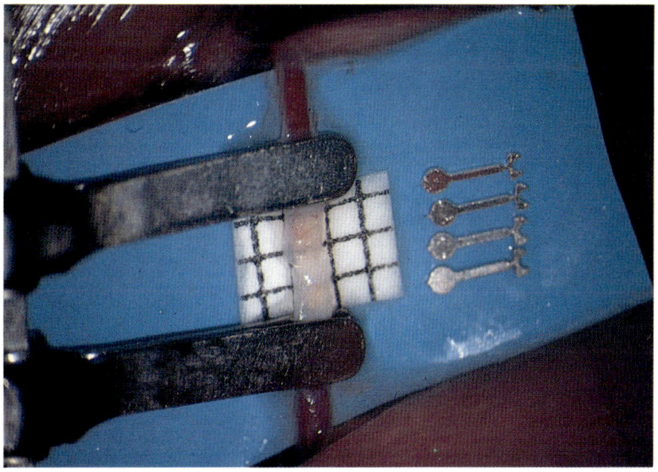

Fig. 10-2

The everting forceps has grasped the opposing adventitial edges and placed them into an everted flanged position. Note the intimal "sandwich" produced by the everting forceps. The pearly, central, intimal appearance indicates the correct intimal-to-intimal apposition.

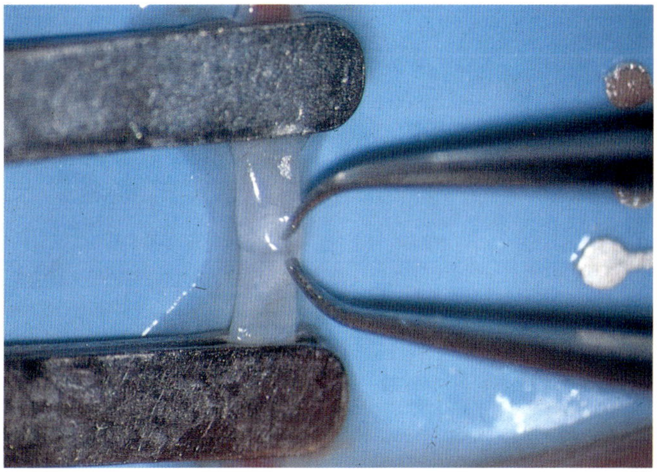

Fig. 10-3

With the everting forceps holding the vessel wall in an everted position, a microclip is applied. The applier approaches the flange at a 90° angle.

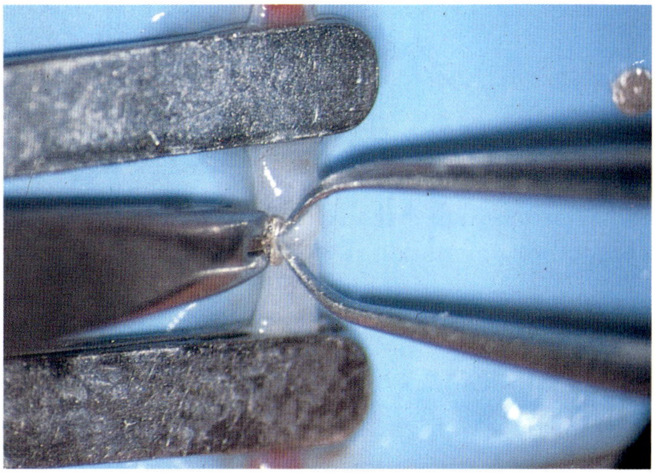

Fig. 10-4

After application of the first clip, the flange has been molded, and successive clips are easier to apply. Another clip is placed in an intermediate position on the front anastomotic line. It is not necessary to either stretch the vessel or place an internal stent. There is no danger of catching the opposite wall with the nonpenetrating clip.

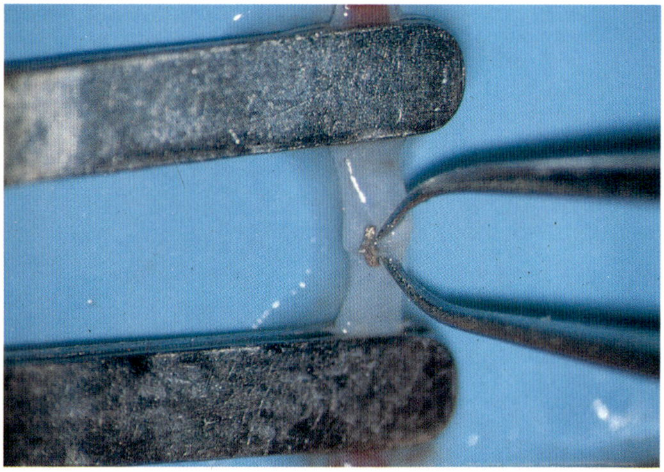

Fig. 10-5

Two clips have been placed on the anterior wall of the vessel. The flanged eversion is apparent as one visualizes the intima-to-intima contact between the clips.

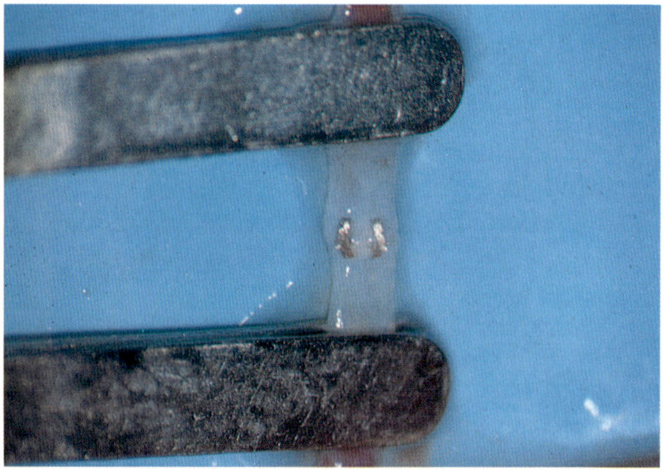

Fig. 10-6

The front wall is sealed with four microclips. The preparation is ready to be turned over to complete the back wall.

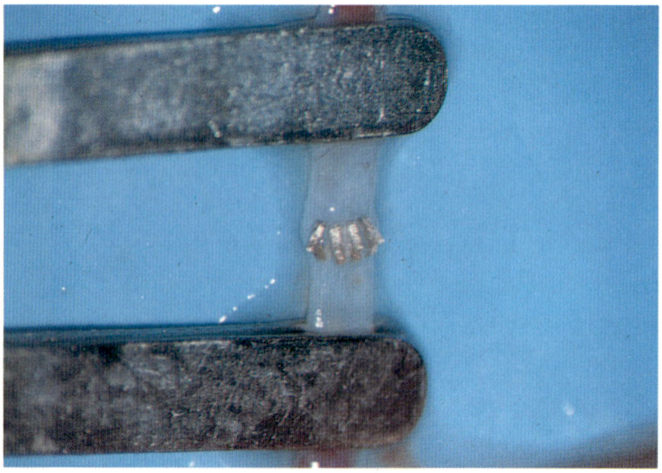

Fig. 10-7

The back wall is exposed. The first clip on the back wall is placed into the middle of the anastomotic line after inspection of the seamless front wall. The weight of clips on the front wall tends to retract the vessel wall away from the wall being anastomosed.

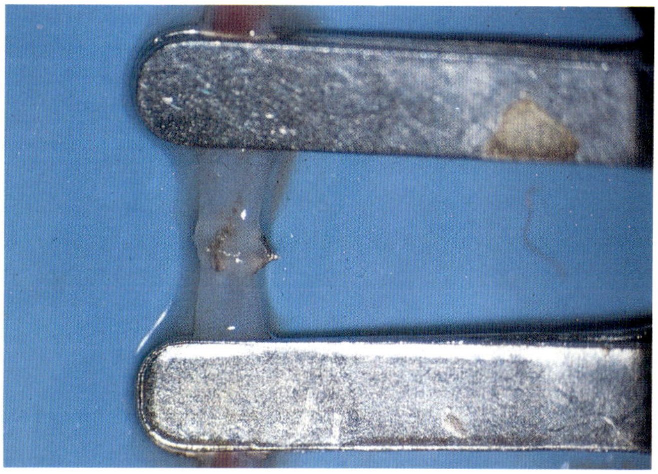

Fig. 10-8

The anastomosis is complete and "blood-tight" at the outset. A total of nine clips were required to complete this anastomosis. Clips have fractured from their neck in a predictable position leaving a smooth tab without sharp projections. This anastomosis can be performed in a physiologic salt solution if desired.

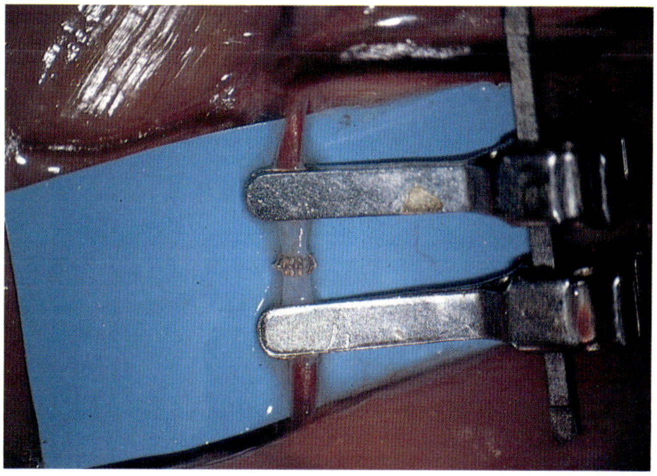

Fig. 10-9

Temporary clips have been withdrawn and the vessel is patent. The speed of this procedure with clips is approximately one third of that required for the use of suture. The intima has not been damaged. In the unlikely event that anastomotic bleeding does occur, it is unnecessary to replace the temporary occluding clips back on the vessel. The everting forceps is used to seal the bleeding point and another clip is applied.

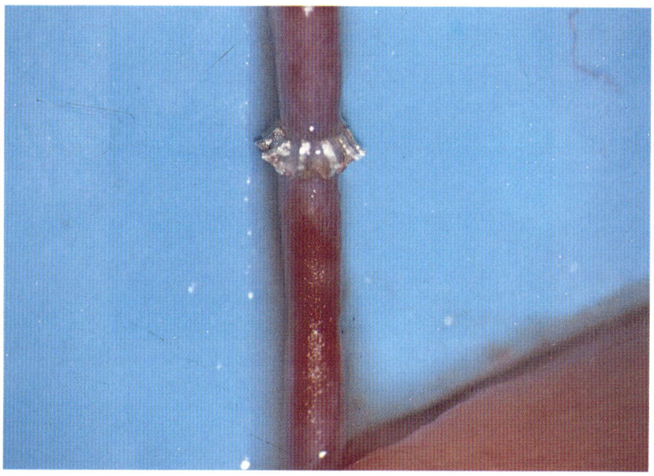

Fig. 10-10

An example of the versatility of the clip anastomotic technique. A 4 mm thin-walled, expanded PTFE vascular prosthesis has been clipped end-to-end to the external jugular vein of the dog and end-to-side into the right common carotid artery. The fistula was "blood-tight." The anastomosis was immediately performed with mezzoclips. This model served as a pilot experiment before proceeding with human vascular access procedures.

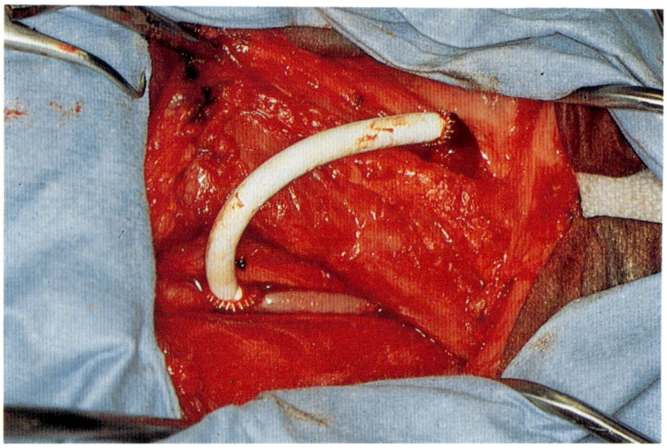

Fig. 10-11

References

1. Lee S. *Experimental Microsurgery*. 1st ed. New York-Tokyo: Igaku-Shoin Medical Publishers, Inc. 1987.
2. Demonstration of the clip at the University of Colorado Medical Center, Department of Surgery, Denver, Colorado, July 1988. Sponsored by Alden Harkin, M.D.

Acknowledgement: We wish to acknowledge and thank Mr. William Tinker, Wild Microscope Company, for his gracious help in obtaining the illustrations in this chapter.

Chapter 11

Morphologic Events During Healing of Microvascular Anastomoses

W.M. Kirsch, MD

Y.H. Zhu, MD

Z. Boukouvalas, MD

R.A. Hardesty, MD

E. LeGrand, DVM, PhD

P. Mann, PhD

There is extensive documentation of the structural response of small arteries and veins to sharp sectioning and subsequent anastomosis. For the most part, these observations have been made on rodent femoral and carotid vessels reconnected without undue tension, trauma, disease or incidental contamination.[1-9] Despite the experimental control feasible with these model systems, artifacts of explantation, preparation, and fixation still cloud experimental results. As improved analytical instruments are applied to the problem, an increasing awareness of artefactual changes has been apparent in published reports.

Comparative histologic studies of microclipped and microsutured rat and rabbit femoral arteries demonstrate remarkable differences. Though medial and elastic laminal damage occur with both suture and clips, the most significant morphologic difference is the thrombogenic and inflammatory response at the anastomotic site. The penetrating needle and suture incite a vigorous and prompt platelet-fibrin reaction at the intial anastomotic site, a reaction more intense in veins than arteries. Within days the sutures are surrounded by inflammatory cells. This thrombogenic response is absent in the clipped microvessels, and correspondingly with reendothelialization is apparent at the anastomotic cleft within 24 hours. Arterial reendothelization after clipping is accompanied by an "intimal hyperplasia" confined to and beginning at the anastomotic cleft. Sutured veins require up to three weeks for anastomotic site reendothelization, whereas microclipped veins are reendothelialized within a week.

The mechanisms for endothelial repair and replacement are a function of vessel diameter. In large vessels, rapid endothelial turnover and replication occur at the ostia of the vasa vasorum and at the margin of endothelial loss. Mechanisms for endothelial repair in 1-2 mm diameter arteries is uncertain. The anastomotic cleft formed by an everted intima-to-intima anastomosis in small caliber arteries and veins can reendothelize without continuity to the advancing edges of endothelial denudation.[11,12] Thus, primary repair of the anastomotic cleft may be due to blood-borne cells recognizing special biochemical signals, or to retained islands of endothelial cells. The transformation of blood-borne cells into endothelium remains speculative and unproven.

Our fine structural studies of clipped arterial and venous anastomoses demonstrate a rapid filling at the denuded anastomotic cleft with bridging endothelial cells interdigitating with one another. These events are occurring within 24 hours after the clipped anastomosis. Considering that one square millimeter of endothelial surface contains 4,000 to 5,000 cells, these "tongue-in-groove" interdigitations could account for the adhesive bonding that characterizes the flange. At higher magnification this endothelial bonding takes the physical form of discrete vesicular cellular interdigitations. These fine structural observations may provide a morphologic explanation for the unusual strength of flanged microvascular anastomoses. This property of relatively rapid anastomotic site reendothelialization has been observed with other mechanical devices (Nakayama Ring, Unilink System). The histologic features common to both systems (Unilink and microsutures) are reendothelization within three weeks for both artery and vein, early intimal and medial inflammatory cell infiltration, and resolution of the inflammatory process by three weeks. The inflammatory response may be secondary to either circumferential tissue crushing of the tissue flange between the polyethylene discs or the steel pin penetration.

In summary, the clipped microarterial and microvenous anastomosis has minimal to no fibrin at the anastomotic line, minimal vessel wall inflammatory reaction, and prompt reendothelization. It is believed that these features are all based on the fact that the intima is not penetrated, thus preventing the access of platelets to subintimal collagen and effectively reducing matrix protein "oxidative" stress.

A longitudinal section of a rat femoral artery 24 hours after microvascular anastomosis with 10-0 nylon, studied by the technique of Acland and Trachtenberg.[12] There is a fibrin clot at the site of the anastomosis and intraluminal suture.

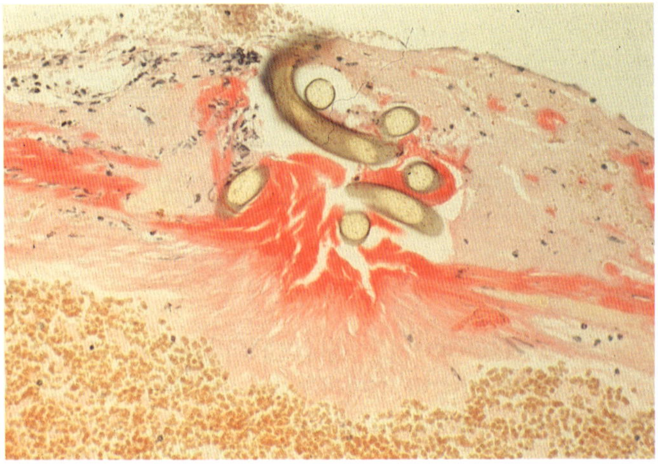

Fig. 11-1

An anastomosed rat femoral vein four days after microsuture. This vein had recanalized and appeared "patent" by conventional "strip and refill" testing.

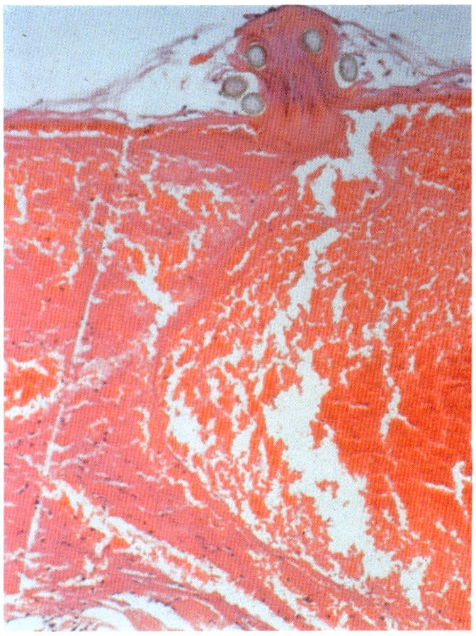

Fig. 11-2

A microclipped rat femoral vein with evidence of endothelial repair four days after anastomosis. There is characteristically minimal evidence of fibrin or thrombosis at the clipped anastomotic site.

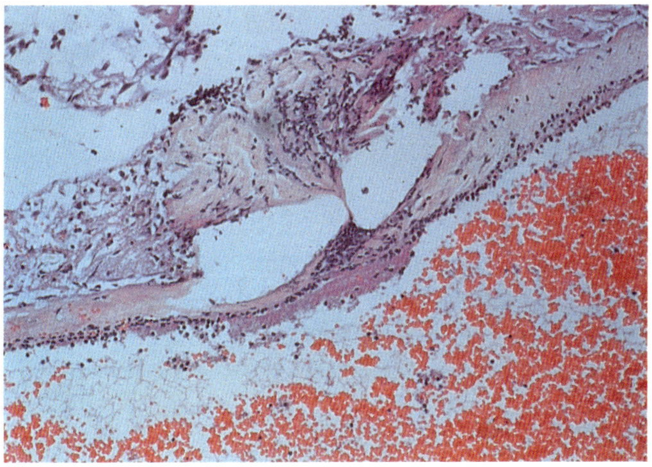

Fig. 11-3

Microclipped rat femoral venous anastomosis four hours post-surgery stained by the Haemotoxylin-Van Giessen method for connective tissue. There is remodeling of the venous wall, absence of clot at the anastomotic site, and a minimal local inflammatory response.

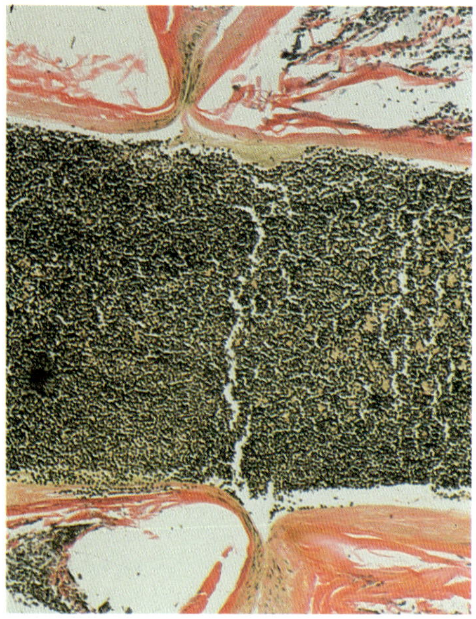

Fig. 11-4

Scanning electron microscopic picture of 1.2 mm microclipped rat femoral vein one week after the anastomosis. Complete reendothelialization of the anastomotic site has occurred.

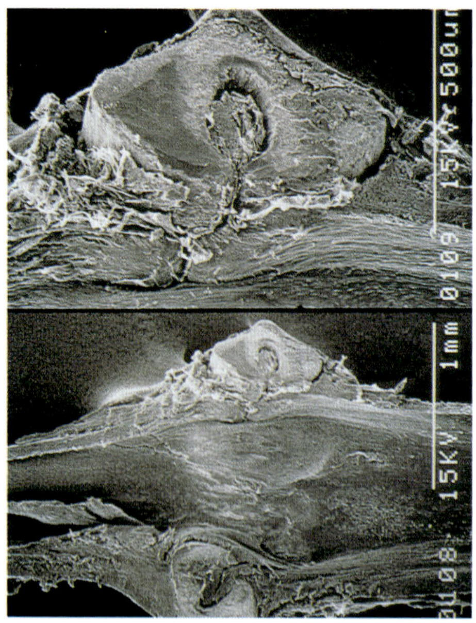

Fig. 11-5

The "zero gap" of the microclip does not penetrate the intima but creates focal adventitial, medial, and endothelial compression and necrosis.

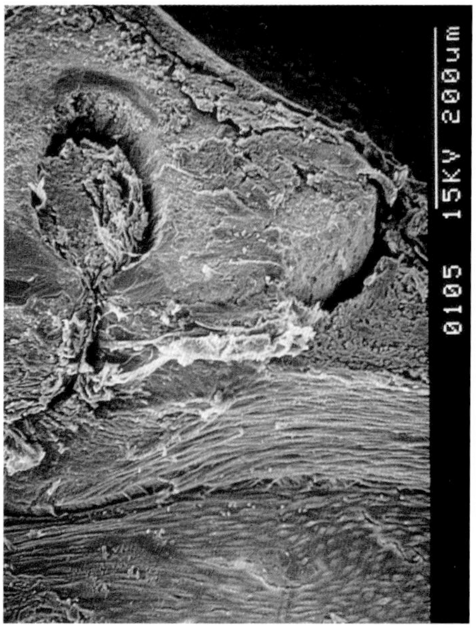

Fig. 11-6

High magnification scanning microscopy of the completely restored endothelial surface one week after clipped anastomosis. This rapid reendothelization has been confirmed in larger venous clipped anastomosis.

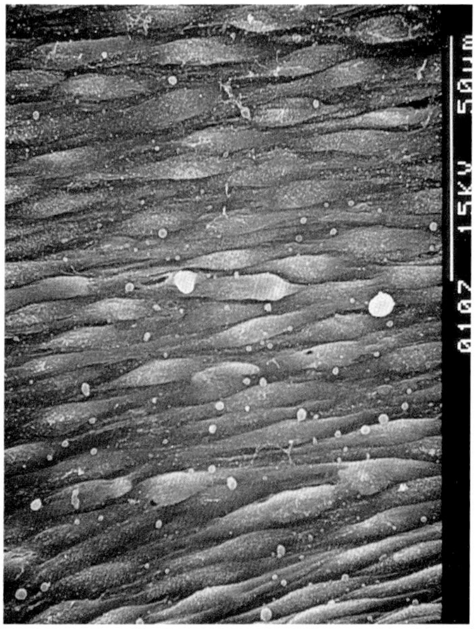

Fig. 11-7

Rat femoral artery sectioned and clip anastomosed. Microclips were removed five hours after the anastomosis and the anastomosis held.

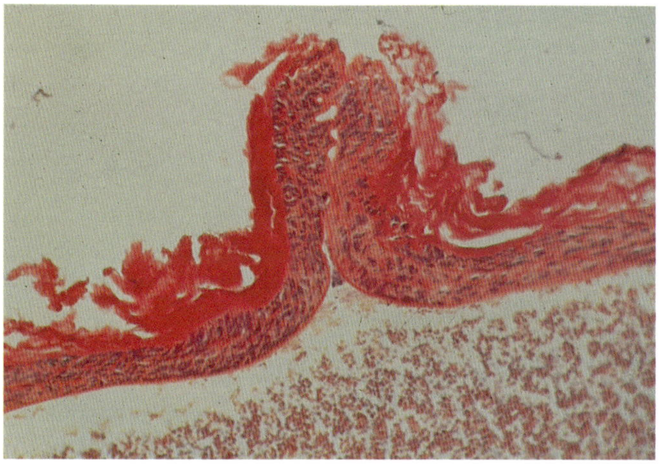

Fig. 11-8

Remodeling of the rat femoral artery wall, absence of anastomotic site fibrin, evidence of endothelialization at three days after a microclipped anastomosis.

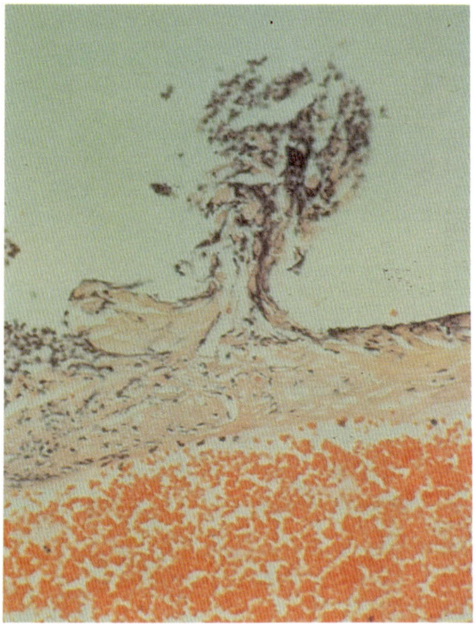

Fig. 11-9

A typical microclipped rat femoral artery one week after anastomosis. The microclips have been removed for histologtical processing. There is evidence for reendothelialization at the anastomotic site.

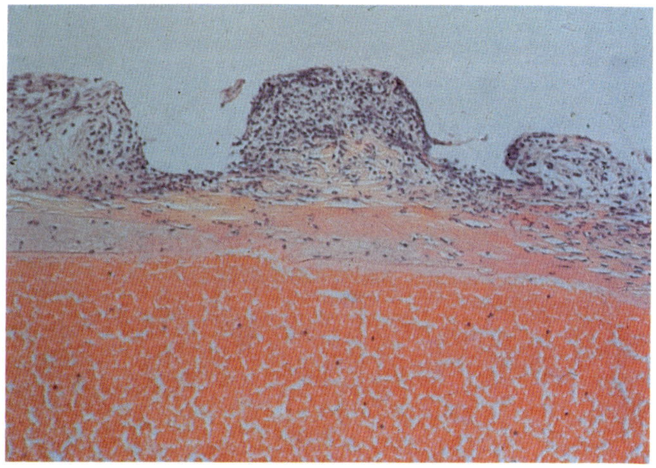

Fig. 11-10

Rat femoral artery to vein end-to-side anastomosis with microclips. Clips were applied for 30 minutes and then removed. The anastomosis remains intact and patent. Healing occurs without aneurysm formation and without immobilizing the leg.

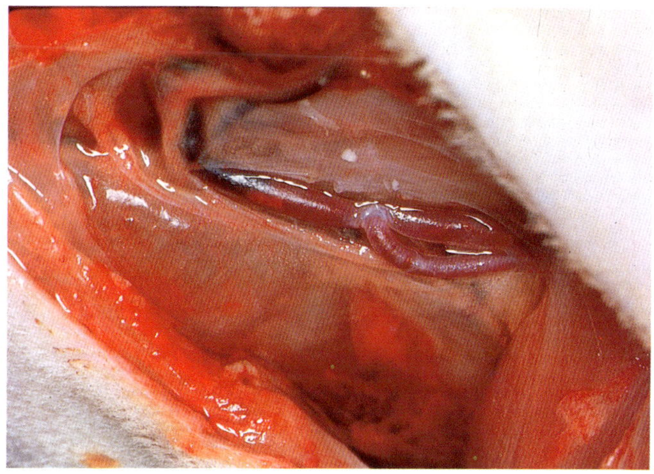

Fig. 11-11

Rat femoral vein re-anastomosed with 10-0 nylon and harvested according to text at one week after surgery. Note the extensive fibrin deposition and inflammatory response at the anastomotic site. The vessel was considered patent by "strip and refill" testing.

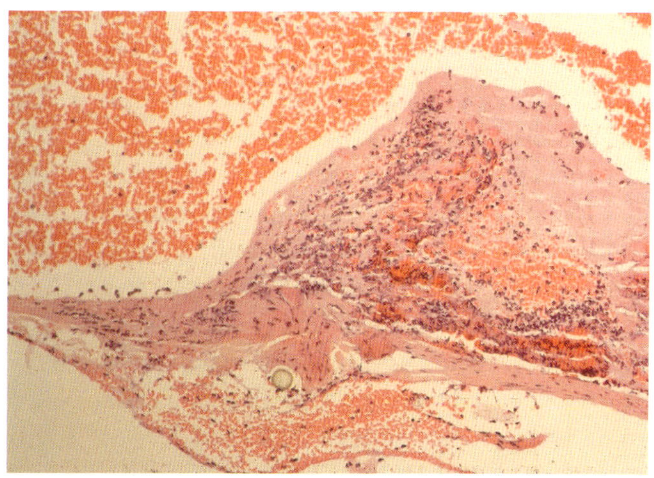

Fig. 11-12

The model system for preparation of the microvascular anastomosis for morphologic study. This idealized diagram shows the specimen configuration and dimensions for the rabbit carotid to jugular end-to-side anastomosis explant.

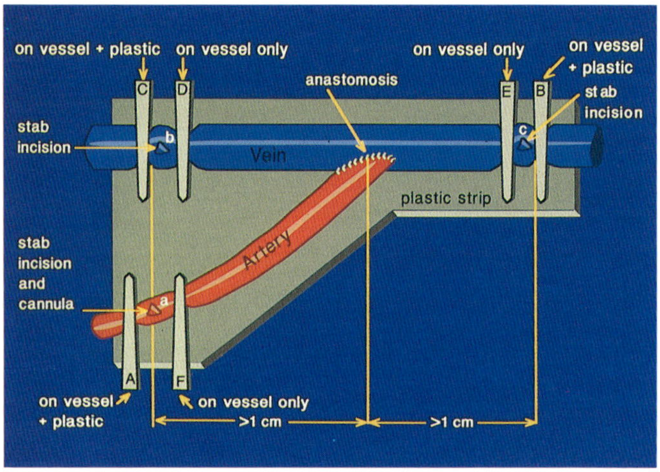

Fig. 11-13

Remodeling of rat femoral vein anastomotic site 140 days after clip anastomosis.

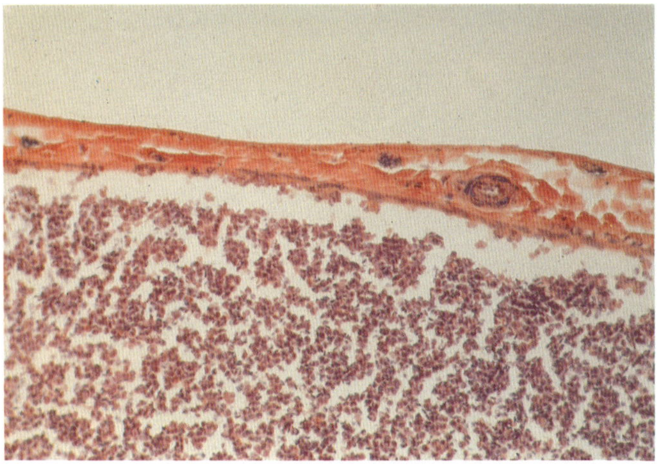

Fig. 11-14

Clinical application of the clips for end-to-end, end-to-side, and vascular mismatch anastomoses in a severe industrial accident. The patient sustained an avulsion fracture of the left arm that necessitated a latissimus dorsi free-flap transfer; donor artery and veins (thoracodorsal artery and associated veins), recipient artery and veins (ulnar artery, vena comitante, superficial forearm vein) (Figs. 11-15 through 11-17).

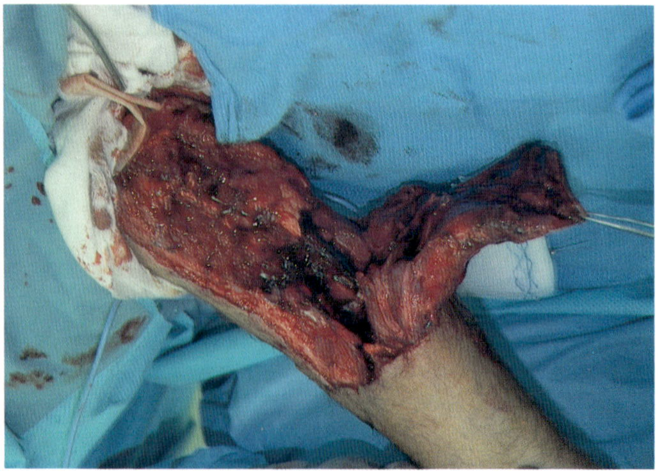

Fig. 11-15

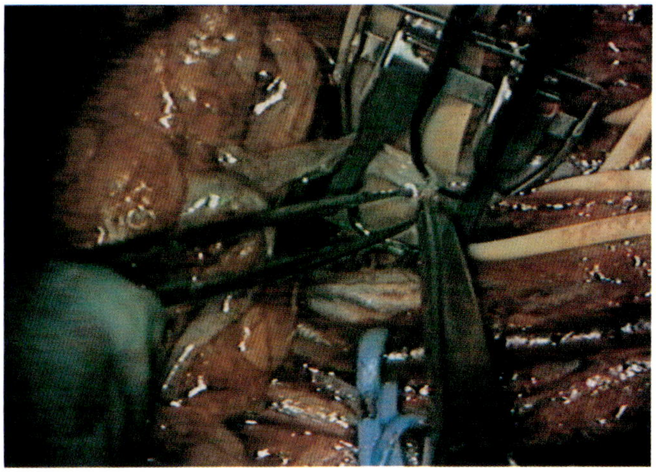

Fig. 11-16

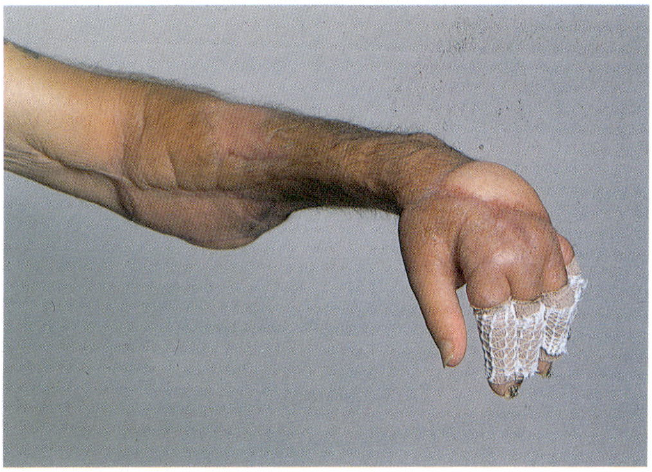

Fig. 11-17

References

1. Horashina T, Fujino T, Watanabe S. The initial healing of microvascular anastomoses. *Plast Reconstr Surg*. 1976;58:608.
2. Zhu YH, Kirsch WM, Cushman R. Comparison of suture and clip for microvascular anastomosis. *Surg Forum*. 1985;36:492.
3. Lidman D, Daniel RK. The normal healing process of microvascular anastomosis. *Scand J Plast Reconstr Surg*. 1981;15:103.
4. Nakayama K, Tamiya T, Yamamoto K, Akimoto S. A simple new apparatus for small vessel anastomosis (free autograft of the sigmoid included). *Surgery*. 1962;52:913.
5. Ostrup LT, Berggren A. The Uni-link Instrument System for fast and safe microvascular anastomosis. *Ann Plast Surg*. 1986;17:721.
6. Gentile F, Lougheed WM, Yoshjima S, Hondolt MB. A technique for rapid non-suture vascular anastomosis. *Can J Neurol Sci*. 1978;14:117.

7. van Gelder PA, Klopper PJ. Healing of microvascular arterial anastomoses as seen on corrosion casts by scanning electron microscopy. *Plast Reconstr Surg*. 1979;1:59.

8. Khodadad G. Histological evaluation of long-term microvascular repair and replacement. *Arch Surg*. 1970;101:503.

9. Longa EZ, Welnstein PR, Chater G. Scanning electron microscopy studies of needle and suture damage in rat carotid and femoral arteries. *Microsurg*. 1984;5:169.

10. Rasmussen LH, Garbarsch, Lorenzen L. Injury and repair of smaller muscular and elastic arteries. *Virschows Arch A*. 1987;411:87.

11. Tanaka A, Hirst AE, Smith LL. Rate of endothelization in venous thrombi. *Arch Surg*. 1982;117:1045.

12. Acland RD, Trachtenberg L. A method for accurately orienting small blood vessels for longitudinal section. *Stain Technology*. 1977;52:2.

Chapter 12

The Nonpenetrating Arcuate-Legged Clip: Clinical Applications

W.M. Kirsch, MD
Y.H. Zhu, MD
R.A. Hardesty, MD
M.H.C. Webster, MD
Z. Boukouvalas, MD
D. Furnas, MD

The nonpenetrating clip has proven useful clinically not only as a vascular anastomosing device but as a unique approximator for other tissues in diverse surgical settings. Clips not only allow speedy, highly reproducible, and patent vascular anastomoses, but are effective for complex dural closures, control of sagittal and cavernous sinus bleeding, and the plication of intracranial arterial aneurysms. The clip has eased the management of complex intracranial tumors, improved the patency rates of arteriovenous (A-V) fistulas for hemodialysis, and shortened the ischemia time associated with free flap transfer. The clip can be used on atherosclerotic arteries and functions as well or better than suture, particularly with A-V access procedures, veins, and intracranial arterial aneurysm walls.[1-4] Other tubular structures have been successfully reconstructed with clips: gut, ureter, Fallopian tube, and vas deferens. The prompt healing afforded by the nonpenetrating arcuate-legged clip has resulted in its use as a suture substitute for endoscopic surgery. This chapter describes clinical experiences from a variety of institutions and surgeons.

Neurosurgical Applications: 52 Cases

The original impetus for developing the microclip stemmed from our dissatisfaction (Kirsch, Zhu) with suturing as the method for anastomosing the superficial temporal artery (STA) to the middle cerebral artery (MCA) branches for the purpose of brain revascularization.[5] Superficial cerebral cortical arteries are small diameter, thin-walled structures that are easily ruined with conventional microneedles, suture, and temporary occluding clips. Ironically, as our confidence with the quality of clipped microvascular anastomosis grew with successful surgical laboratory experiments and progressive improvements in instrumentation, the popularity and frequency of the cerebral "bypass" operation waned. A large, cooperative clinical trial failed to prove uniform merit for the procedure.[6] The procedure is justified, however, for selected cases of cerebral ischemia with very specific indications, and the clip has been applied successfully in two of these special cases. *In our opinion, the entire STA-MCA issue warrants reexamination using an anastomotic technique other than needle-and-suture.* This technical consideration has been completely overlooked in interpreting the results of the cooperative study. A high flow rate, microsutured arterial anastomotic line is an active source for emboli.[7] The poor results of the sutured "bypass" anastomoses could well be due to persistent showers of emboli into the brain's microcirculation. Despite the angiographic appearance of anastomotic "patency," microinfarcts in the cerebral circulation leading to progressive neurologic deterioration are a conceivable cause for the lack of effectiveness of the sutured STA-MCA anastomoses.

Two patients have had "bypass" procedures performed with clips for cerebral ischemia. The first patient, a 68-year-old woman with bilateral internal carotid and left vertebral artery occlusions, had only the left vertebral artery as the major artery supplying her brain. Her collateral circulation via the external carotids was decompensating and resulting in frequent transient ischemic attacks manifested by speech disturbance and weakness. A right STA-MCA anastomosis was performed in June, 1989 with microclips. A 10-0 suture was placed at the "heel" and "toe" of the anastomosis prior to the application of microclips because the clip tips were too small to encompass the everted edges at these points. The STA, despite papaverine, measured 1 mm (O.D.) and the MCA branch 2 mm (O.D.). Though microclips were too small for the "heel" and "toe" and the mezzoclips too large, a successful anastomosis was created with microclips for both sides of the end-to-side anastomosis. Two sutures were necessary, one for the "heel," and the other for the "toe." The patient has subsequently improved and the anastomosis is open by transcranial Doppler and MR angiography (Figs. 12-1, 12-2, and 12-3). As a consequence of this case, the miniclip was constructed, a clip intermediate in size between mini and mezzo that functions well for cerebral vessels 1.0-2.5 mm (O.D.). This clip with a slightly larger mouth has worked well in a second bypass case, for two cerebral arterial reconstructions, and achieving hemostasis from the cavernous sinus during the course of subtotal meningioma removal.

Clips have proven useful in the surgical management of eleven complex intracranial aneurysms. The first human application of the nonpenetrating Kirsch clip occurred in September, 1986 to achieve intraoperative hemostasis during the course of resecting a giant vertebral artery aneurysm (Fig. 12-4). The aneurysm was "trapped" but continued to back-bleed from collateral channels despite presumed proximal and distal control. Bleeding from the opened and diseased left vertebral artery could not be controlled by balloon catheters. Hemostasis was achieved by sealing the opened artery with a large pericardial patch graft secured by macroclips (Figs. 12-5, 12-6, and 12-7). The clip's ability to control hemorrhage in this awkward anatomical situation warranted further use. Among the eleven cases have been the successful plication of a dissecting right vertebral artery aneurysm (macroclips); plication of a traumatic right internal carotid, medially presenting, infraclinoid internal carotid artery aneurysm (macroclips); the intraoperative reconstruction of the basilar bifurcation and posterior circle of Willis after intraoperative rupture of a large, sessile, basilar aneurysm (mezzoclips); and resection of a megagiant (9 cm diameter) aneurysm with an interpositional internal carotid-to-MCA bifurcation 15 mm saphenous vein graft (miniclips).

The megagiant aneurysm patient presented with severe acute neurologic deterioration; transtentorial and transfalcine herniation. The interpositional graft thrombosed 24 hours postoperatively. There are a number of technical factors that in retrospect may have contributed to the acute graft failure. These include damage to the proximal atherosclerotic middle cerebral artery by a temporary occluding Satinsky clamp, severe postoperative hypotension that was persistent, and the fact that the patient was not treated with volume expanders or anticoagulants. A balloon angioplasty of the proximal middle cerebral artery may have been advantageous to maintain patency. The patient was relieved of his mass effect that was producing transtentorial and transfalcine herniation, but was hemiplegic and aphasic.

Clips have been used for complex dural closures as well as base-of-skull tumors (thirty-six cases) (Fig. 12-8). Mezzo clips enabled a flanged, "water-tight," craniotomy closure in one case in the absence of available dura. A 68-year-old woman with a large pituitary tumor and severe hyperostosis frontalis had a right frontal craniotomy. The frontal dura was atrophic and nonexistent in some areas, but the inner table of frontal bone was soft and evertable. The dural prosthesis was macroclipped directly to this edge and her craniotomy healed uneventfully. The clip very effectively controls bleeding from torn dural sinuses, as established by application to the bleeding sagittal and cavernous sinuses (three cases).

Vascular Access Surgery: 16 Cases

The first systematic controlled clinical trial of the clip for a specific surgical procedure took place at the Nephrology Center of Lower Saxony, Germany (Prof. Dr. F. Quellenhorst, Director) under the auspices of Dr. Winfred Schott, Chief of the Department of Urology and Transplantation and Dr. Jurt Rohwher. The vascular access procedure was selected for study because of the relatively high rate of early thrombosis (10% immediate, 14 to 20% within the first year), minimal threat to life or limb, and the ease of noninvasive monitoring for fistula dimensions and flow rate. Access surgeons have an increasing appreciation of the need to apply microsurgical techniques to the procedure to achieve better results. The macro and mezzoclip were designed specifically for this procedure on the basis of multiple measurements of human brachial arteries and cephalic veins at surgery and formalin-fixed histological sections. The study was initiated on August 2, 1988 with three surgeons performing all access procedures, clipped and sutured. Most of the procedures were performed on patients whose A-V access procedures had failed on at least one occasion with conventional suture. Between August 2, 1988 and December 1989, a total of 79 A-V fistulas were performed on 64 patients: 16 by clip, the remainder by conventional suture (Fig. 12-9).

All but one of the 16 clipped fistulas have so far remained patent and in steady use for hemodialysis. One patient had acute shunt thrombosis. This patient had advanced and severe atheroschlerosis. In another case (basilic vein to a brachial artery), a postoperative subcutaneous hematoma required draining 24 hours after surgery. The fistula was noted to be blood-tight at reexploration and bleeding was from a subcutaneous vessel not involved in the anastomosis. The only complication of note in this series has been the slow and progressive growth of two clipped fistula sites that increased the minute shunt volume to the point of creating a peripheral "steal" syndrome. In these two cases it was necessary to reexpose the fistula and narrow the anastomosis with suture. Spontaneous narrowing of a clipped anastomosis has not yet been observed. This phenomenon of progressive fistula growth observed with clips may be beneficial when utilizing clips for anastomoses in the distal forearm or creating angio access in small diameter (1 mm) vessels of children (Figs. 12-13 and 12-14).

In the same period of time (August, 1988 to December, 1989), 57 A-V fistulas were created by conventional suture, 42 at the wrist (Brescia-Cimino) and the remainder at the brachial level. Early thrombosis (within six months) was noted in nine patients, or 14%, an acute failure rate consistent with previous reports. This study remains in progress, with results under continuous review.

Free Flap Reconstruction: 15 Cases

The transposition of large composite tissue blocks for coverage of extensive body defects is based on the surgical advance of microvascular reconstructions—both arterial and venous. The clip technique enables the rapid assembly of venous and arterial vascular connections, thereby reducing the warm ischemia time of the transposed tissue. A total of fifteen cases have been performed, and these experiences will be described. The first application of the clip technology to free-flap transfer was conducted by Dr. Martyn Webster at the Canniesburn Hospital, Glasgow, Scotland. Though his initial experiences were positive (eight free-flap transfers without failure), he encountered mechanical difficulties with a prototype clip applier. These difficulties were associated with electrolytic changes in the cams, causing the applier to malfunction. These problems were promptly remedied by reassembling the appliers with electrocorrosion-resistant materials. Dr. Webster feels that the clips offers significant advantages in terms of speed of the anastomotic procedure, thus shortening the warm ischemia time. Other free flaps have been performed at the University of California, Irvine (Dr. David Furnas) and Loma Linda University (Dr. Robert Hardesty).

Details of Dr. Hardesty's (Cases 1, 2) and Dr. Furnas's (Case 3) cases are given below to illustrate other clinical experiences.

Clinical Applications of the Nonpenetrating "Kirsch" Clip

Case #1

A 68-year-old diabetic woman with an 8 cm by 7 cm ulcerated osteomyelitic lesion of the left tibia and fibula had transfer of a rectus abdominous muscle flap to cover the defect. The anterior tibial artery and two vena comitantes were isolated in the leg and joined end-to-side to the epigastric artery and to the vena comitantes of the rectus abdominus muscle. Warm ischemia time for the flap was ninety-eight minutes, suturing time: tibial to epigastric artery, thirty minutes; one posterior tibial vena comitante to one rectus vena comitante, twenty-five minutes; the third anastomosis of the post-tibial and rectus vena comitante was done with mezzoclips, eight minutes. The muscle was covered with split skin. The flap remains viable.

Comment

This case illustrates the advantage offered by the clips in shortening the duration of the anastomotic procedure, particularly for the venous anastomoses. This reduction of warm ischemia time can contribute to flap survival, but more importantly, the troublesome venous anastomosis is simplified.

Cases #2

A 72-year-old male with metastatic squamous carcinoma of the right buccal cavity with dissemination into the mandible had been previously treated with a right radical neck dissection, mandibulectomy, and 5000 rads of local irradiation. The ensuing extensive ulcerating lesion was debrided with a right radical neck dissection. Reconstruction of the oral cavity and neck was attempted with a transverse rectus abdominous myocutaneous flap. The right common, internal, and external carotid artery were profoundly atherosclerotic and diseased secondary to irradiation. The superior thyroid artery was opened and found to be totally occluded. The flap was placed into position and a venous anastomosis between the rectus vena comitantes was promptly established by mezzoclips end-to-side to the right internal jugular vein. The end-to-side clip anastomosis of veins required six minutes. The markedly atheromatous, and almost totally occluded, external carotid stump was then clipped end-to-end to the rectus arterial supply. Flow through the flap was adequate for fifteen minutes and then stopped. The arterial anastomotic site was occluded with fresh thrombus, particularly proximally. The arterial anastomosis was then restructured with 8-0 nylon and blood flow was temporarily restored to the flap with excellent venous drainage. The arterial anastomosis thrombosed again after a ten minute interval. A third attempt to establish an arterial supply to the free flap was made by attempting a microsutured anastomosis end-to-side to the right common carotid artery. The artery was severely atheroschlerotic and a limited endarterectomy was performed before establishing a microsutured anastomosis. Perfusion was restored to the flap for about ten minutes with excellent venous drainage, but again the arterial anastomosis thrombosed. The free flap was then abandoned and coverage was accomplished by a pectoral flap.

Comment

Case #2 demonstrates the futility of attempting to access an exceedingly diseased arterial supply to a free flap. The external carotid artery should have been endarterectomized at its origin, or an interpositional venous graft should have been placed. The remarkable fact is that the clipped venous anastomoses did not occlude and reopen with arterial perfusion. This event would be unusual in a sutured venous anastomoses.

Case #3

A 47-year-old woman with leiomyosarcoma invading the right middle fossa, orbit, and maxilla incontinuity had a radical "base of skull" tumor resection after unsuccessful local irradiation and chemotherapy. She sustained a massive infratemporal-orbital craniofacial resectional defect that included the right hemimaxilla with palate and nasal septum, right orbit, orbital floor and orbital contents, right zygomatic body and arch, right pterygoid processes and right pterygoid portion of the floor of the middle cranial fossa. Closure of this large defect was accomplished by procurement and transfer by microvascular anastomosis of segmented right serratus anterior osteo-cutaneous free flap. The vascular anastomoses consisted of subscapular artery to facial artery (end-to-side with Kirsch clips), and subscapular vein to facial vein (end-to-end with Kirsch clips). The facial artery was extensively atherosclerotic secondary to local radiation and required an endarterectomy. The arterial anastomoses required eighteen messo clips and twenty minutes. Immediate pulsative flow was noted with release of the occluding temporary clamps, and the rcconstructed veins filled immediately. The anastomoses were blood tight at the outset and the flap has remained viable for the past two years (Figs. 12-11 through 12-16).

Comment

Case #3 presented a similar clinical problem as noted in Case #2, but in this case it was solved by the performance of an extensive endarterectomy with adequate arterial perfusion pressure. This anastomosis was essentially adventitia-to-adventitia mediated by clip and demonstrates the utility of the system even in the face of diseased arteries.

MR angiogram of a superficial temporal-to-middle cerebral artery anastomosis performed with microclips. Superficial temporal artery 1 mm, recipient middle cerebral branch 2 mm. The patient's clinical status improved subsequent to the procedure. Figure 12-1 demonstrates the right STA entering the intracranial circulation.

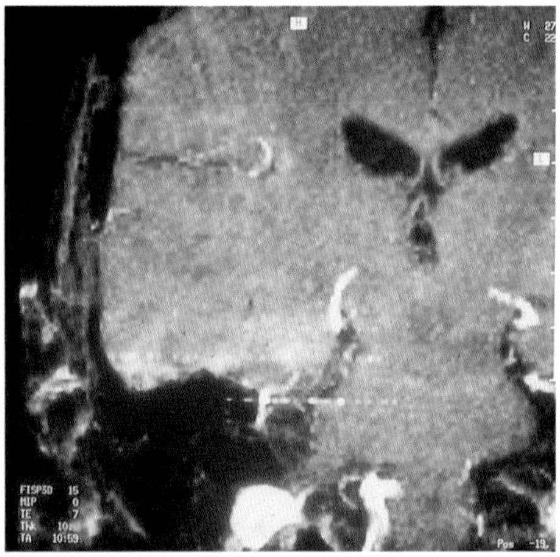

Fig. 12-1

Figures 12-2 and 12-3 demonstrate the patent end-to-side anastomosis at high resolution (arrows).

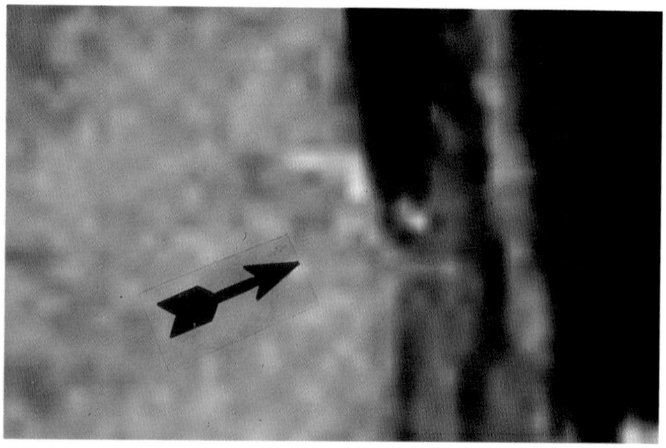

Fig. 12-2

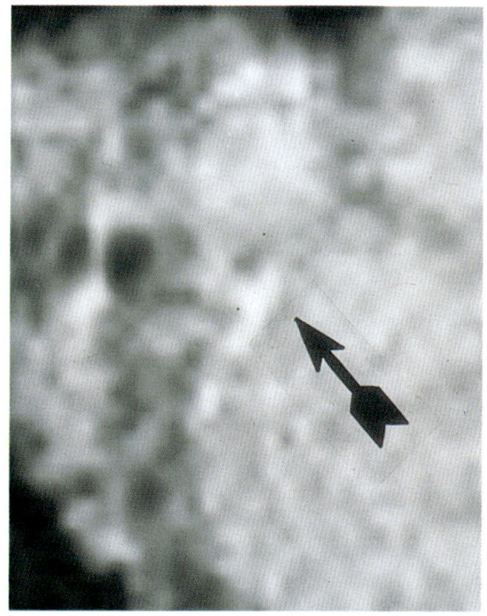

Fig. 12-3

Sagittal MRI demonstrating large left vertebral artery aneurysm markedly deforming and dorsally displacing the medulla. The flow void within the aneurysm is the residual left vertebral artery that was reconstructed with a pericardial patch and macroclips.

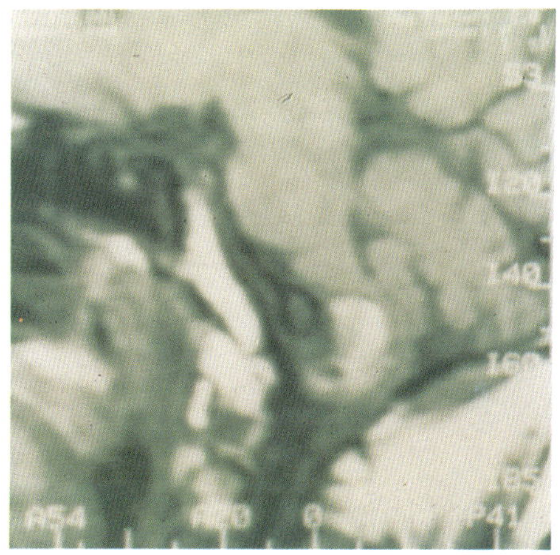

Fig. 12-4

Postoperative angiogram demonstrating repair of the giant left vertebral artery aneurysm using clips and a pericardial patch. Trapping of the artery was accomplished, but persistent back-bleeding from the interposed segment could not be controlled by balloons. Back-bleeding was eventually controlled by the clip application of a pericardial patch (Shiley), reconstructing the artery wall.

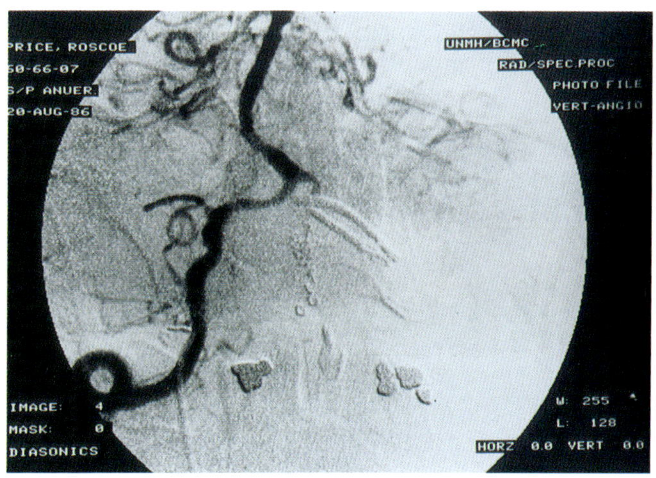

Fig. 12-5

Postmortem specimen demonstrating the clipped patch repair of the trapped left vertebral artery segment. There is a smaller right vertebral fusiform aneurysm that was obscured by the giant left-sided lesion.

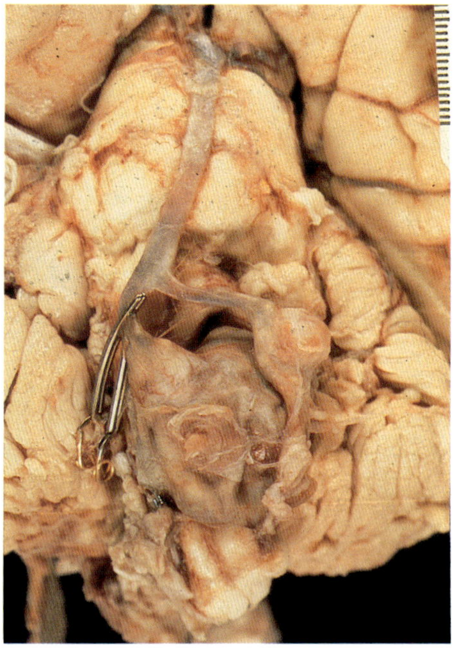

Fig. 12-6

Patch graft of the calcified, open left vertebral artery after aneurysm resection. Attempts at hemostasis by balloon occlusion and conventional aneurysm clips failed to control back bleeding. Hemostasis secured with patch and macroclips. Clips are visible.

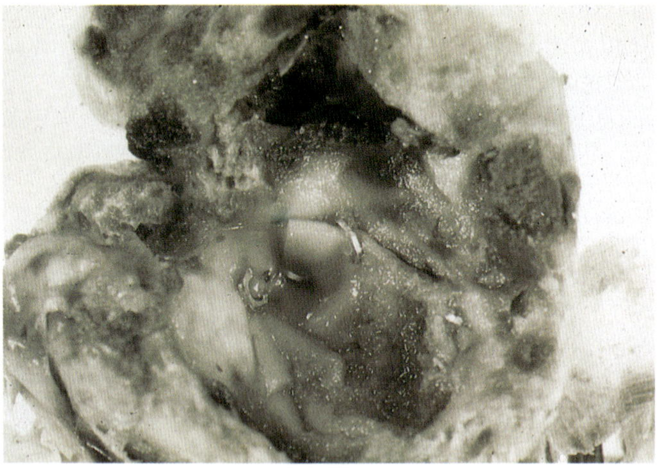

Fig. 12-7

Dural closure with macroclips. The patient underwent a craniotomy for large internal carotid aneurysm. A dural substitute of Edwards pericardium was secured for a "water-tight" closure using macroclips. The clip provides a rapid and safe dural closure without the danger to the brain of a blind needle passage. The clip has proven useful for the control of dural sinus bleeding secondary to trauma.

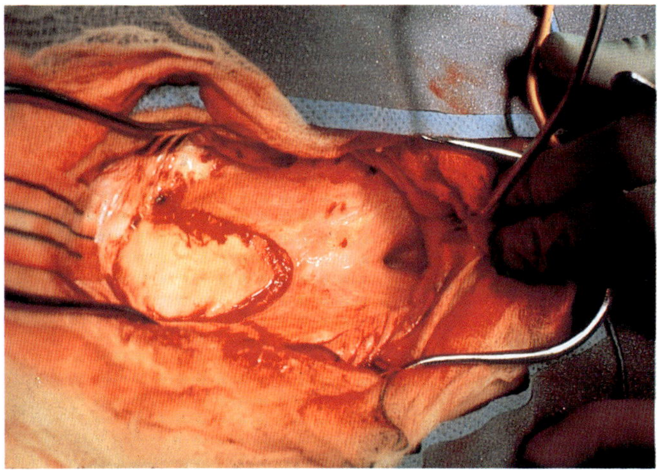

Fig. 12-8

The use of mezzoclips to construct an expanded PTFE arteriovenous fistula for hemodialysis in the upper extremity in a patient with advanced vascular and renal disease. The brachial artery is exceptionally atherosclerotic. The eversion forceps are manipulated to place the first clip at the "heel" of the end-to-side anastomosis. After completion of the "heel" flange, attention is directed to the "toe" to apply a clip, and then both sides completed with clips. The surgeon can provide the eversion and the assistant can apply the clips (Figs. 12-9 A and B).

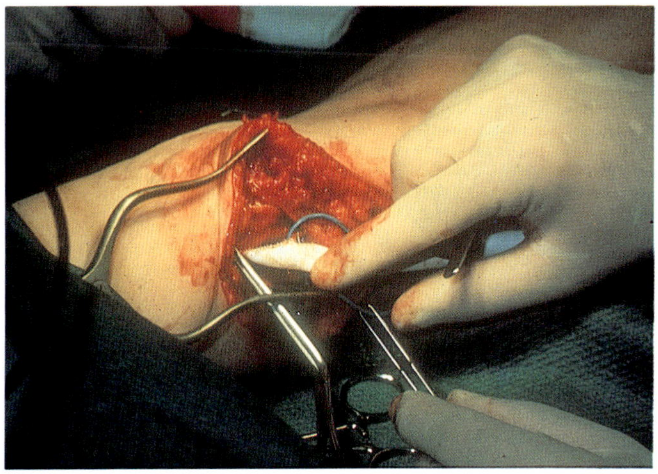

Fig. 12-9 A

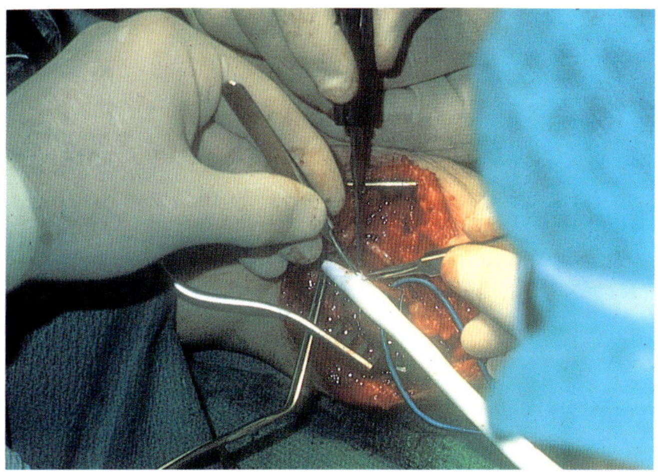

Fig. 12-9 B

Rectus abdominous muscle transfer to an ulcerated lesion over the right tibia. Two venae comitantes were anastomosed, one by suture, the other by clip. The sutured venous anastomosis required twenty-five minutes; the clipped venous anastomosis seven minutes. This free flap remains viable. The arterial anastomosis was done with suture.

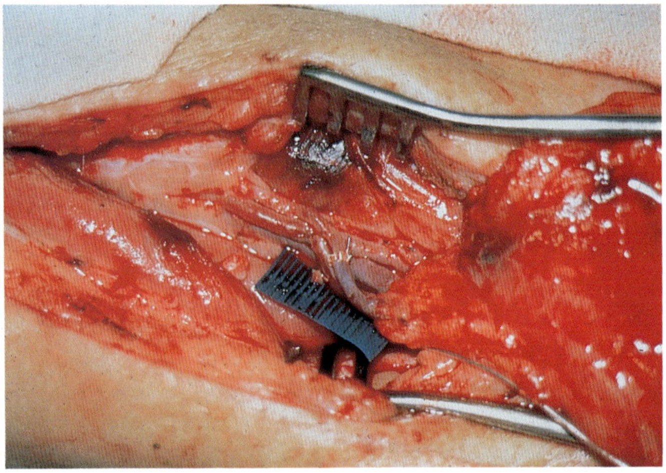

Figs. 12-10.

Craniofacial defect secondary to leiomyosarcoma resection to include orbit, maxilla, and zygomatic arch. Acrylic palatal prosthesis visible. This defect was in a previously irradiated field.

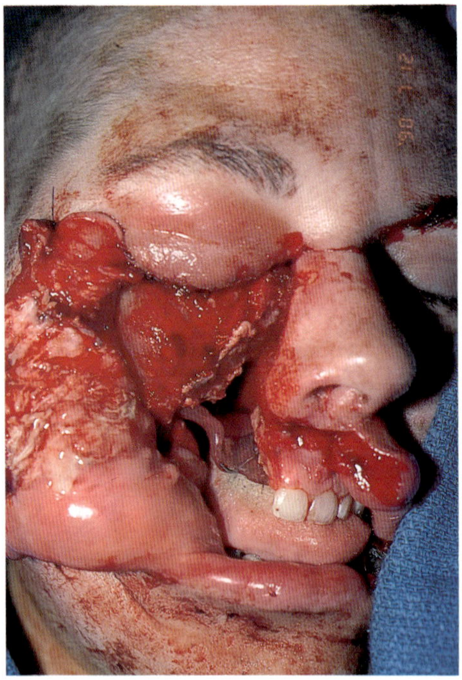

Fig. 12-11

A right serratus anterior bilobed free-flap was harvested with adjacent 7th rib to fill the defect. The subscapularis artery and vein are visible.

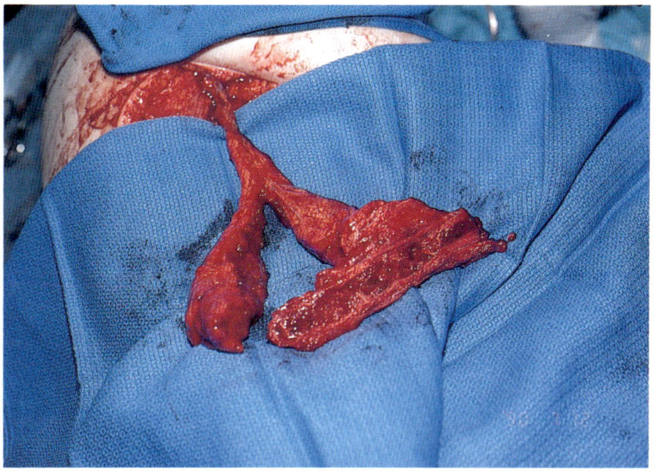

Fig. 12-12

The clipped arterial and venous anastomoses for the serratus anterior free flap. The venous anastomosis end-to-end in the facial vein required eight minutes. The arterial anastomosis to a diseased facial artery required fifteen minutes after an endarterectomy.

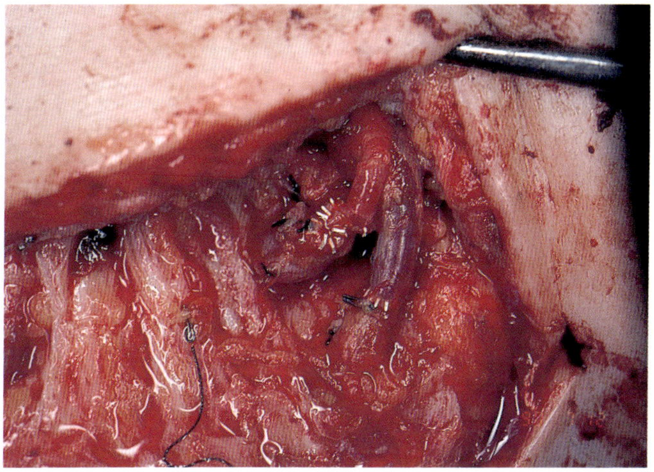

Fig. 12-13

Immediate postoperative demonstration of muscle perfusion. The flap has remained viable.

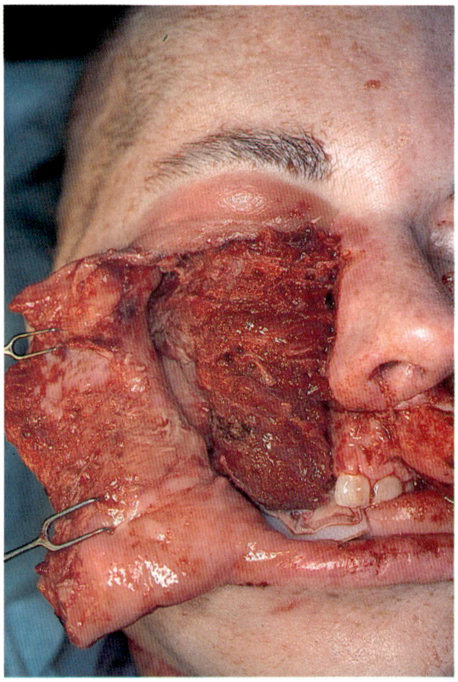

Fig. 12-14

MRI angiogram demonstrating patency of facial-subscapular arterial anastomoses—end-to-side. One year postoperatively.

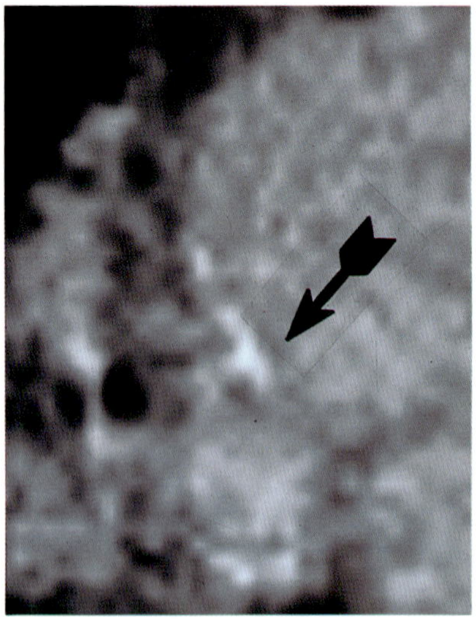

Fig. 12-15

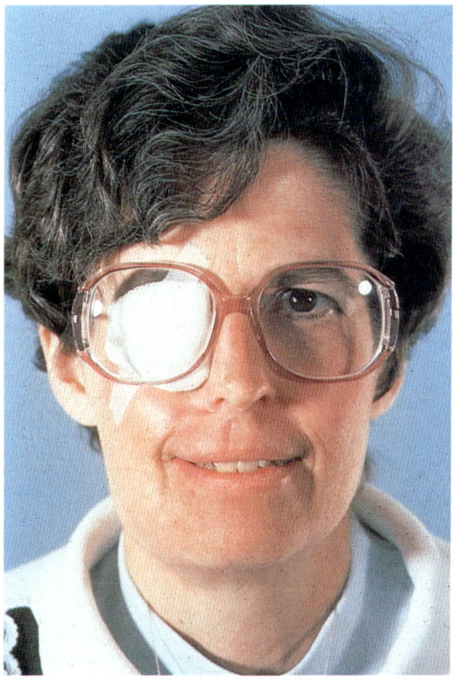

Fig. 12-16

Patient's appearance eighteen months postoperatively.

References

1. Wilson NM, Rutt DL, Browse NL. Venous valve replacement: A new technique. *Brit J Surg*. 1991;78:595-600.
2. Gaskill D, Stewart S, Kirsch WM, Zhu YH, Thompson K. Sutureless vasovasotomy: A new technique demonstrating an experimental microclip using a rat model. *Urology*. In press, 1992.
3. Kirsch WM, Zhu YH, Hardesty RA, Chapolini R. A new method for microvascular anastomosis: Report of experimental and clinical research. *Amer Surgeon*. In press, 1992.
4. Kirsch WM, Zhu YH, Gaskill D, Stewart S, Hardesty RA, Lyons TL. Tissue reconstruction with non-penetrating arcuate-legged clips: Potential endoscopic applications. *J Reproductive Med*. In press, 1992.
5. Comforti P, Tomasello F, Albanese V. *Cerebral Revascularization By Microneurosurgical Bypass*. Padora, Italy: Piccin Nuova Libraria, S.P.A., 1984.
6. The EC/IC Bypass Study Group. Failure of extracranial-intracranial arterial bypass to reduce the risk of ischemic stroke: Results of an international randomized trial. *N Engl J Med*. 1985;313:1191-1200.
7. Barker JH, Anderson GL, Wyllie FJ. Acland RD. Formation of Platelet Emboli at the Site of Surgical Repair of a Severed Artery is Blood Flow Dependent. *FASEB Journal*. Feb. 15, 1989;3(4):A1379.
8. Kootstra EG, Jorning PJG. *Access Surgery. Proceedings of the First International Congress on Access Surgery*. Boston: MTP Press Ltd., 1982.

Section III

Reconstructive Microsurgery

Chapter 13

Free Fibula Osteoseptocutaneous Flap For Mandibular Reconstruction

Fu-Chan Wei, MD

The free fibula osteoseptocutaneous flap is an ideal reconstructive option for a major mandibular defect, especially when either oral inner lining or external soft tissue defects are associated with such a defect. The vascularized fibula provides enough bone to reconstruct any length of mandibular defect. It is easy to contour with multiple osteotomies. Excellent esthetic results are consistently achieved.

Case Example

A 62-year-old man suffered from epidermoid carcinoma of oral mucosa involving the left mandible from the angle to the symphysis. Simultaneous reconstruction of the oral inner lining and the mandibular defect was accomplished with a composite free fibula osteoseptocutaneous flap after radical excision of the lesion and neck dissection. The fibula was osteotomized at two sites to create a suitable contour for mandibular reconstruction. The skin portion was used to reconstruct the oral inner lining. The postoperative course was uneventful. Both skin and bone of the fibula osteoseptocutaneous flap survived completely.

Preoperative view of the epidermoid carcinoma of the oral mucosa.

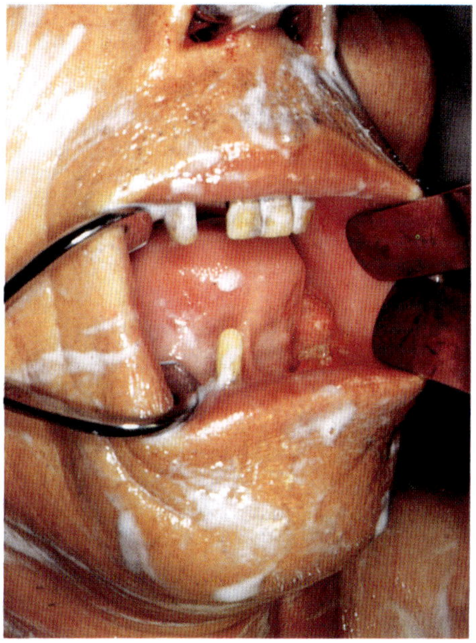

Fig. 13-1

Surgical specimen containing the epidermoid carcinoma in the oral mucosa and a segment of mandible.

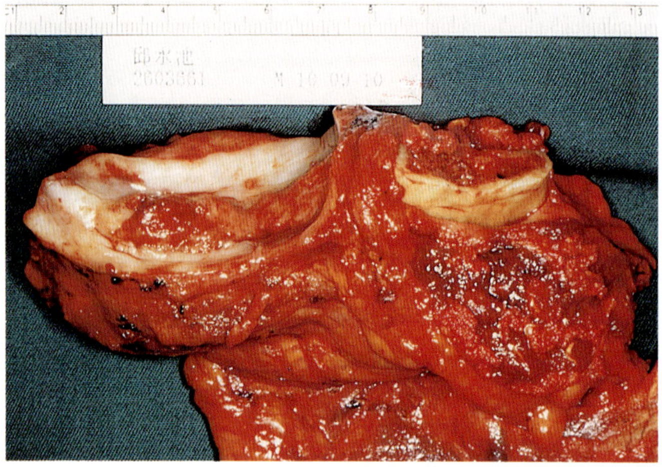

Fig. 13-2

Defect of the oral inner lining and the mandible.

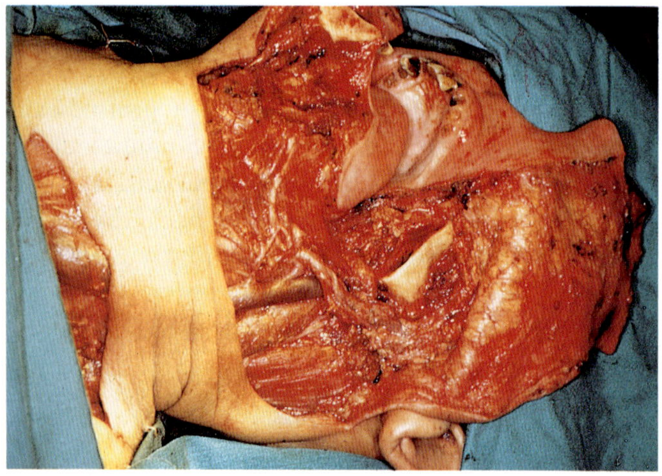

Fig. 13-3

Design of a fibula osteoseptocutaneous flap.

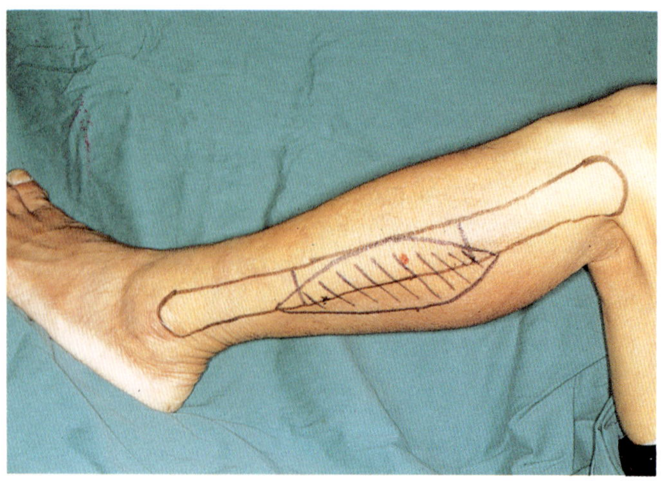

Fig. 13-4

Demonstration of the septocutaneous branches of the peroneal artery supplying the skin island of the fibula osteoseptocutaneous flap.

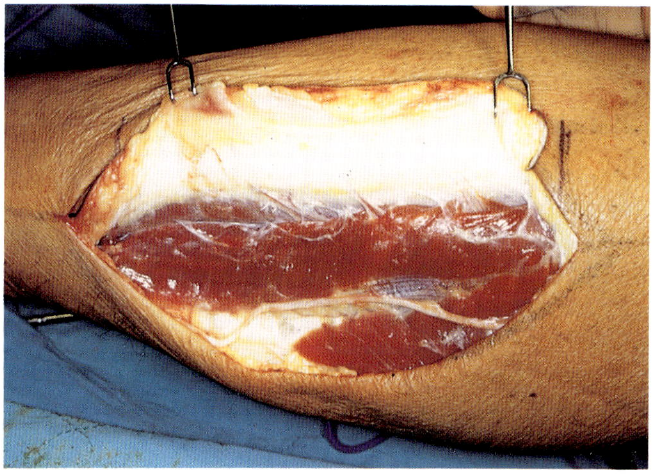

Fig. 13-5

Good circulation in both bone and skin of the fibula osteoseptocutaneous flap based on the peroneal vessel.

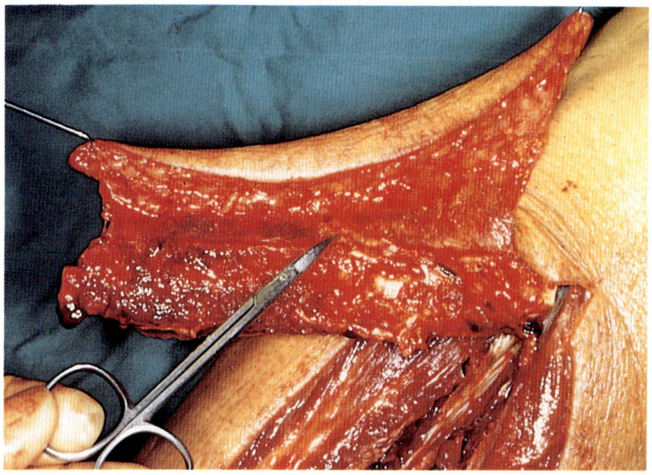

Fig. 13-6

Harvested fibula osteoseptocutaneous flap.

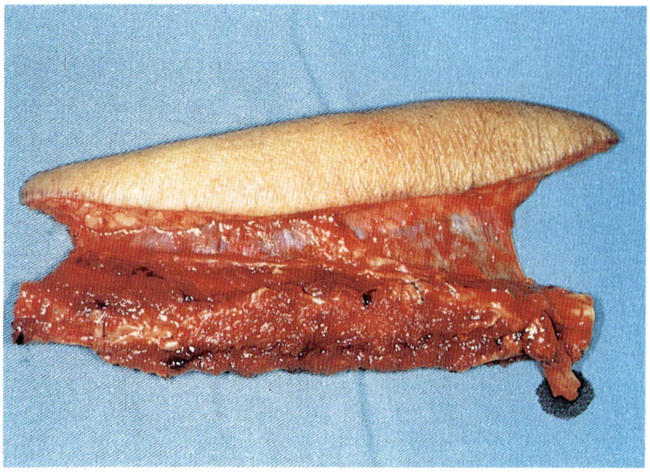

Fig. 13-7

Hemicircumferential periosteal elevation, preparation for two site osteotomies.

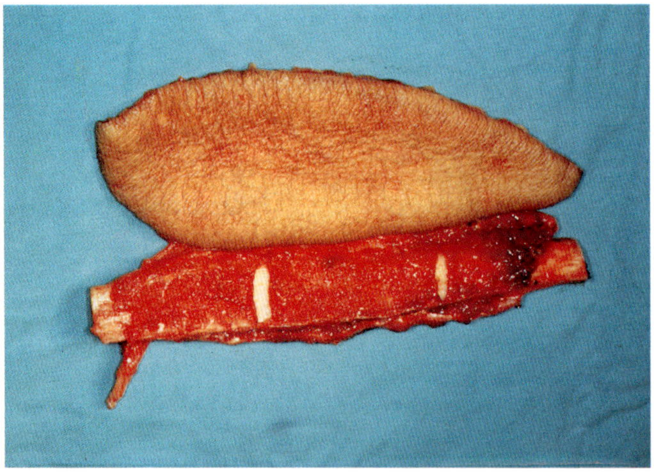

Fig. 13-8

Osteotomies accomplished and fibula contoured.

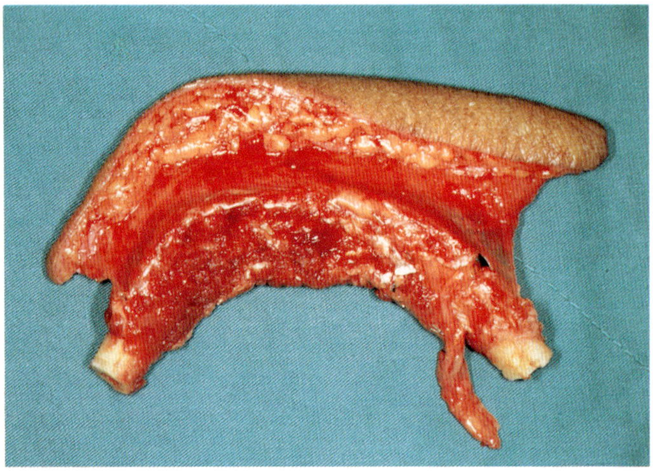

Fig. 13-9

Fibula osteoseptocutaneous flap inset. Note the cutaneous portion inside the oral cavity.

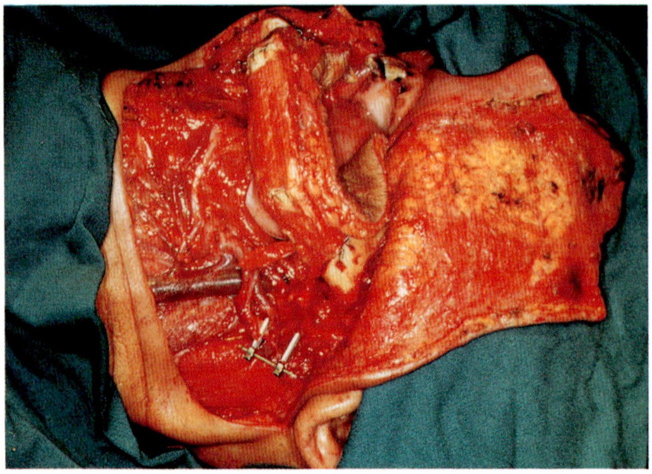

Fig. 13-10

Immediate postoperative appearance.

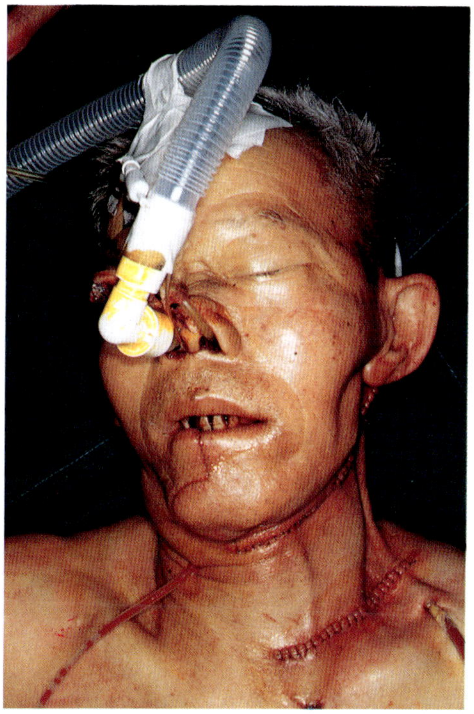

Fig. 13-11

X-ray of the mandible: Preoperative (above), Postoperative (below).

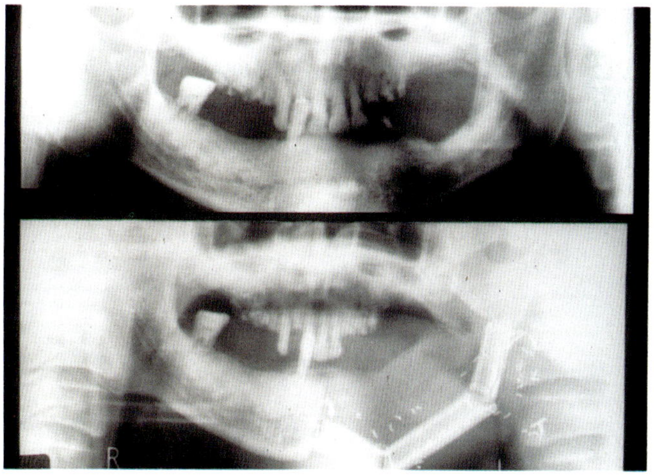

Fig. 13-12

Suggested Reading

Hidalgo DA. Fibula free flap: a new method of mandible reconstruction. *Plast Reconstr Surg*. 1989;84:71.

Wei FC, Chen HC, Chuang CC, Noordhoff MS. Fibular osteoseptocutaneous flap: anatomic study and clinical application. *Plast Reconstr Surg*. 1986;78:191.

Chapter 14

Thumb Reconstruction with a Great Toe Wrap-around Flap

Fu-Chan Wei, MD

Thumb reconstruction with a microsurgical great toe wrap-around flap and iliac bone graft was originally described by Morrison. It was once considered the ideal technique for an esthetic thumb reconstruction at any level, provided the basal joint was mobile. Lack of joint motion, swiveling of the wrap-around flap, iliac bone fracture and reabsorption have unfortunately limited its clinical application. At the present time, it is best suited for those thumbs with circumferential soft tissue and nail loss, or distal phalangeal amputations in which a reasonable range of motion in the interphalangeal and metacarpophalangeal joints is still maintained.

Case Example

A 25-year-old man sustained an unreplantable right thumb amputation at the distal phalangeal level. The interphalangeal joint, flexor pollicis longus and extensor pollicis longus were all intact. A great toe wrap-around flap was used for primary reconstruction.

Right thumb amputation (crushed) at the distal phalangeal level.

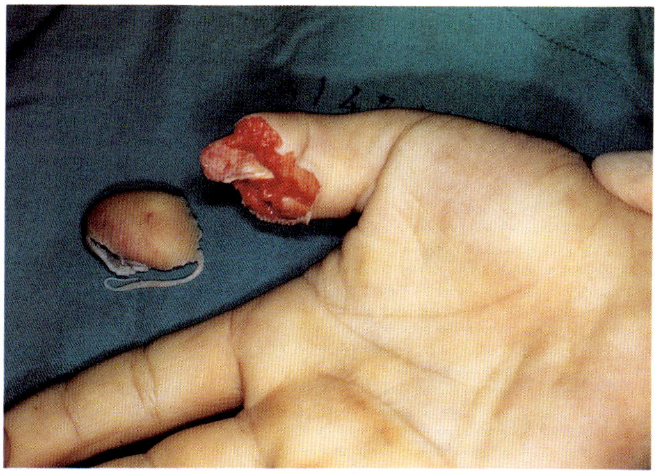

Fig. 14-1

Design of a wrap-around flap from the left great toe.

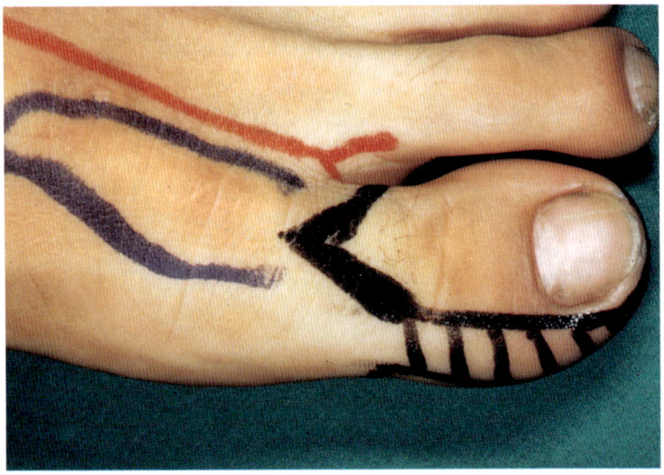

Fig. 14-2

Great toe wrap-around flap (including distal phalanx) harvested.

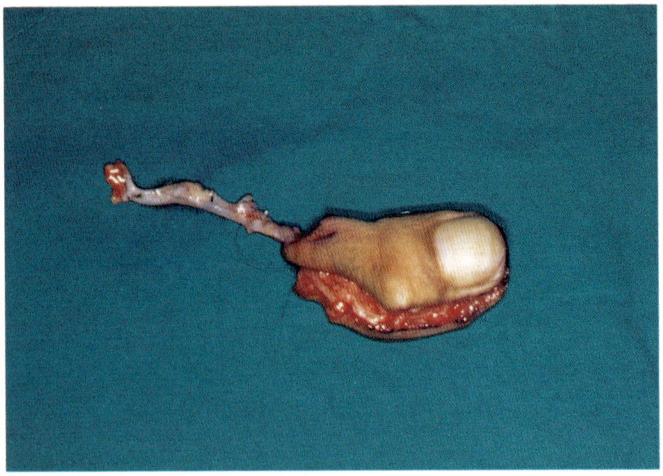

Fig. 14-3

Appearance and function six months after reconstruction (Figs. 14-4 through 14-7).

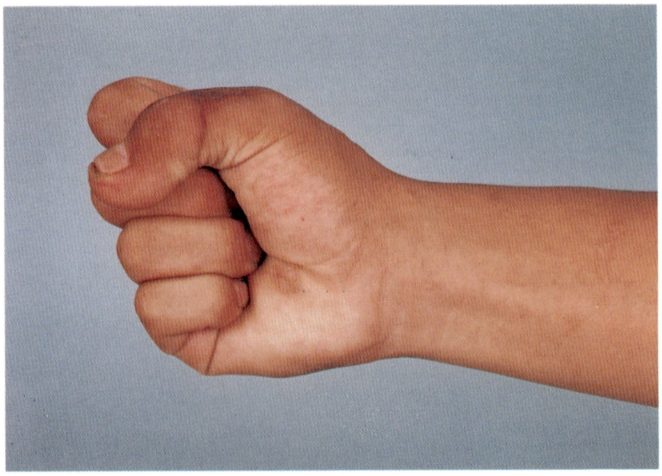

Fig. 14-4

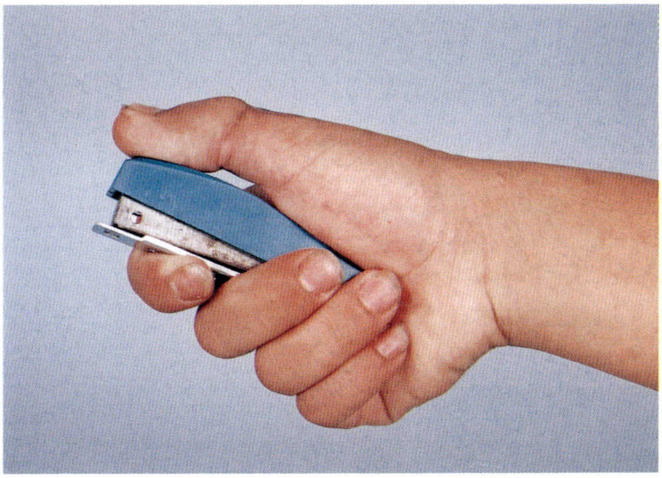

Fig. 14-5

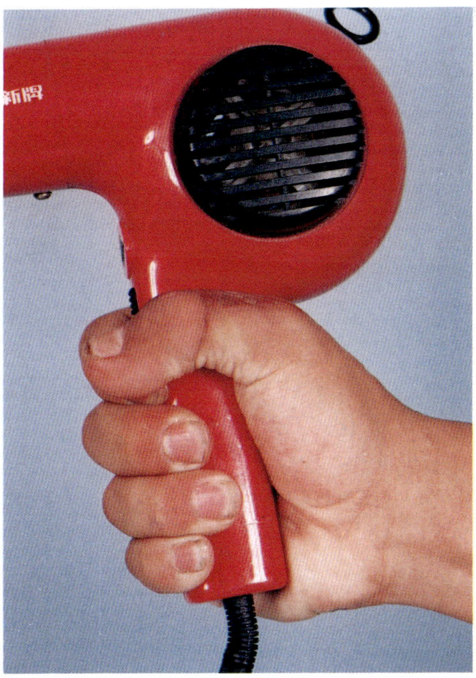

Fig. 14-6

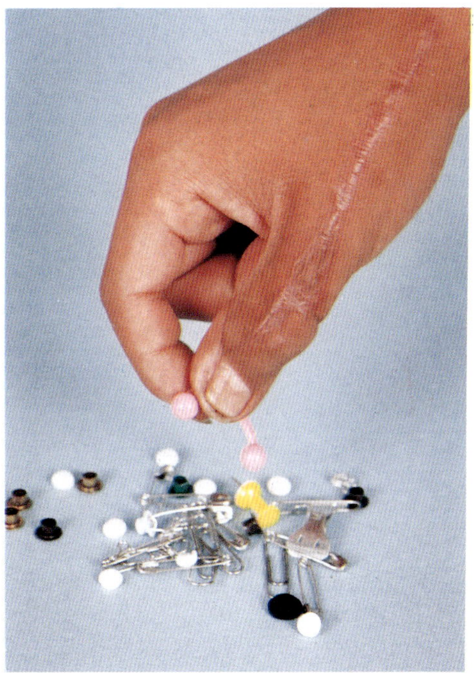

Fig. 14-7

Donor foot appearance (Figs. 14-8 and 14-9).

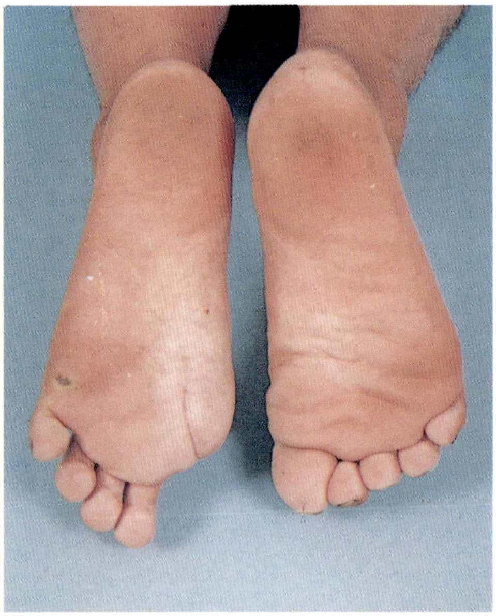

Fig. 14-8

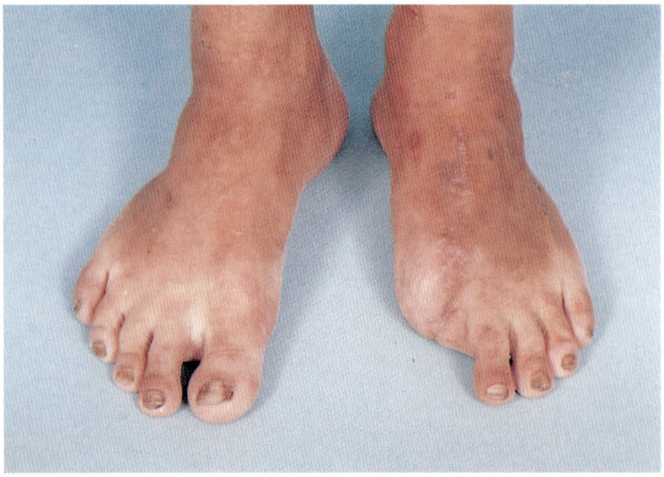

Fig. 14-9

Suggested Reading

Morrison WA, O'Brien B, Macleod AM. Thumb reconstruction with a free neurovascular wrap-around flap from the big toe. *J Hand Surg*. 1980;5:575.

Chapter 15

Thumb Reconstruction with Microsurgical Trimmed Great Toe Transfer (T.T.T.)

Fu-Chan Wei, MD

The trimmed great toe transfer technique was first developed by Wei. It combines the mobility of a total great toe transfer with the tailored appearance of the great toe wrap-around flap. Therefore, it is best used for reconstruction of an esthetic, mobile thumb at the metacarpophalangeal joint or proximal phalangeal level. The maintenance of interphalangeal joint motion is useful for nail pinch and fine manipulation.

Case Example

A 25-year-old man was referred to the author after an attempted left thump replantation failed. The bone amputation occurred at the head of the proximal phalanx, and skin at the base of the proximal phalanx. A trimmed left great toe was used for reconstruction in the subacute stage.

Left thumb amputation at the proximal phalangeal level.

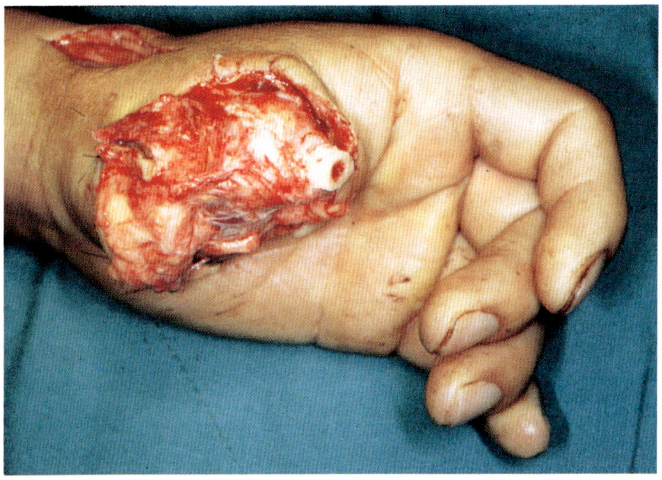

Fig. 15-1

Design of the trimmed great toe in the left foot.

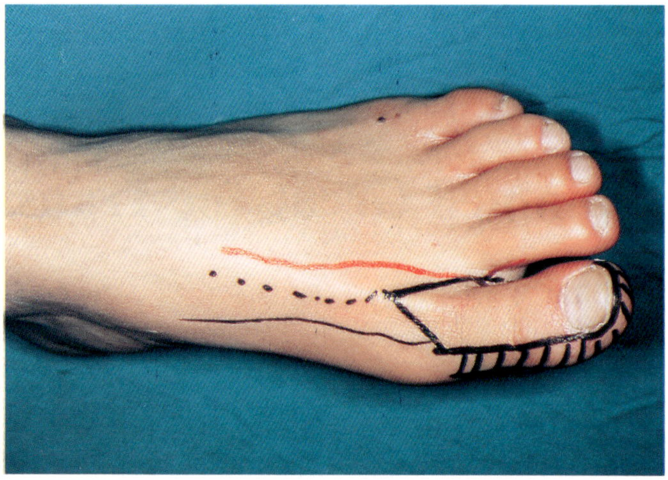

Fig. 15-2

Elevation of a medial skin strip.

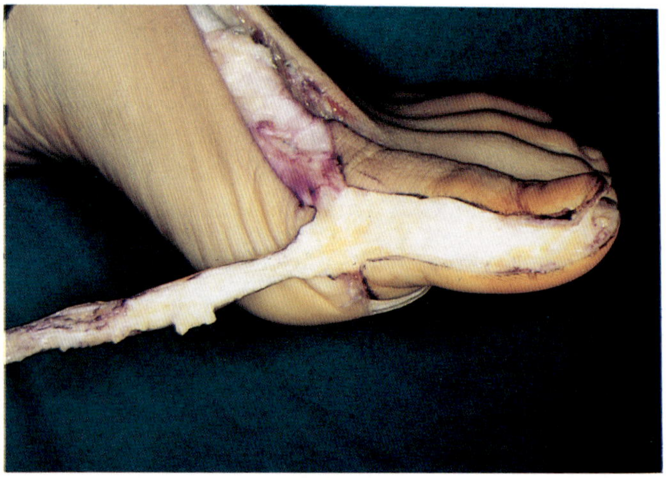

Fig. 15-3

Elevation of an inferiorly based hemicircumferential joint flap.

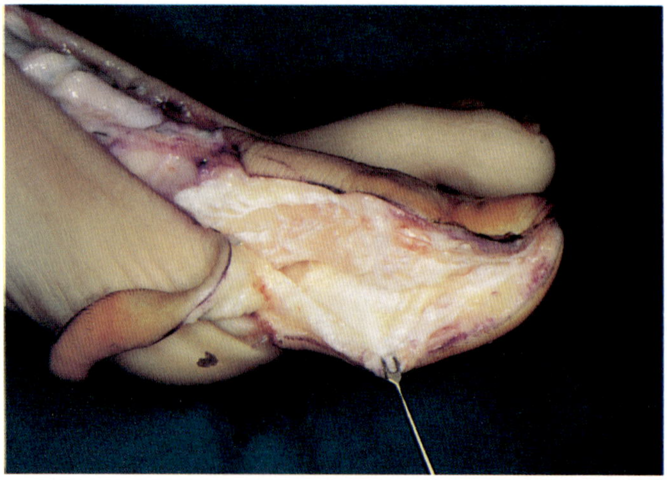

Fig. 15-4

Longitudinal osteotomy of the phalanges and the interphalangeal joint.

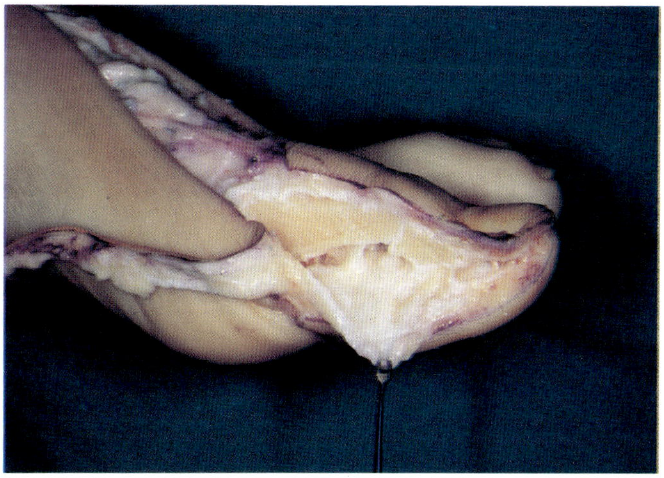

Fig. 15-5

Repair of the joint flap.

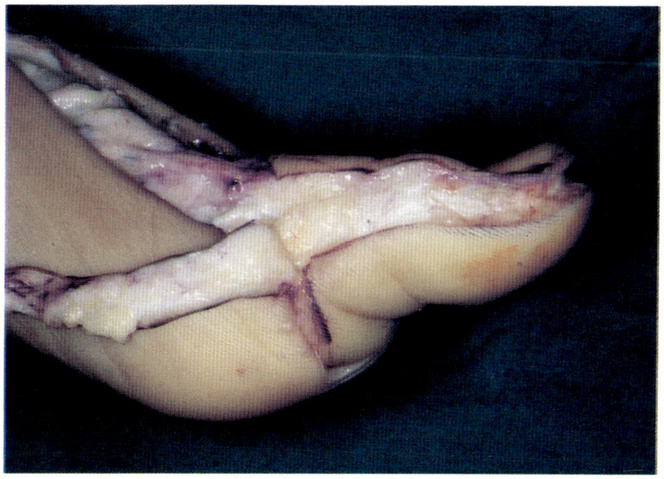

Fig. 15-6

Closure of the trimmed toe wound before transfer.

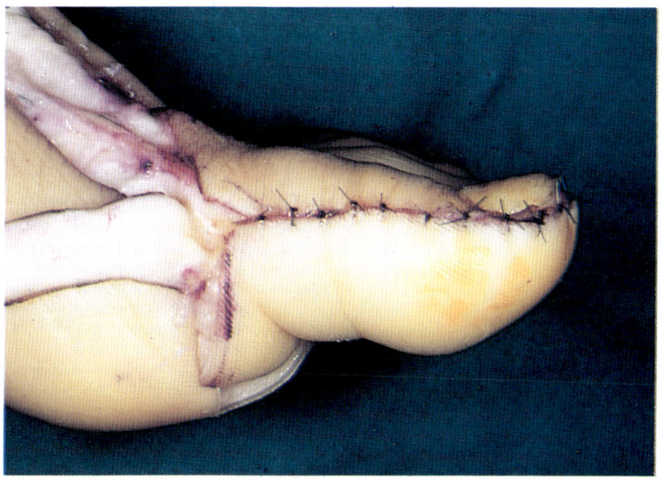

Fig. 15-7

Appearance and function one year after reconstruction (Figs. 15-8 through 15-12).

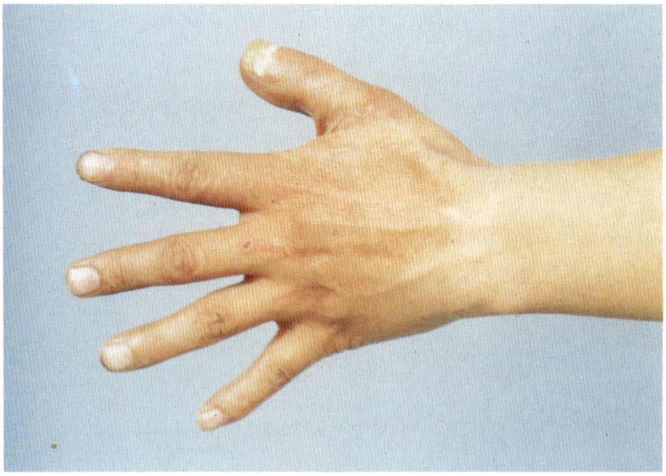

Fig. 15-8

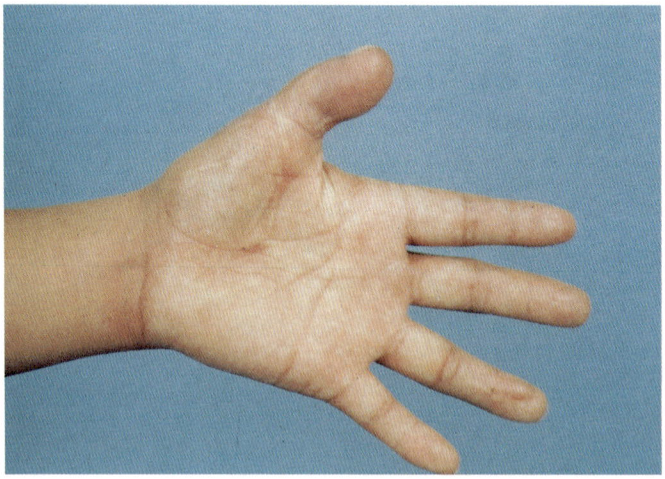

Fig. 15-9

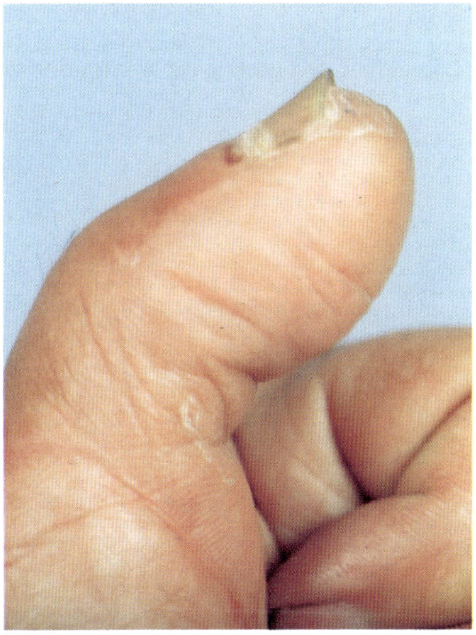

Fig. 15-10

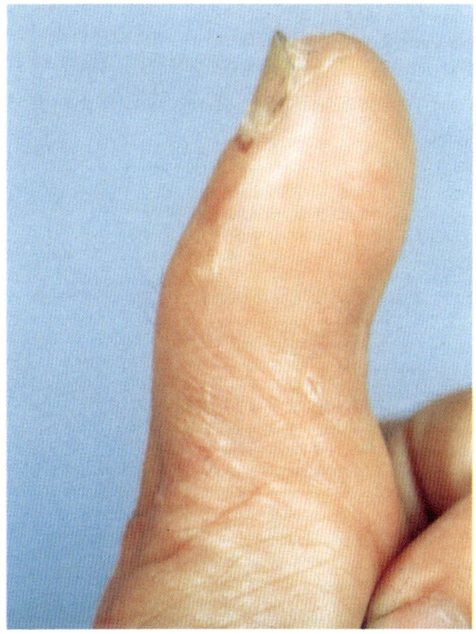

Fig. 15-11

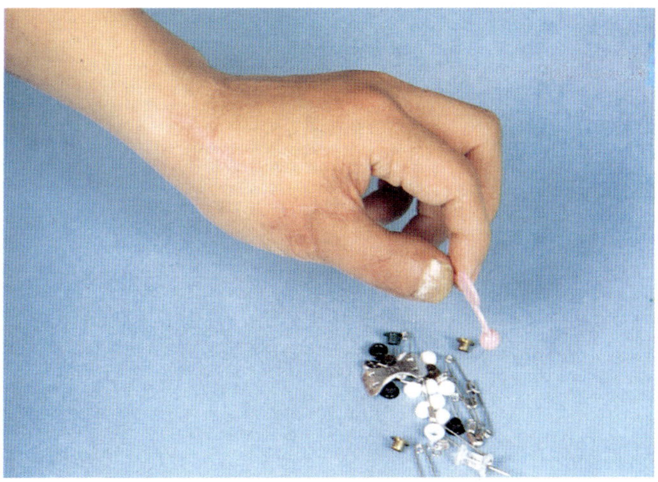

Fig. 15-12

Suggested Reading

Wei FC, Chen HC, Chuang CC, Noordhoff MS. Reconstruction of the thumb with a trimmed-toe transfer technique. *Plast Reconstr Surg*. 1988;82:506.

Chapter 16

Second Toe Wrap-Around Flap

Fu-Chan Wei, MD

The second toe wrap-around flap is most suitable for finger reconstruction when the distal half of the finger has circumferential loss of skin and the nail and while the proximal interphalangeal joint and tendons are still intact. This is similar to the great toe wrap-around flap for thumb reconstruction. The esthetic appearance of the reconstructed finger is generally good, and functional recovery is fast and satisfactory.

Case Example

A 23-year-old man suffered a right index finger tip amputation with the loss of pulp and nail. A second toe wrap-around flap was used for immediate reconstruction.

Right index finger tip crush amputation with loss of pulp and nail (Figs. 16-1 and 16-2).

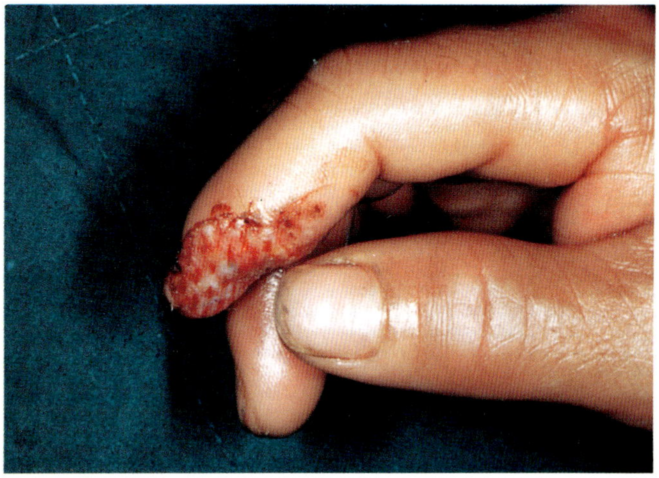

Fig. 16-1

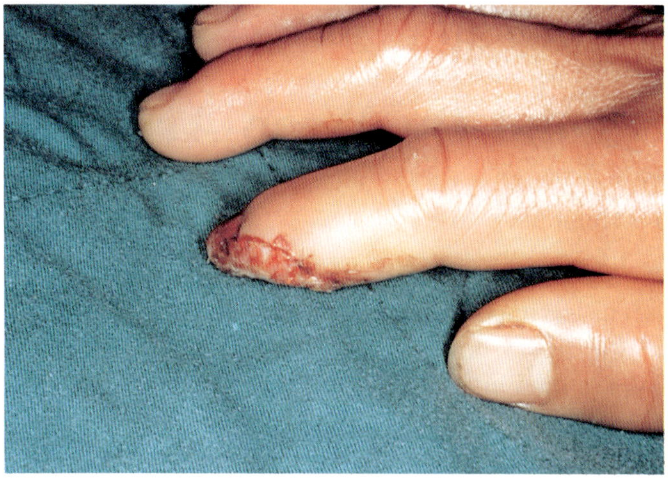

Fig. 16-2

A wrap-around flap from the left second toe was designed.

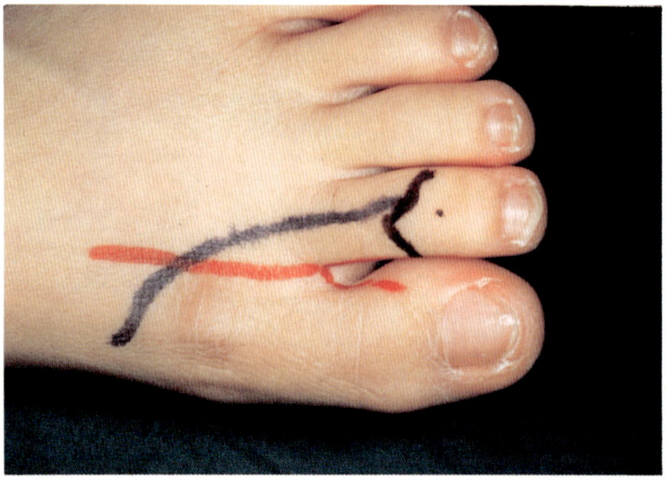

Fig. 16-3

Harvested left second toe wrap-around flap (including distal interphalangeal joint and distal phalanx) based on the first dorsal metatarsal vessel.

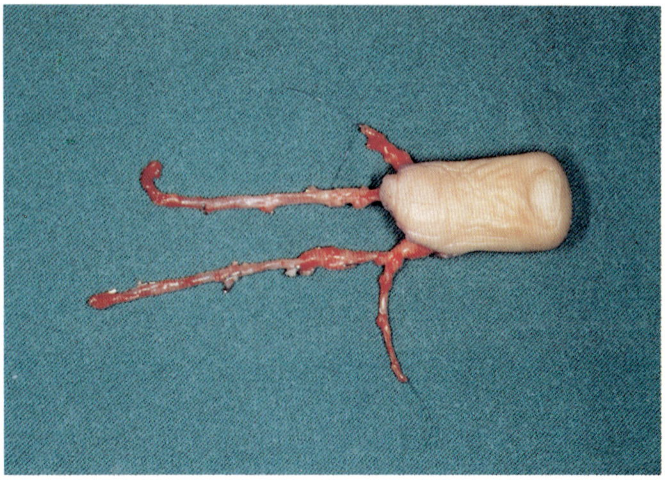

Fig. 16-4

Preparation of the distal phalanx of the index finger and the harvested second toe for bone doweling (Figs 16-5 and 16-6).

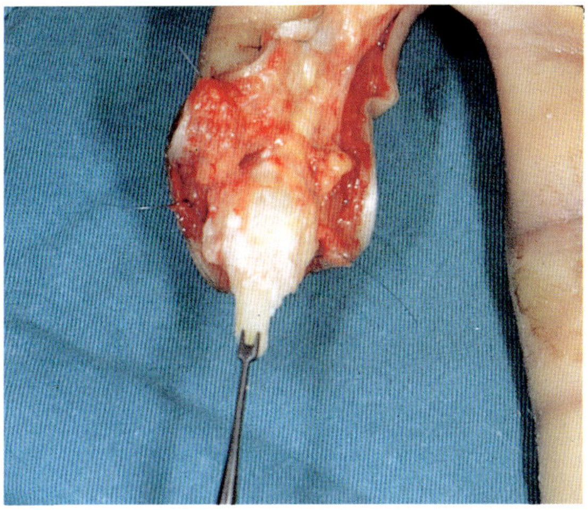

Fig. 16-5

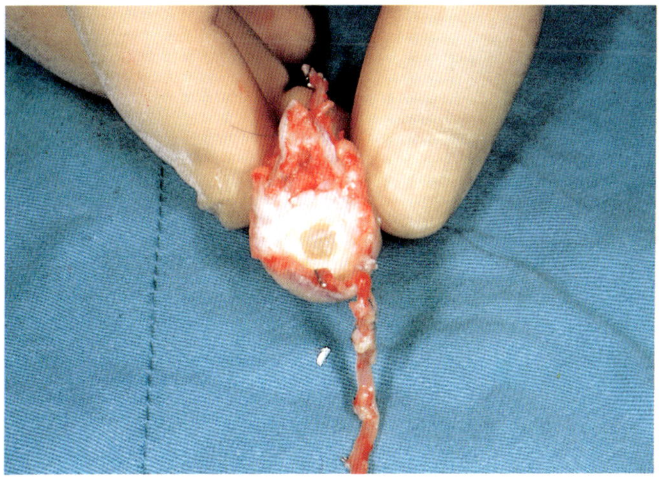

Fig. 16-6

Appearance and function one month after reconstruction (Figs 16-7 through 16-10).

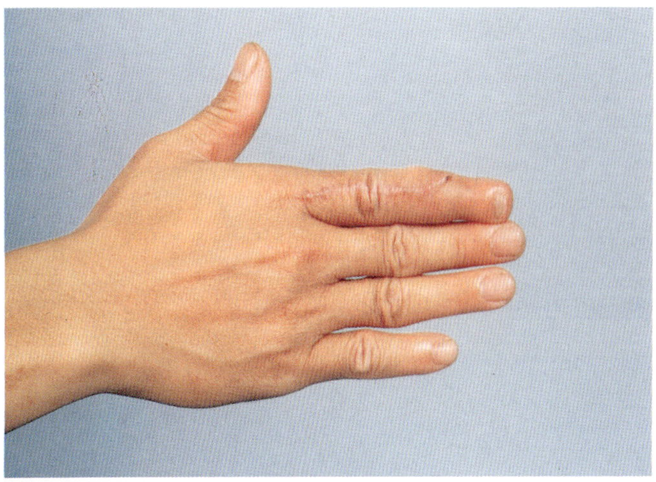

Fig. 16-7

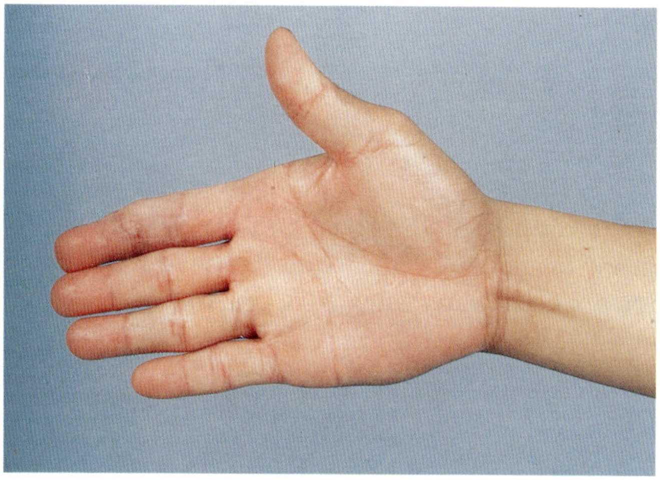

Fig. 16-8

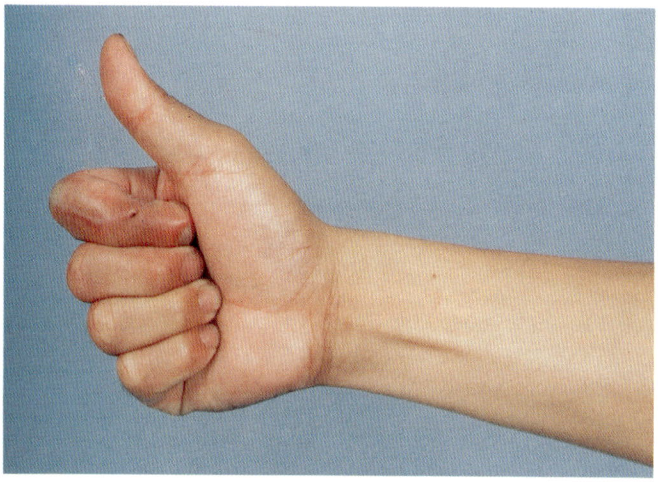

Fig. 16-9

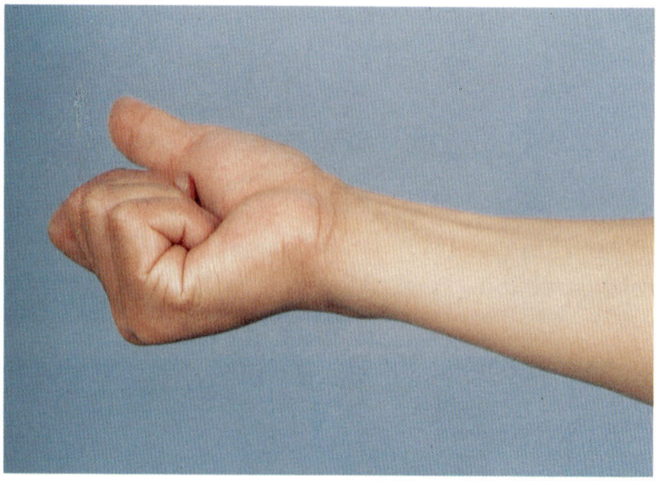

Fig. 16-10

Appearance of donor foot one month after surgery.

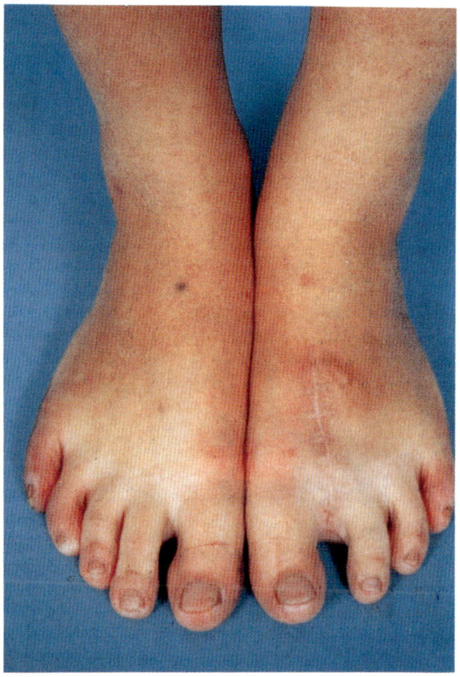

Fig. 16-11

Suggested Reading

Wei FC, Colony LH. Microsurgical reconstruction of opposable digits in mutilating hand injuries. *Clin Plast Surg*. 1989;16:491.

Wei FC, Colony LH. Microsurgical restoration of distal digital function. *Clin Plast Surg*. 1989;16:443.

Chapter 17

Microsurgical Toe Pulp Transfer

Fu-Chan Wei, MD

The total pulp or hemipulp from either the great toe or lesser toe are good reconstructive options for resurfacing volar digital soft tissue losses. These flaps can restore good stability and sensibility.

Case Example

A 25-year-old man was referred to the author four days after a traumatic loss of the pulps of his left middle and ring fingers. There was exposure of the flexor digitorum profundus tendons and the distal interphalangeal joints. Simultaneous two pulp flaps from the second toes of both feet were used for reconstruction.

Left middle and ring finger pulp defects with exposure of flexor digitorum profundus tendons and distal interphalangeal joints.

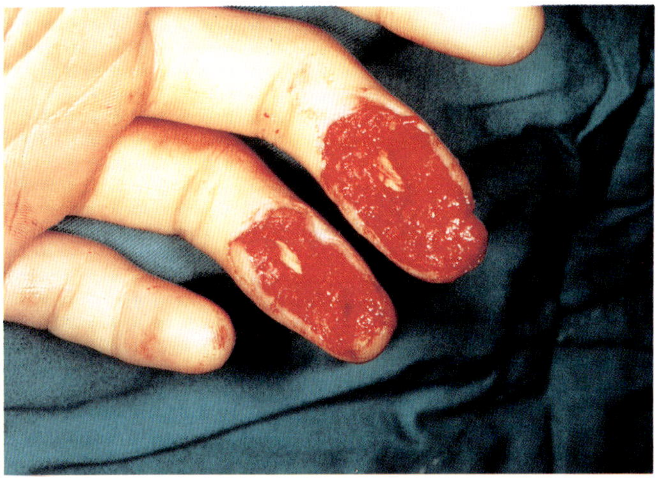

Fig. 17-1

Pulp flaps designed on the second toes of both feet.

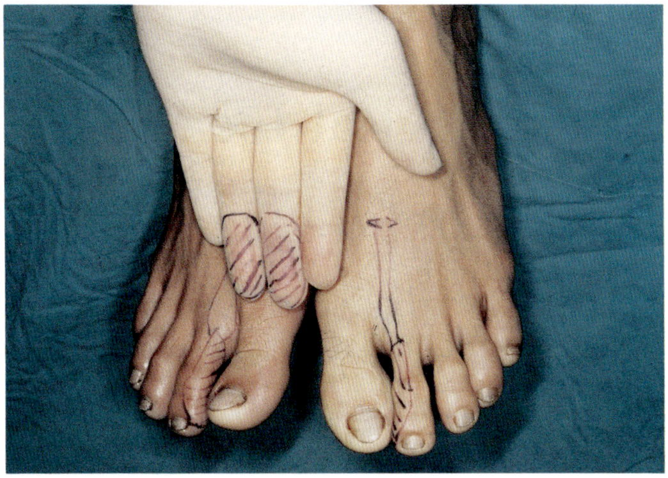

Fig. 17-2

Harvested second toe pulp flap based on plantar digital artery.

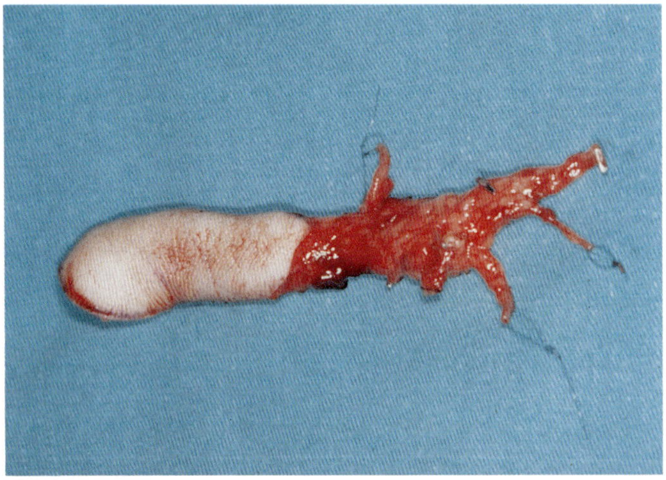

Fig. 17-3

Appearance immediately after revascularization of the transferred pulp flaps.

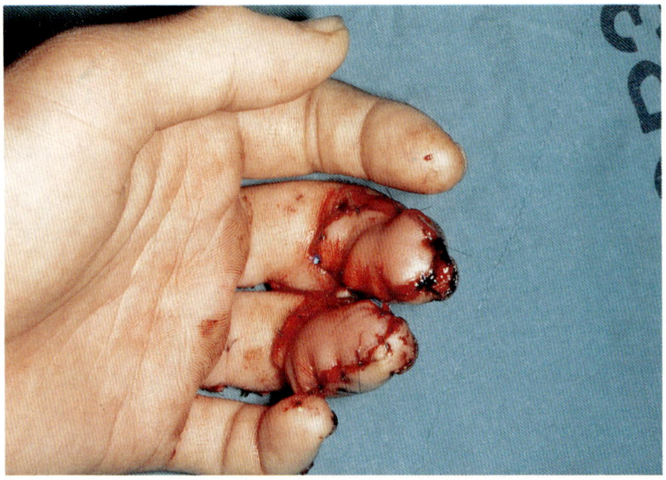

Fig. 17-4

Appearance and function of reconstructed middle and ring fingers after one year (Figs. 17-5 through 17-9).

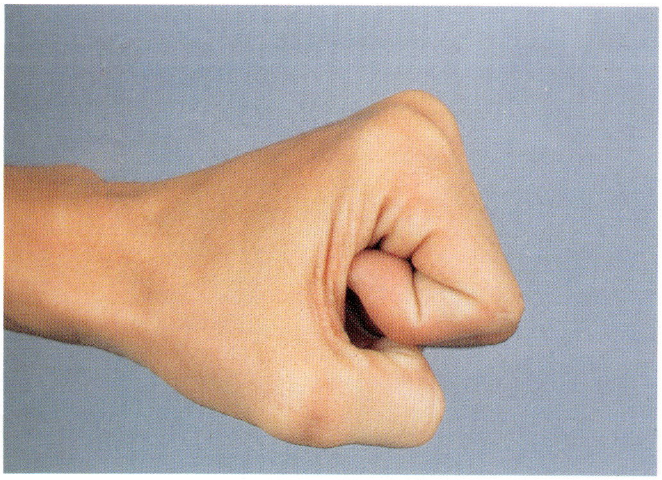

Fig. 17-5

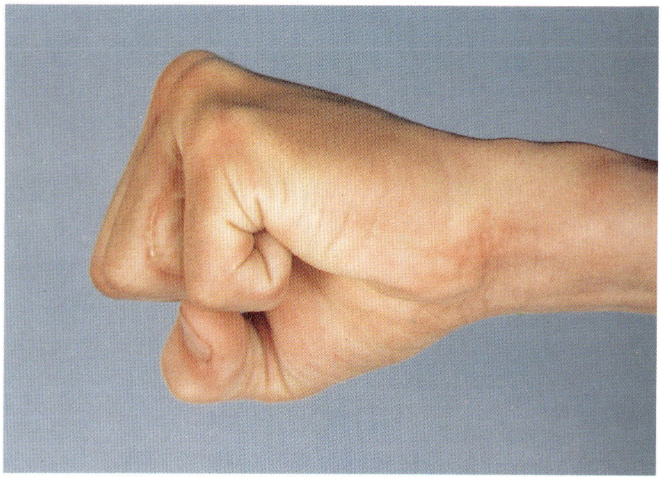

Fig. 17-6

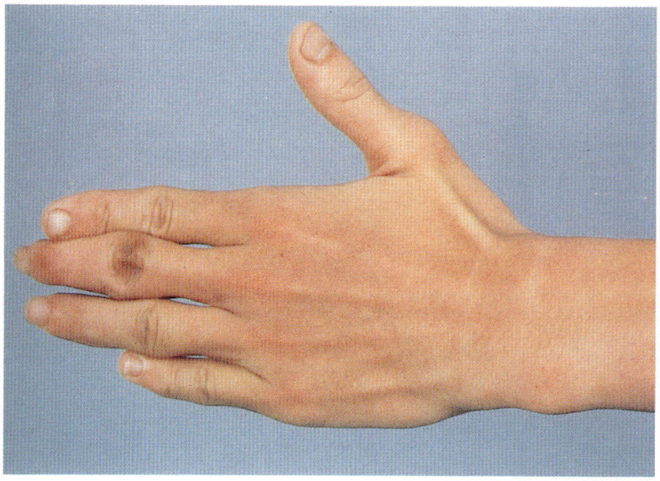

Fig. 17-7

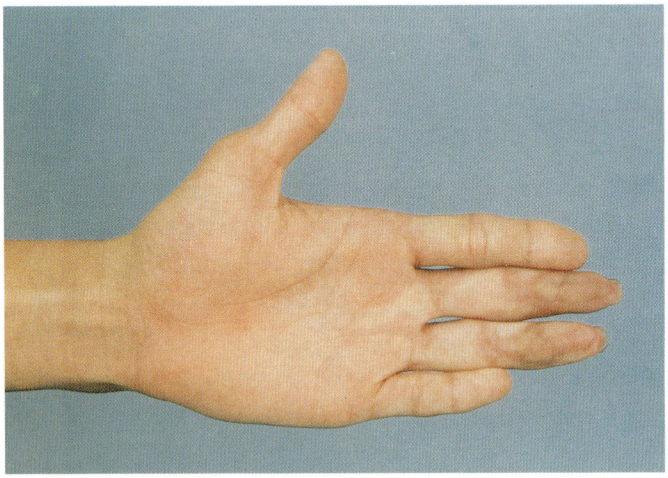

Fig. 17-8

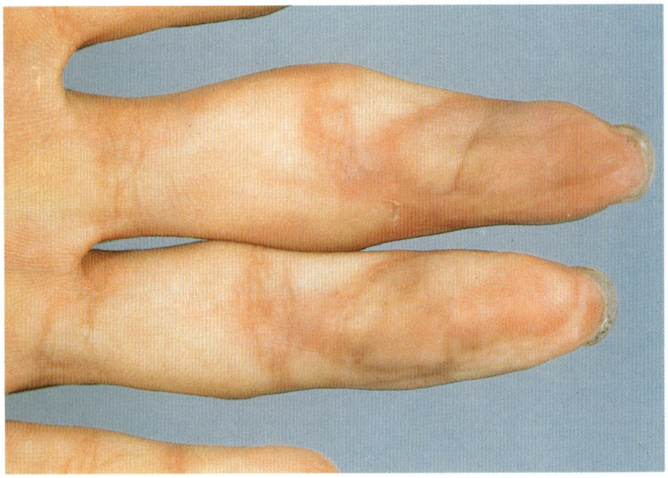

Fig. 17-9

Appearance of donor sites (Figs. 17-10 and 17-11).

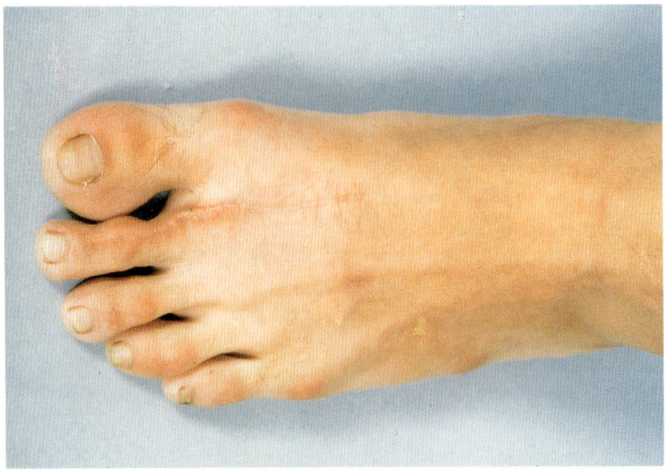

Fig. 17-10

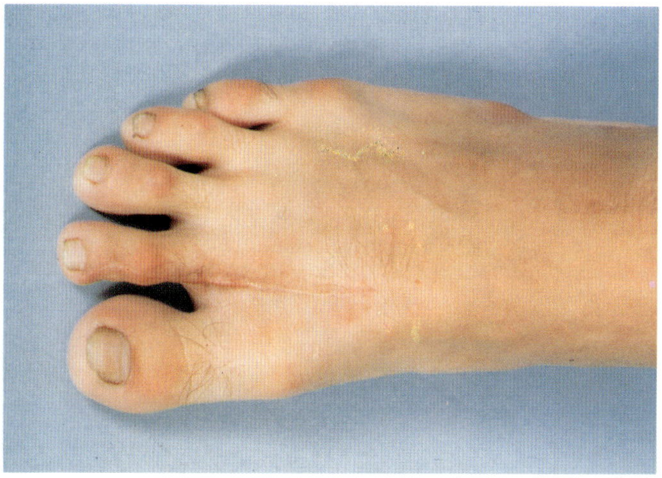

Fig. 17-11

Suggested Reading

Foucher G, Merle M, Maneaud M, et al. Microsurgical free partial toe transfer in hand reconstruction: a report of 12 cases. *Plast Reconstr Surg*. 1980;65:616.

Wei FC, Colony LH. Microsurgical restoration of distal digital function. *Clin Plast Surg*. 1989;16:443.

Chapter 18

Combined Second and Third Toe Transfer

Fu-Chan Wei, MD

The second and third toes can be harvested as a block on a single vascular pedicle for reconstruction of a hand with adjacent finger amputations proximal to the web space. The remaining finger should be no longer than the little finger. With refinement in surgical planning and technique, this single stage microsurgical procedure can restore prehensile function, improve the appearance of the hand, and preserve near-normal donor foot function.

Case Example

A 23-year-old man sustained a traumatic amputation of his left index through little fingers at the metacarpal level. A groin flap was used for coverage in the acute stage. A combined second and third toe unit from the left foot was employed for reconstruction of the middle and ring fingers two months later. Transmetatarsal amputations of the second and third toes were carried out and the donor wound was closed directly.

Amputation of index through little fingers at the metacarpal level of the left hand.

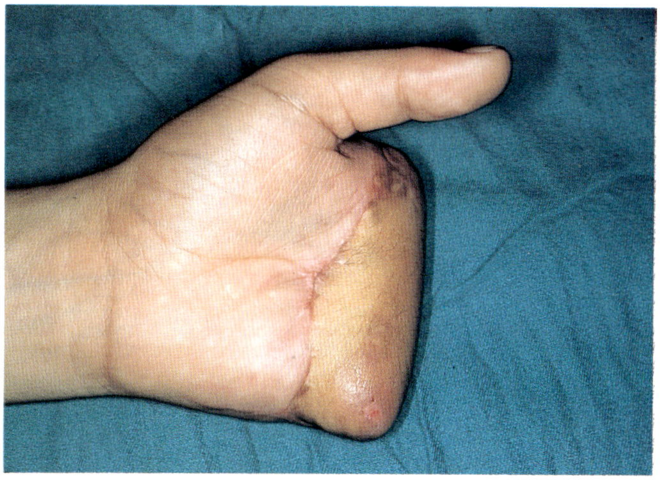

Fig. 18-1

Design of a combined second and third toe unit based on a single vascular pedicle (pedis dorsalis vessel).

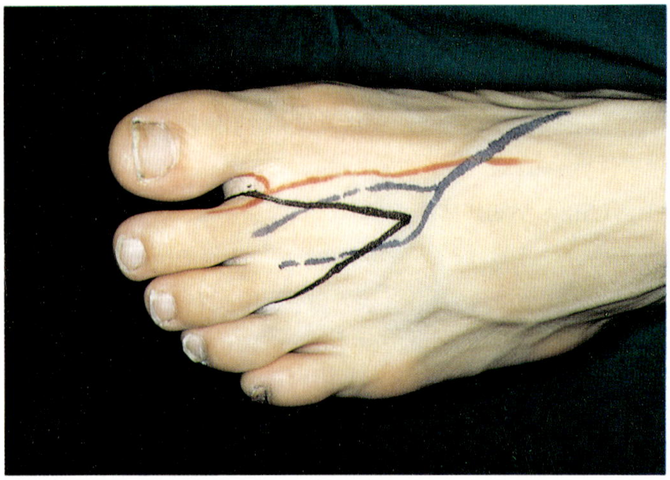

Fig. 18-2

Dissection of the first dorsal metatarsal artery (distal continuation of the pedis dorsalis artery).

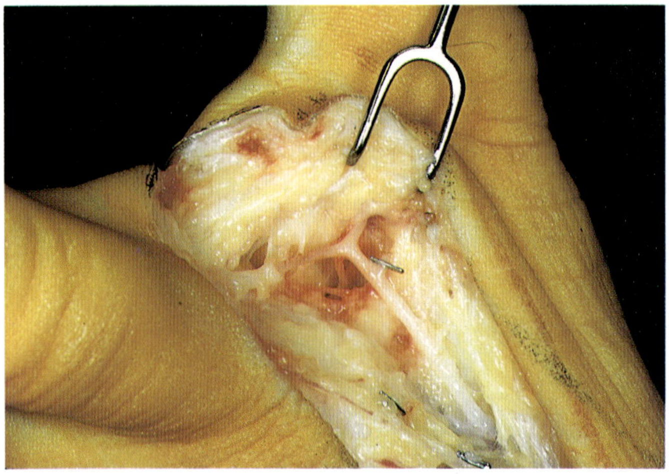

Fig. 18-3

Elevated combined second and third toe unit attached to the foot with vascular pedicle only.

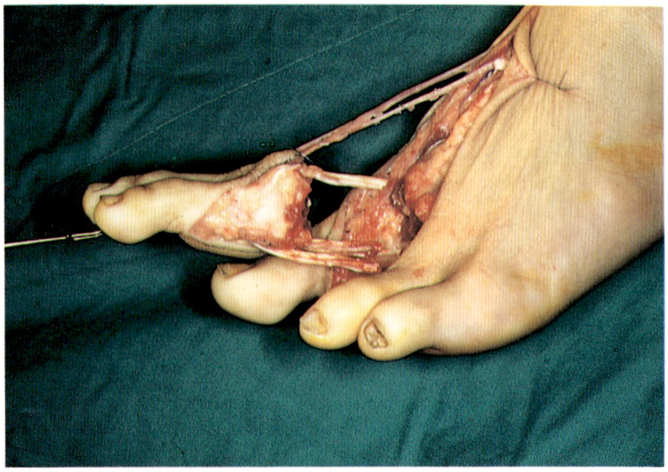

Fig. 18-4

The harvested combined second and third toes.

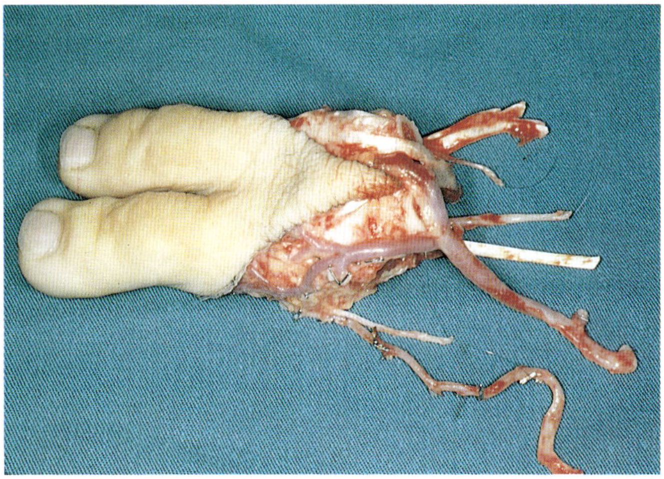

Fig. 18-5

The donor site before wound closure.

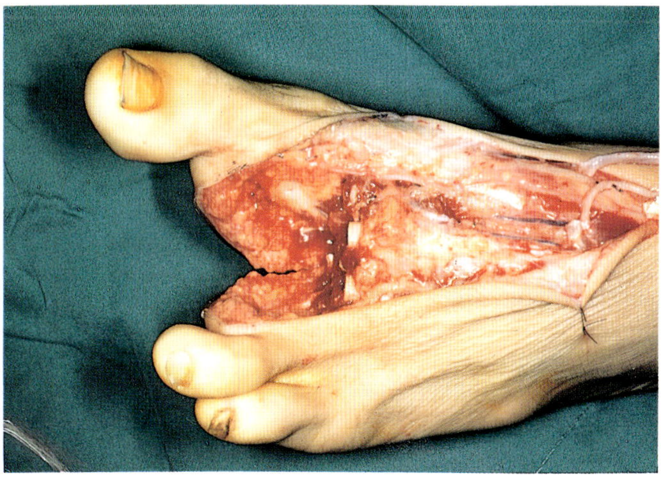

Fig. 18-6

Appearance and function one year after reconstruction (Figs. 18-7 through 18-12).

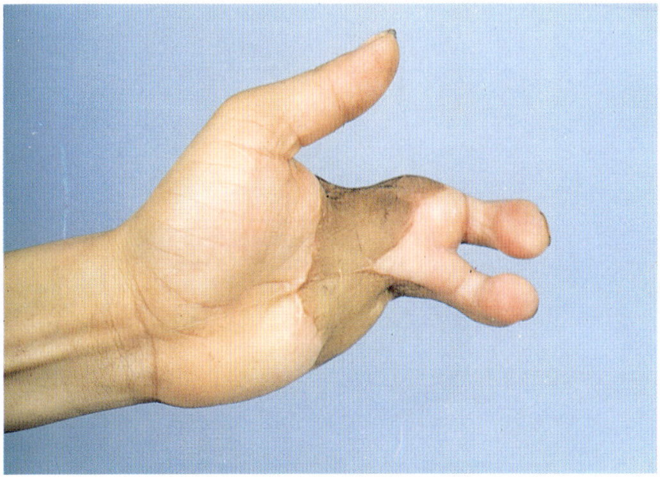

Fig. 18-7

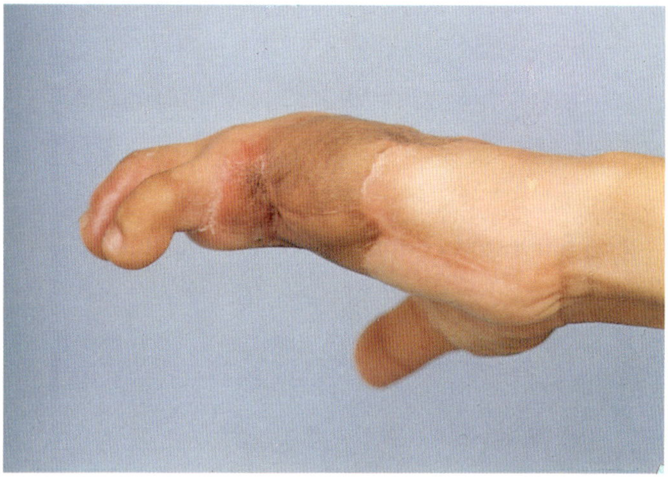

Fig. 18-8

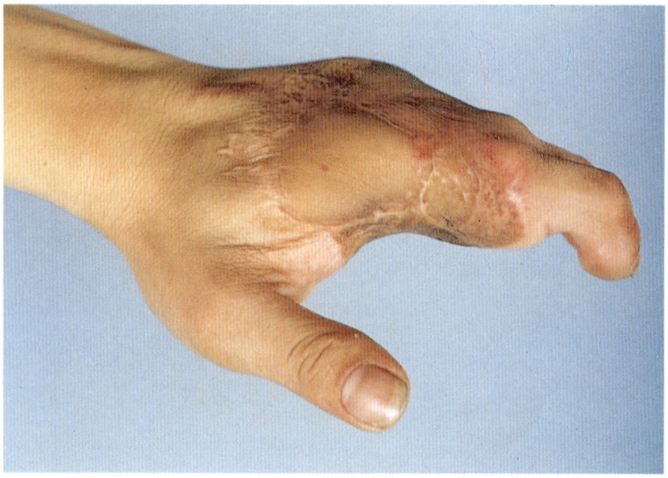

Fig. 18-9

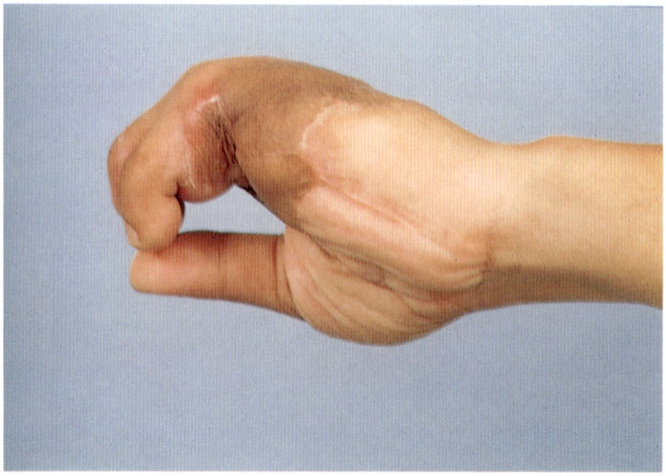

Fig. 18-10

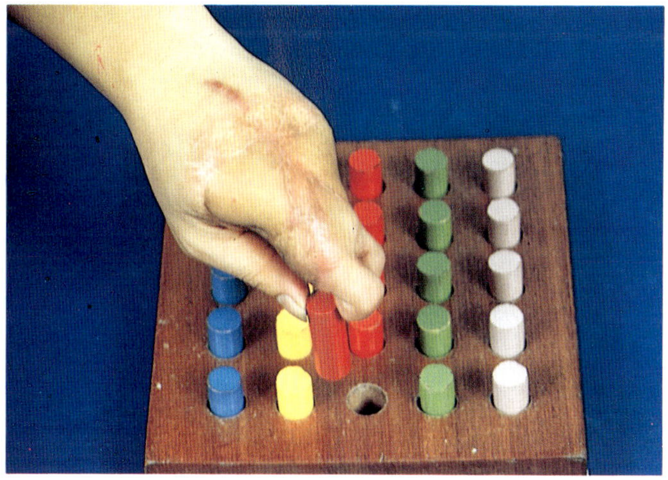

Fig. 18-11

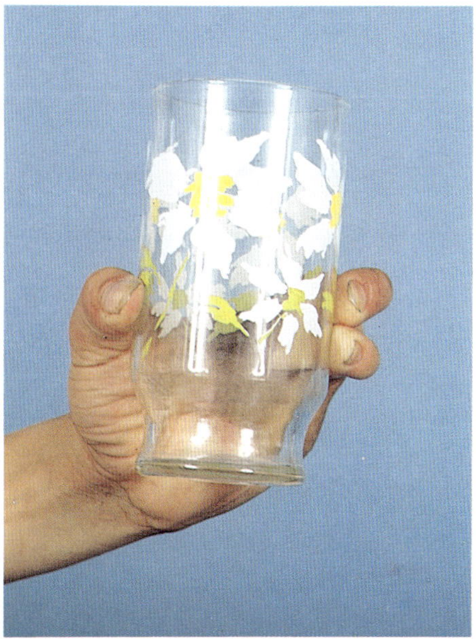

Fig. 18-12

Appearance of the donor site.

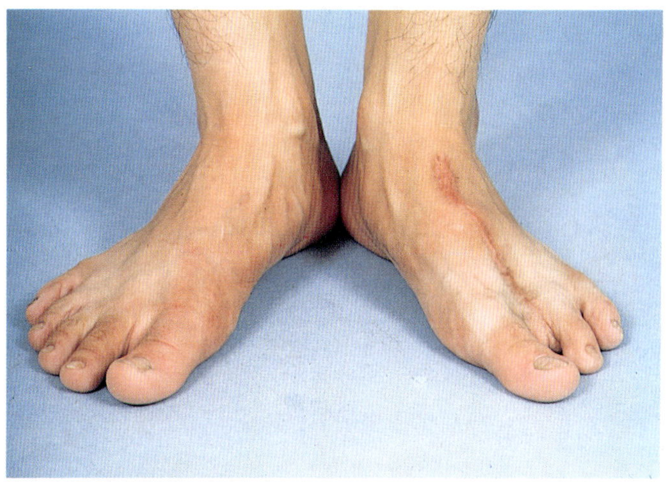

Fig. 18-13

Gait analysis.

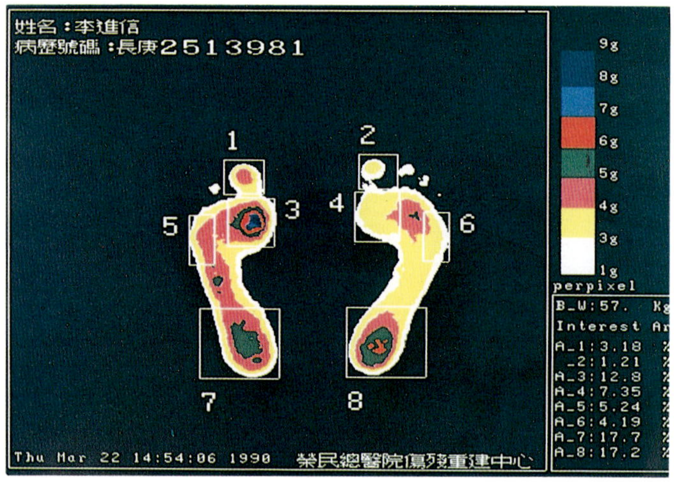

Fig. 18-14

Suggested Reading

Tsai TM. Second and third toe transplantation to a transmetacarpal amputated hand. *Ann Acad Med Singapore*. 1979;8:413.

Wei FC, Colony LH, Chen HC, Chuang CC, Noordhoff MS. Combined second and third toe transfer. *Plast Reconstr Surg*. 1989;84:651.

Chapter 19

Iliac Crest Osteocutaneous Flap

Jonathan W. Jones, MD

The iliac crest and overlying skin based on the deep circumflex iliac vessels provide vascularized bone and soft tissues for single stage reconstruction of tibia and mandible defects.

Case Examples

Case #1

A 22-year-old male was crushed between the bumpers of two cars. Loss of the proximal tibia and overlying soft tissues resulted. The deep circumflex iliac artery and veins were anastomosed to the anterior tibial artery stump and accompanying veins. Additional cancellous grafts were later placed. A stable closure resulted.

Right leg proximal tibia wound with necrotic tissues overlying remaining intact posterior tibial vessels.

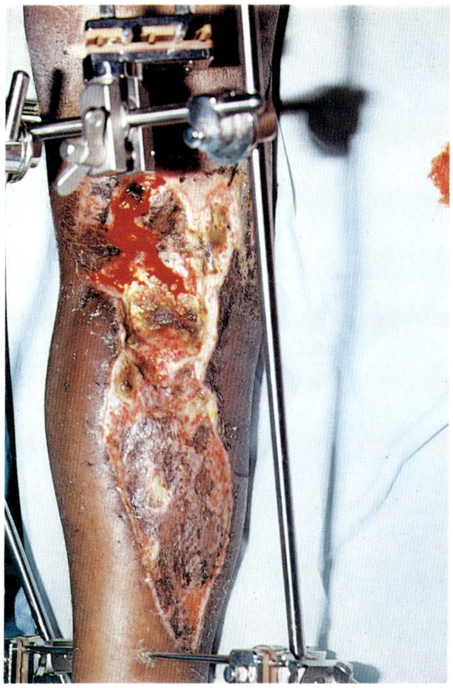

Fig. 19-1

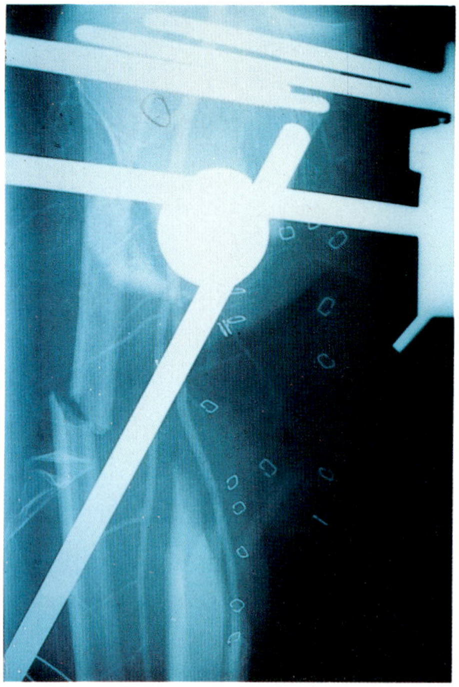

Fig. 19-2

Arteriorgram of leg showing anterior tibial stump, posterior tibial artery, and peroneal artery.

Landmarks for iliac crest dissection.

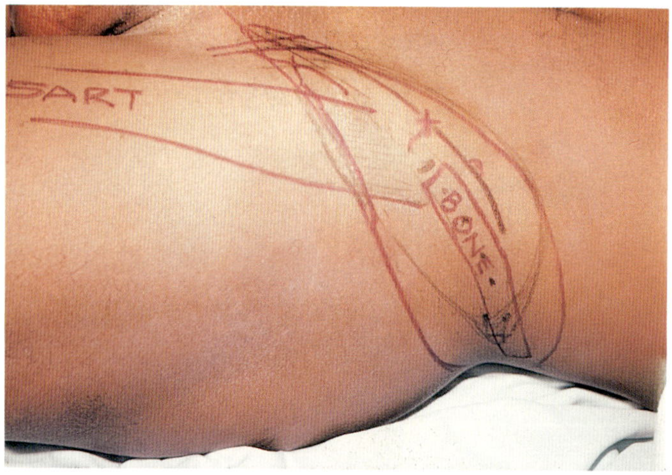

Fig. 19-3

Left iliac crest dissection.

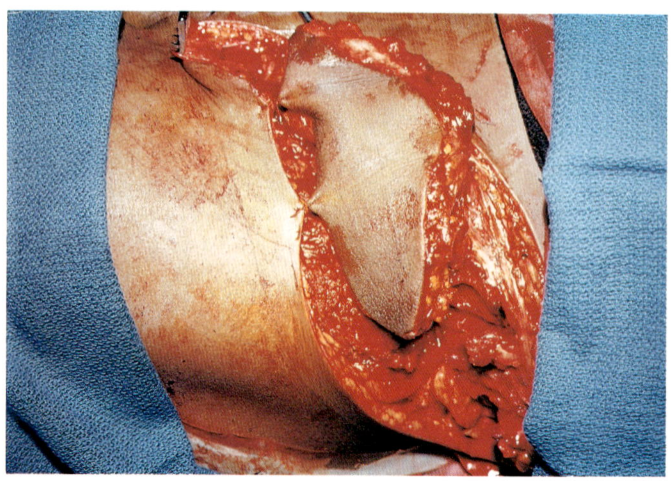

Fig. 19-4

Osteocutaneous flap in place.

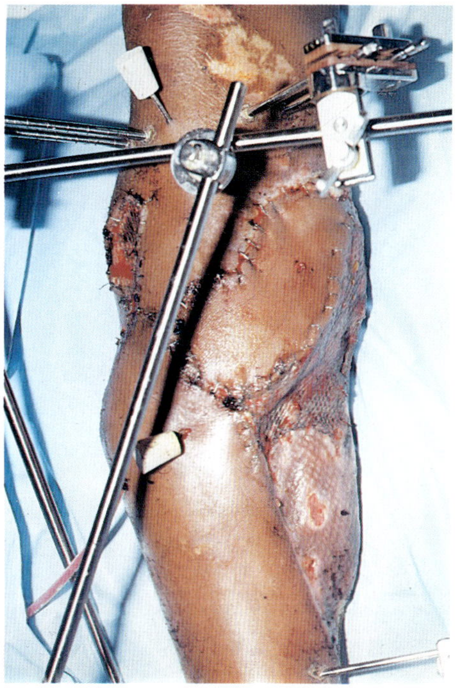

Fig. 19-5

Radiograph of vascularized iliac crest spanning tibia defect.

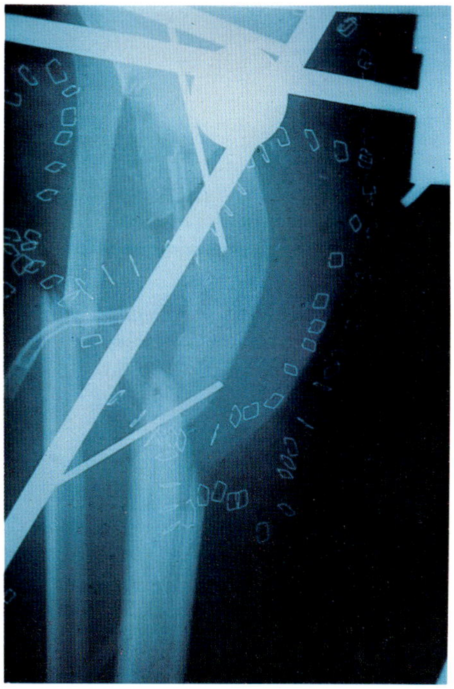

Fig. 19-6

Right leg one year following transplant.

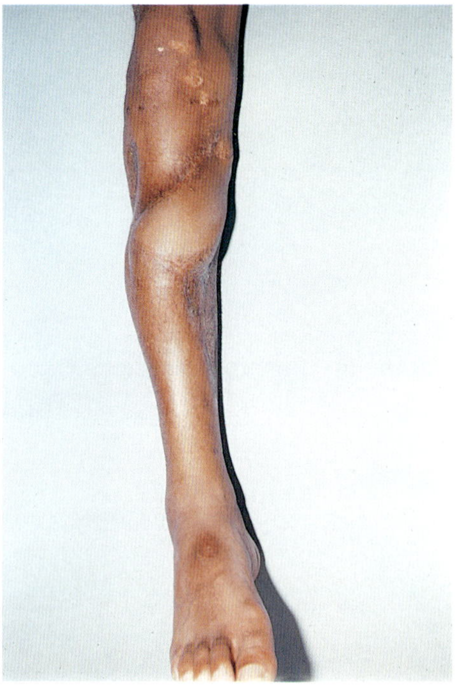

Fig. 19-7

Radiograph of healed tibia after one year.

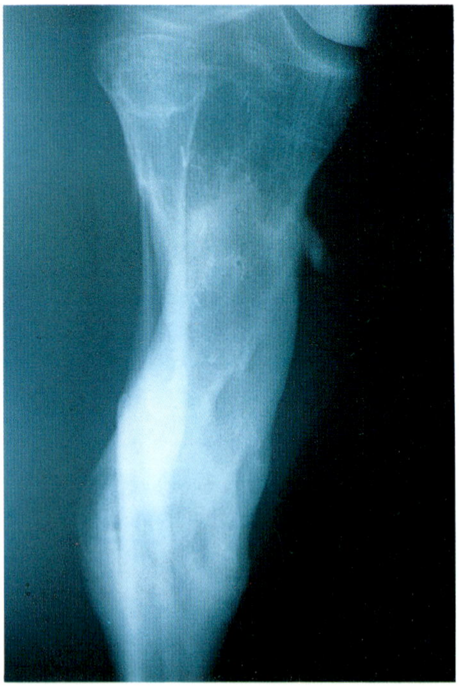

Fig. 19-8

Donor site scar.

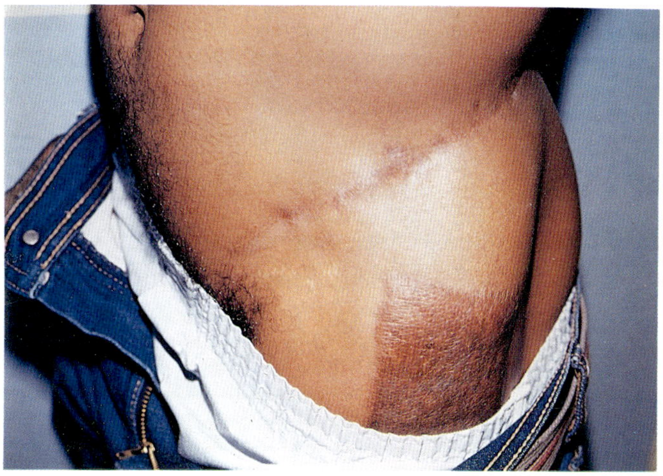

Fig. 19-9

Case #2

A patient with a gunshot wound to the mandible underwent hemimandible reconstruction with vascularized iliac crest graft. Another patient received an iliac crest osteocutaneous graft following oral tumor resection.

Hemimandible sculptured from iliac crest.

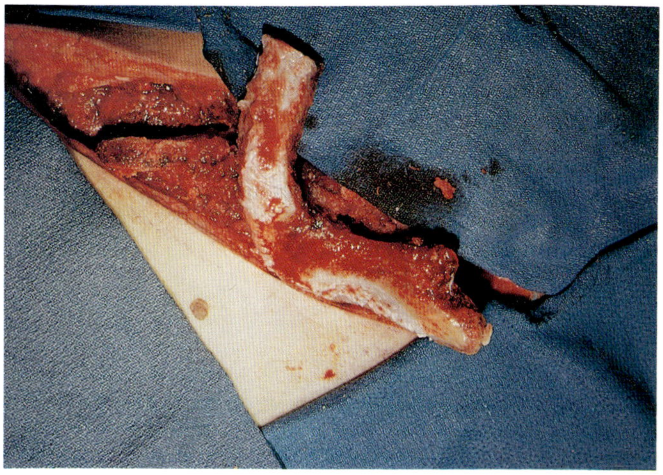

Fig. 19-10

Small iliac crest free flap for segmental defect of mandible, also requiring oral lining.

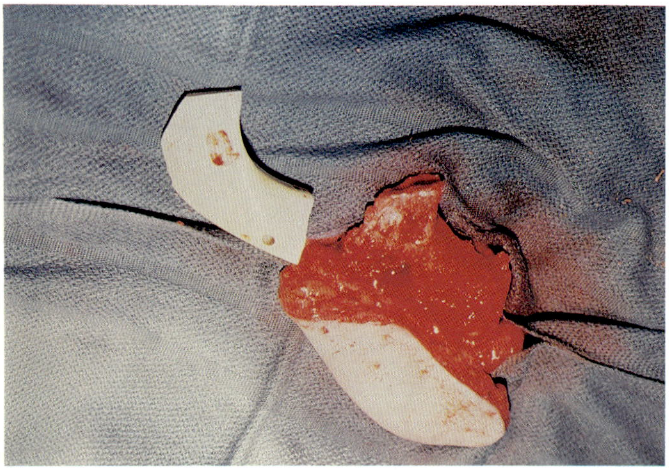

Fig. 19-11

Suggested Reading

Taylor GI, Townsend P, Corlett R. Superiority of the deep circumflex vessels as the supply for free groin flaps: clinical work. *Plast Reconstr Surg*. 1979;64:745-759.

Taylor GI. Reconstruction of the mandible with free composite iliac bone grafts. *Ann Plast Surg*. 1982;9:361-375.

Chapter 20

The Superficial Circumflex Iliac Artery-Based Groin Flap

Jonathan W. Jones, MD

Contour defects which traditionally have been filled with dermal fat grafts may be more reliably and permanently corrected when the transplanted tissues are immediately revascularized. The superficial circumflex iliac vessels of the de-epithelialized groin flap are anastomosed to the facial artery and vein for the correction of hemifacial defects.

In thin patients, the groin flap may also be used to cover avulsion injuries where tendon exposure has resulted. Tendons will more easily glide through fatty tissues than through the fascia or muscle of other free flaps.

Case Examples

Case #1

A 34-year-old male developed progressive atrophy of the subcutaneous tissues of the right side of his face over a two-year period. The condition remained unchanged one year prior to referral. A groin flap was used to replace the lost tissues. The flap was elevated in a lateral-to-medial direction including a portion of the sartorius fascia so as to protect the overlying superficial circumflex iliac vessels. Following secondary debulking of the flap, adequate contour correction resulted.

Right hemifacial atrophy.

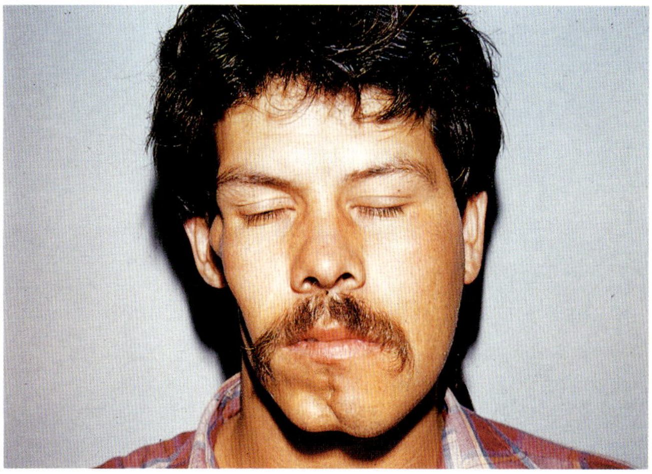

Fig. 20-1

Oblique view of facial contour defect.

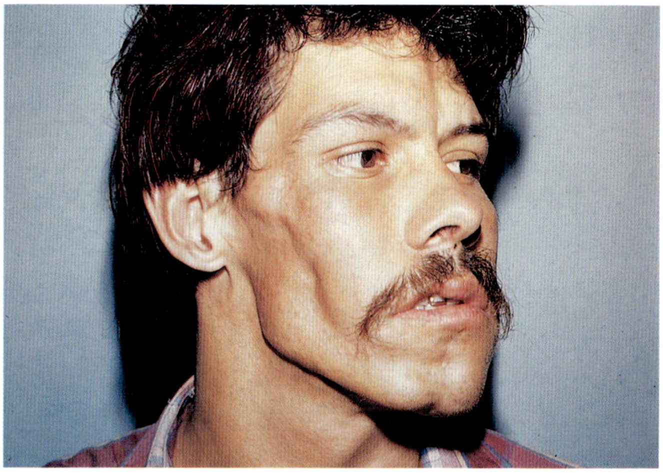

Fig. 20-2

Landmarks for groin flap dissection.

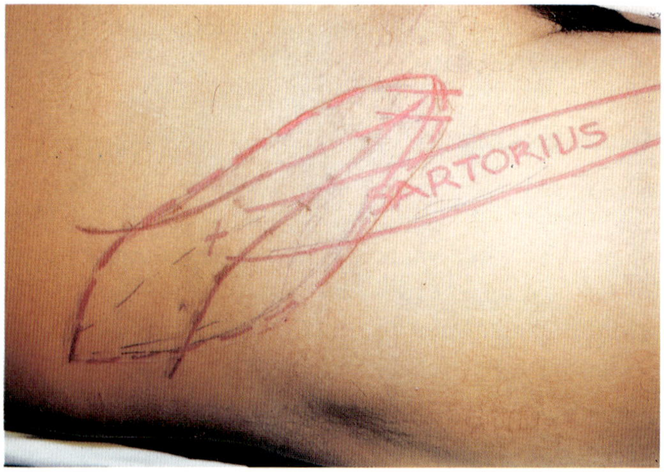

Fig. 20-3

Vascularized groin flap placed beneath cheek flap.

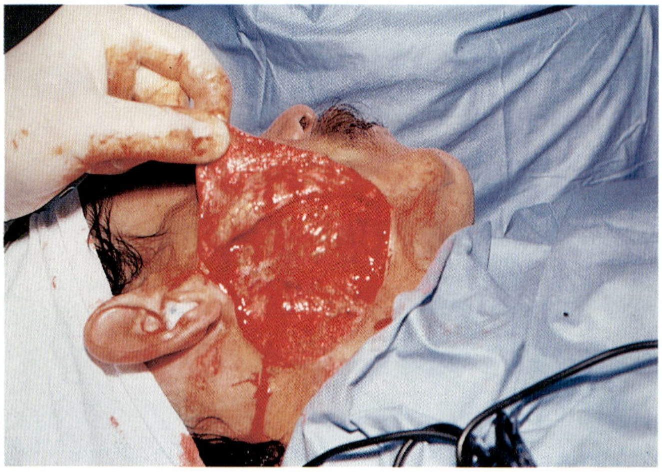

Fig. 20-4

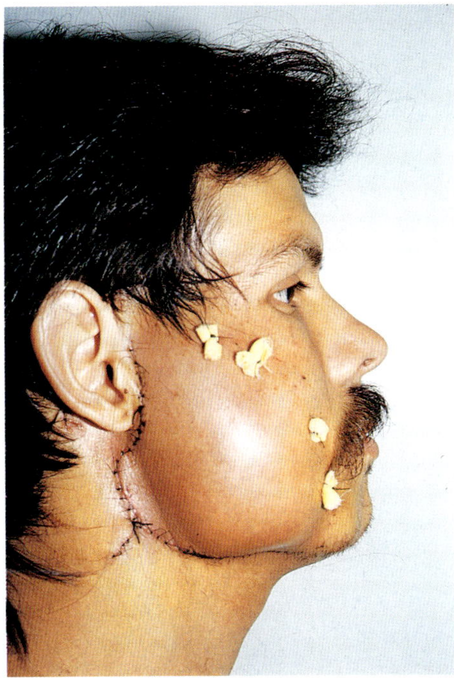

Fig. 20-5

Swelling is common in the early postoperative period.

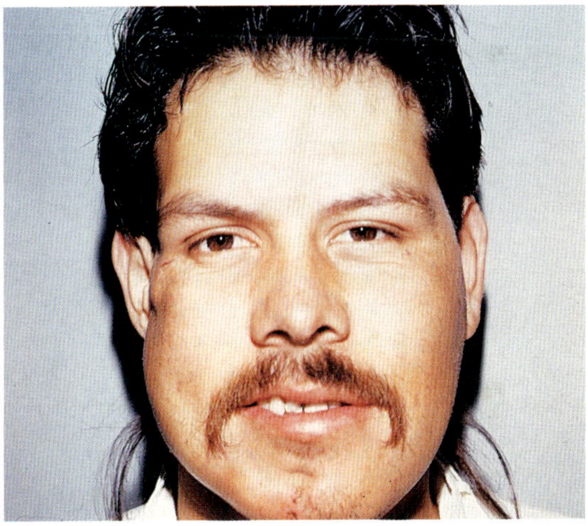

Fig. 20-6

Appearance following secondary debulking of flap (Figs. 20-6 and 20-7).

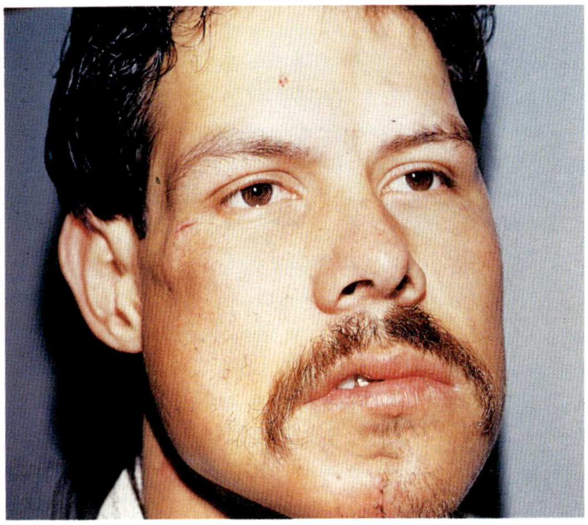

Fig. 20-7

Case #2

A 37-year-old male sustained an avulsion injury to his right foot. The thin unstable skin graft over the tarsal bones was replaced with a free groin flap.

Unstable skin graft over tarsal bones (Figs. 20-8 and 20-9).

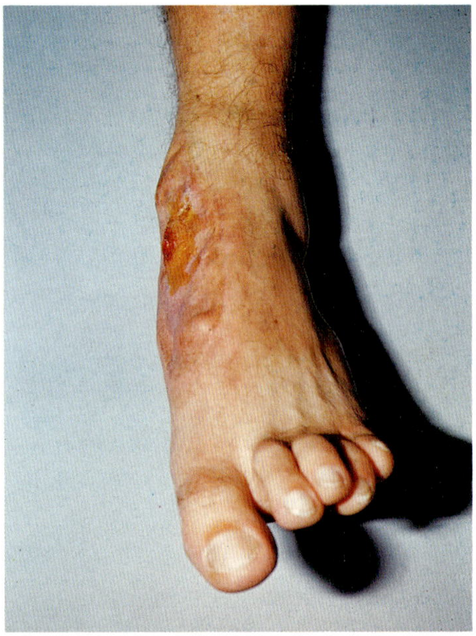

Fig. 20-8

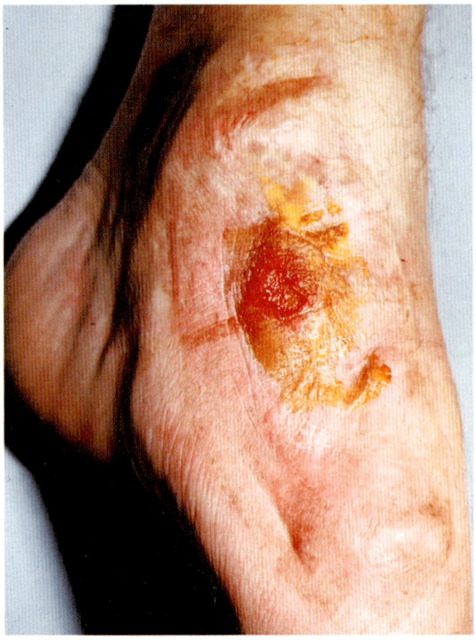

Fig. 20-9

Groin flap with anastamoses to anterior tibial vessels.

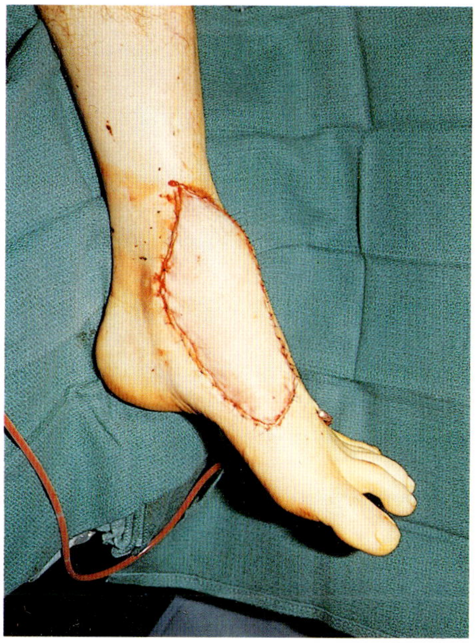

Fig. 20-10

Stable wound closure following secondary defatting of groin flap.

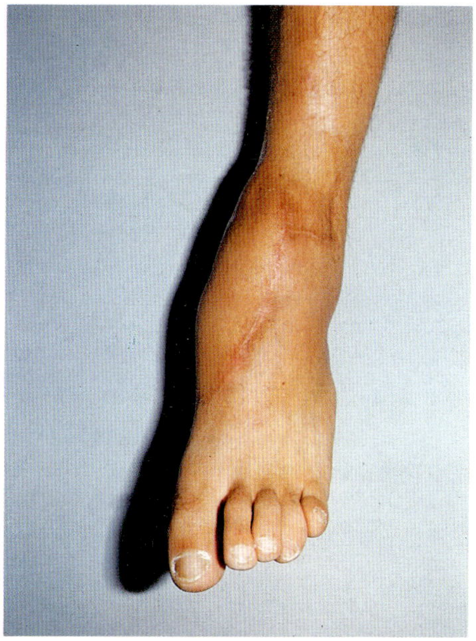

Fig. 20-11

Suggested Reading

Daniel RK, Taylor GI. Distant transfer of an island flap by microvascular anastomoses: a clinical technique. *Plast Reconstr Surg*. 1973;52:111.

Harii K, Omari K, Shuher T, et al. Free groin skin flaps. *Br J Plast Surg*. 1975;28:225.

McGreggor I, Jackson I. The groin flap. *Br J Plast Surg*. 1972;25:3.

Chapter 21

Omentum

Jonathan W. Jones, MD

First used for resurfacing cranial defects, the omentum remains a good option for filling irregular contour defects such as the orbit. The gastroepiploic vessels nourishing the omental fatty tissues may be passed beneath a cheek flap into the neck for anastomosis to large caliber vessels distant from scarred or radiation-damaged tissues.

Case Examples

Case #1

A 63-year-old man underwent resection of a recurrent meningioma. A fascia graft alone separated the brain from the orbital exenteration defect and nasal cavity. The gastroepiploic vessels were anastamosed to the lingual artery and a branch of the internal jugular vein. A skin graft was applied to the exposed portion of the omentum within the orbit.

Orbital defect with exposure of sinuses, frontal.

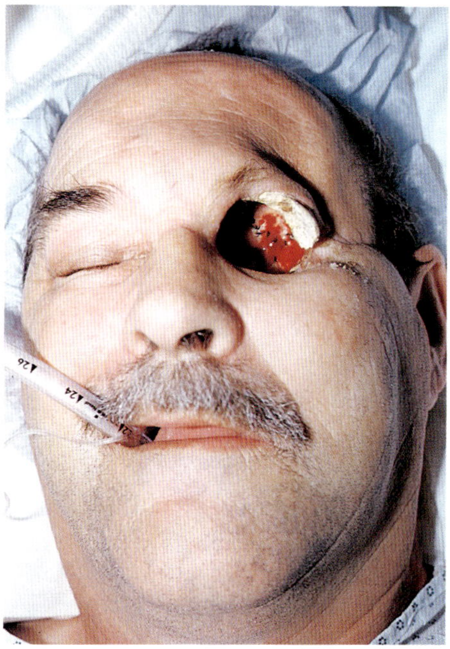

Fig. 21-1

Omentum with gastroepiploic vessels intact.

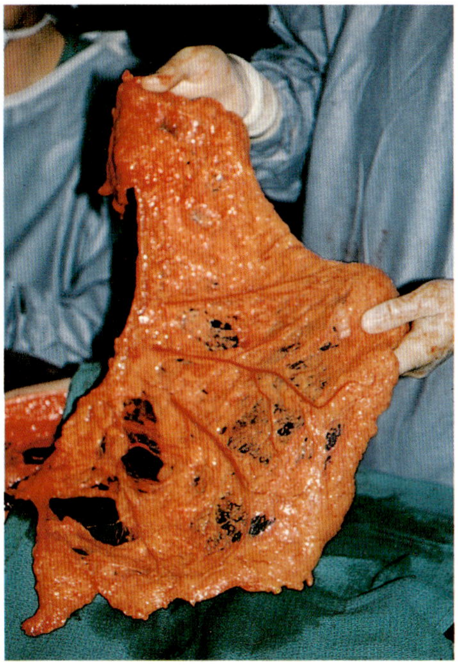

Fig. 21-2

Skin-grafted omentum and photoplethysmograph probe used to monitor circulation in transplanted tissues.

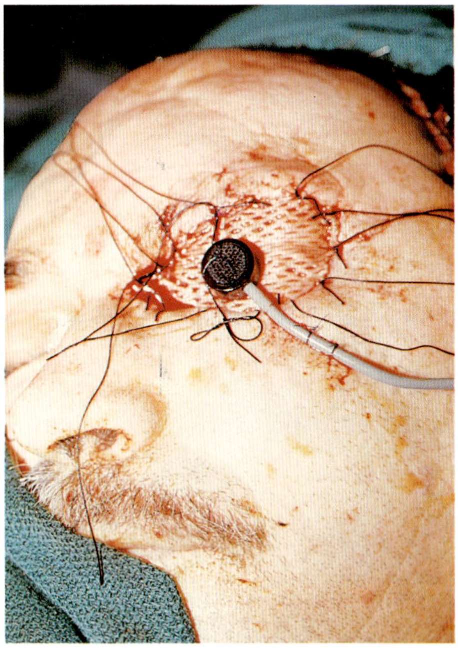

Fig. 21-3

Lateral view of transplanted omentum.

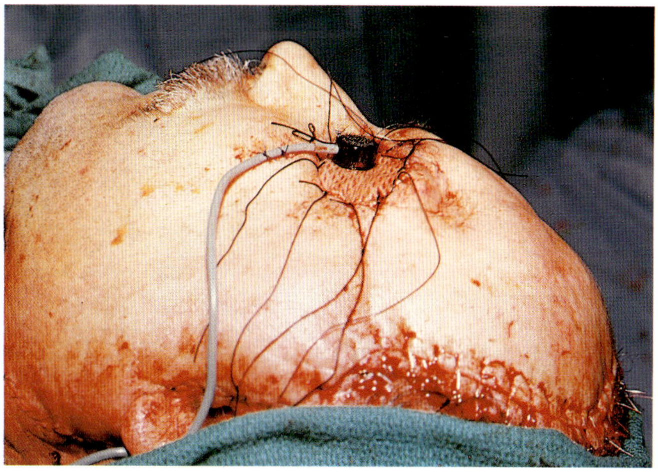

Fig. 21-4

Healed skin graft over omentum.

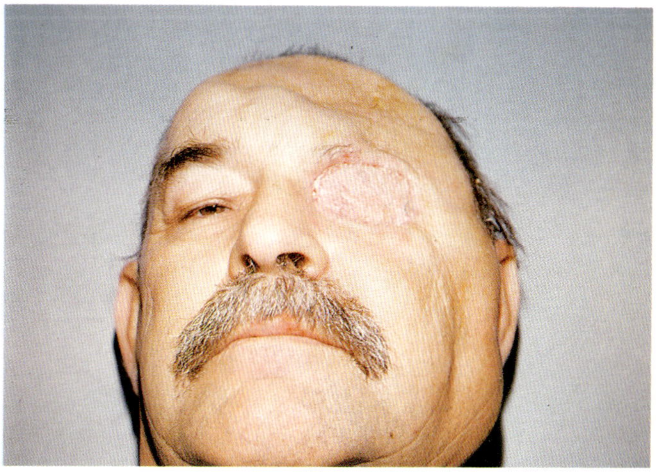

Fig. 21-5

Glasses and hat allow comfortable excursions in public.

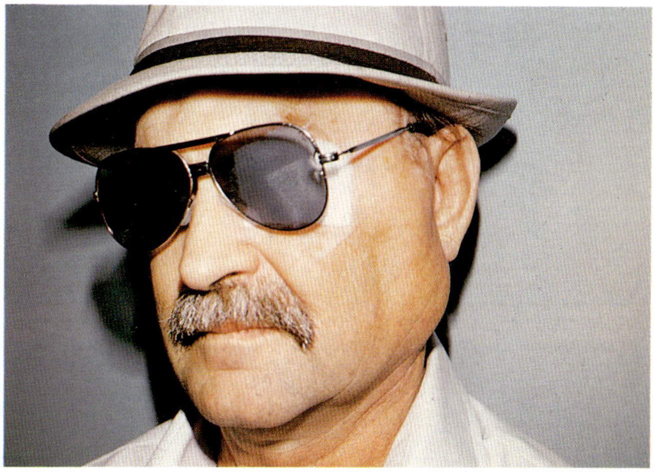

Fig. 21-6

Case #2

A 32-year-old woman with metastatic adenoidcystic carcinoma underwent omental transfer. This wound closure permitted her to confortably travel, swim, and visit with friends before she ultimately succumbed to her disease.

Defect following tumor resection.

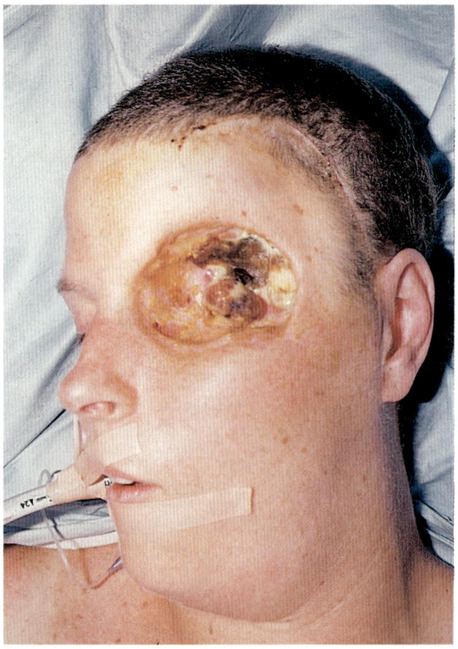

Fig. 21-7

Omentum filling orbital defect.

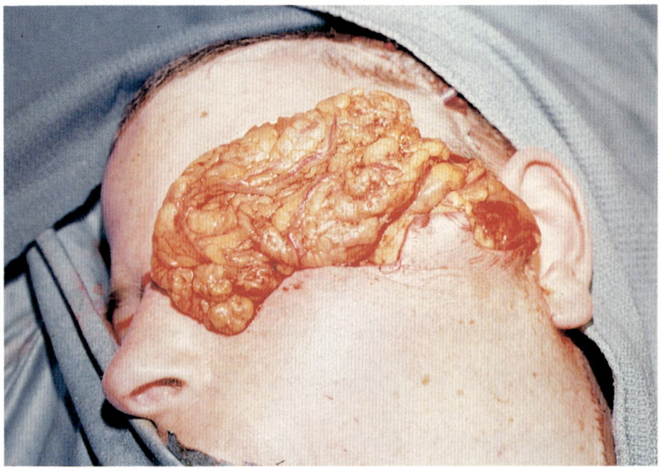

Fig. 21-8

Orbital defect sealed with omental transplant.

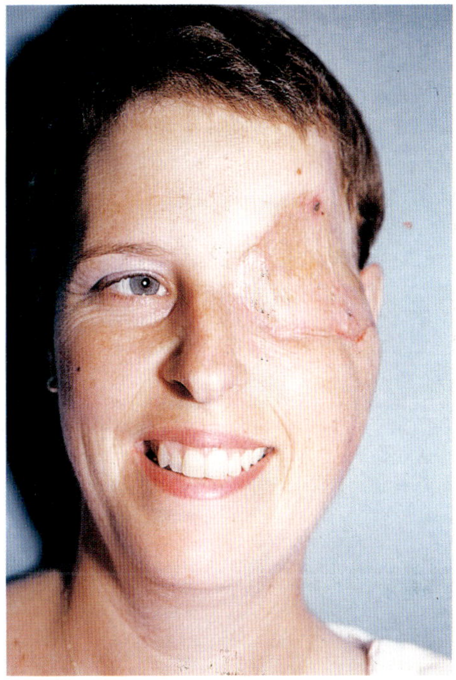

Fig. 21-9

Suggested Reading

Jurkiewicz MJ, Wahal F. The omentum: its use as a free vascularized graft for reconstruction of the head and neck. *Ann Surg*. 1982;195:756-764.

McLean DH, Bunke HJ, Jr. Autotransplantation of omentum to a large scalp defect, with microvascular revascularization. *Plast Reconstr Surg*. 1972;49:268-274.

Chapter 22

Circumflex Scapular-Based Flaps

Jonathan W. Jones, MD

The scapular and parascapular fasciacutaneous free flaps based on transverse and oblique perforating branches of the subscapular artery and veins enable resurfacing of large wounds without sacrificing functional muscle units. As the circumflex scapular artery ascends through the triangular space, branches are given off to the lateral border of the scapula; this enables concurrent transplantation of a vascularized scapular bone graft.

Circumflex scapular artery-based flaps and thoracodorsal artery-based latissimus flaps may be transplanted together on the same subscapular pedicle.

Case Examples

Case #1

A 35-year-old male sustained extensive facial injuries in a roll-over automobile accident. He was driving a convertible at a high speed. An anesthesiologist and an emergency medical technician witnessed the accident and intubated the patient. Loss of the left mandible, maxilla, and adjacent soft tissues resulted. Oral lining, bone support, and outer cover were provided with a bilobed osteocutaneous free flap.

Appearance of face following roll-over injury.

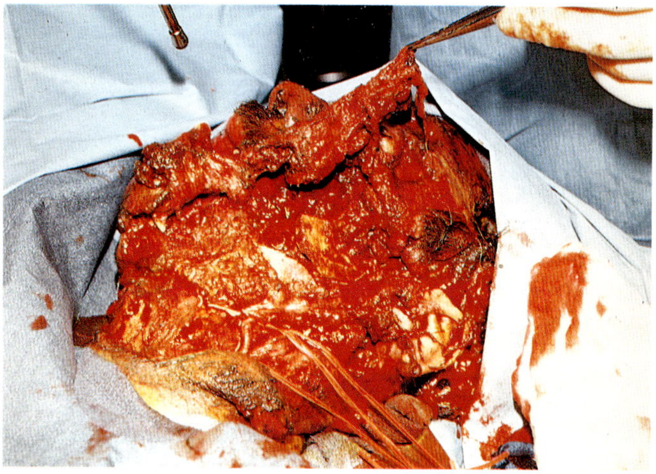

Fig. 22-1

Scarred contracted facial defect following temporary skin graft placement.

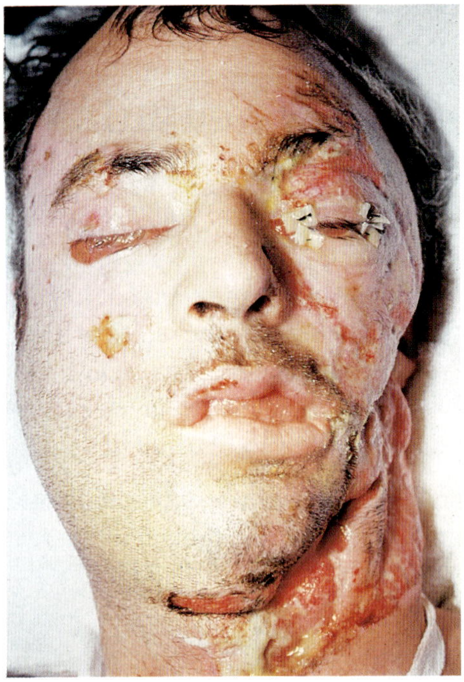

Fig. 22-2

Cheek defect following scar release.

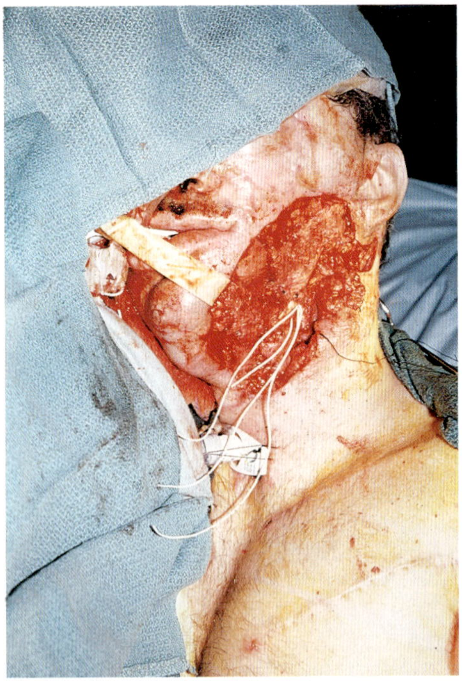

Fig. 22-3

Bilobed scapular region flap.

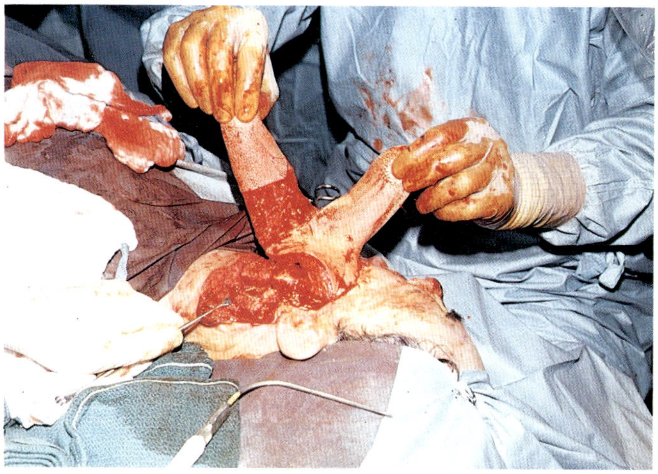

Fig. 22-4

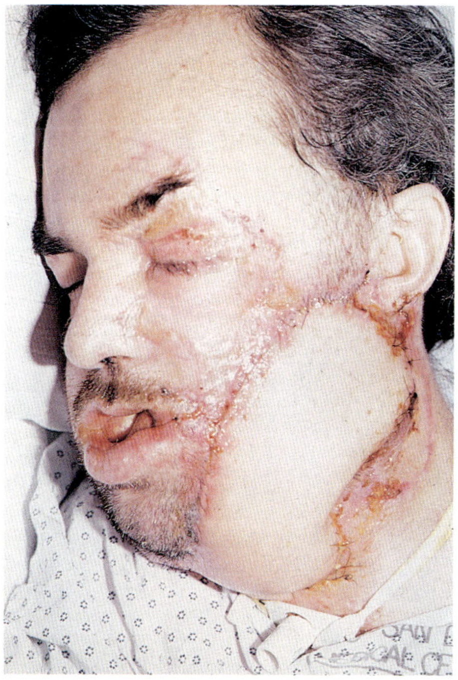

Fig. 22-5

Early appearance of flap.

Radiograph of face showing bar and bone graft.

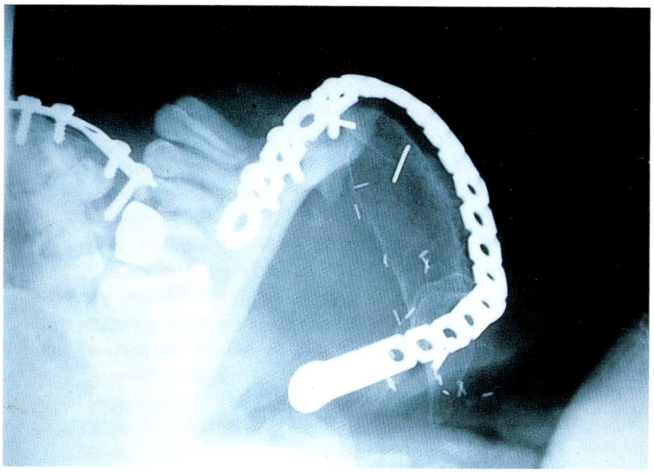

Fig. 22-6

Early appearance of flap with folded over portion visible at left oral commissure.

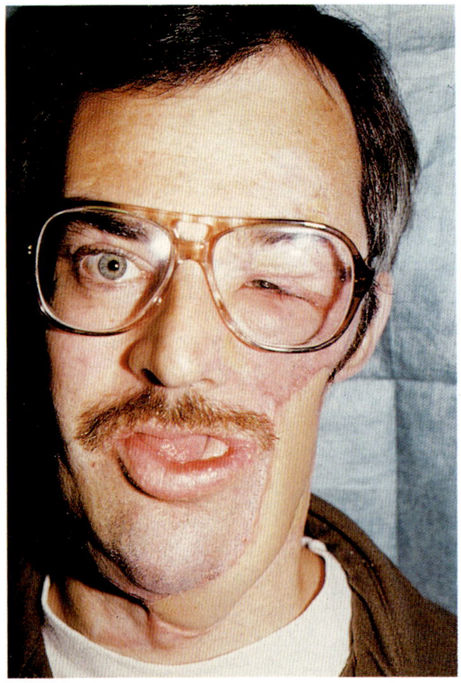

Fig. 22-7

Appearance following recontouring of flap.

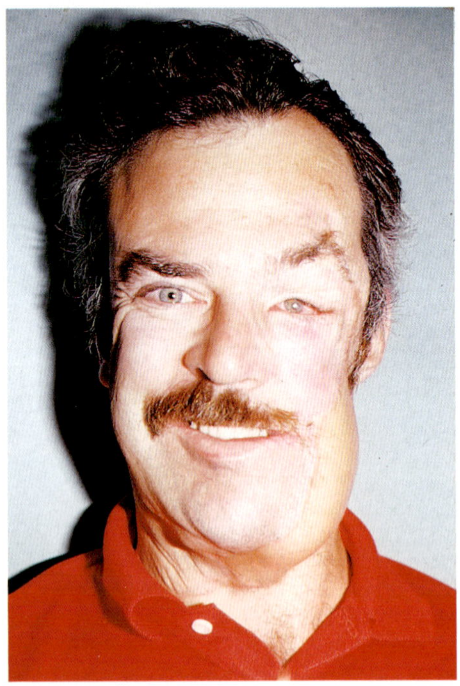

Fig. 22-8

Case #2

A 13-year-old child was run over by a car and sustained tibia fractures and an open ankle joint. A parascapular free flap and skin grafts provided stable coverage.

Child's leg defect.

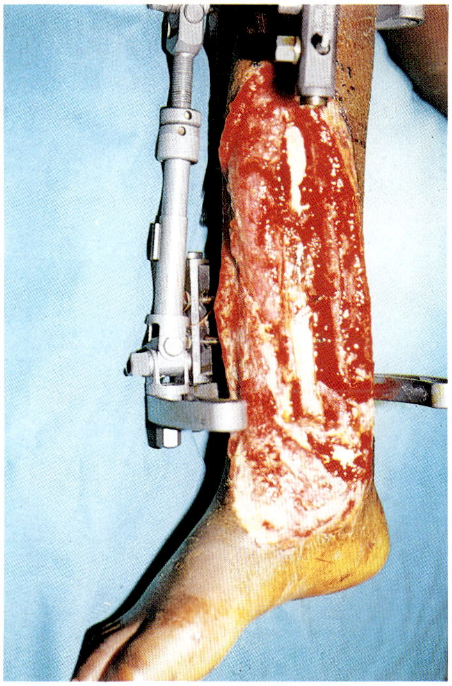

Fig. 22-9 A

Parascapular flap prior to skin grafting.

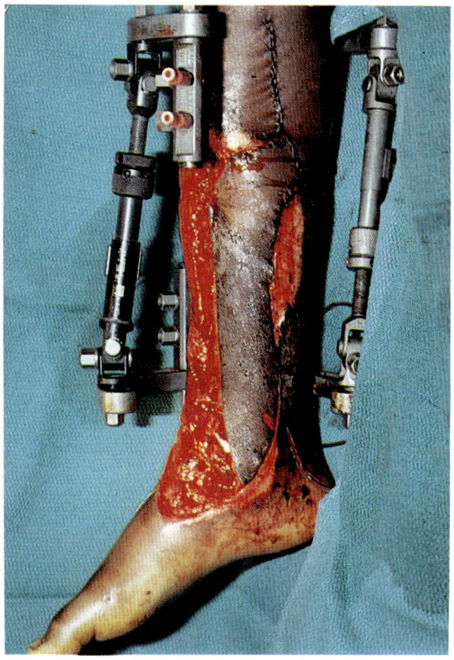

Fig. 22-9 B

Defect sealed with parascapular flap.

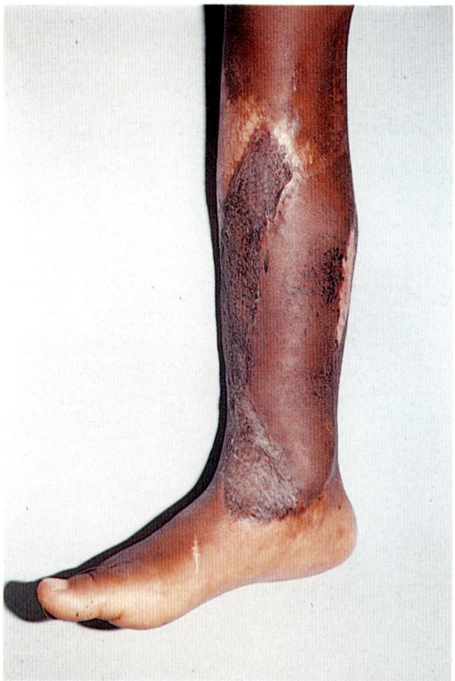

Fig. 22-10

Case #3

A 24-year-old nursery worker sustained injuries from a fertilizer mixing machine. A large parascapular free flap provided stable coverage.

Leg defect following avulsion injury.

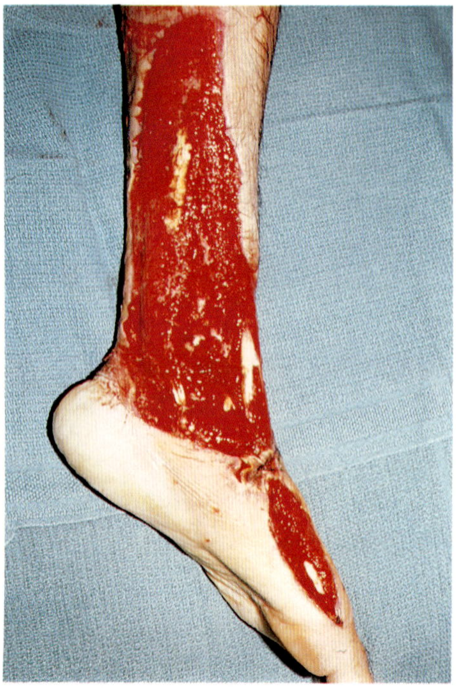

Fig. 22-11

Outline of flap.

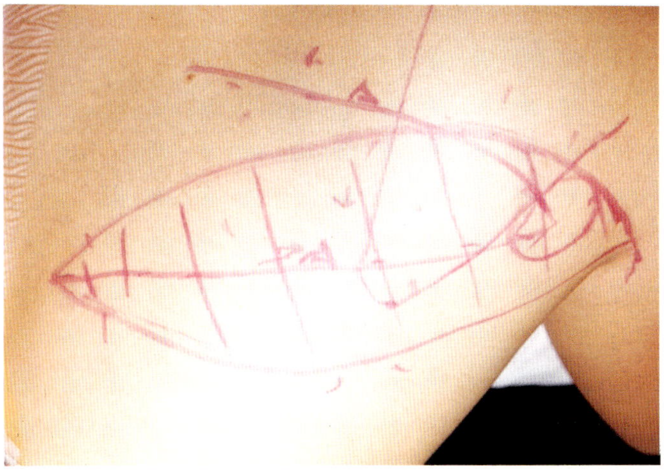

Fig. 22-12

Transplanted parascapular flap.

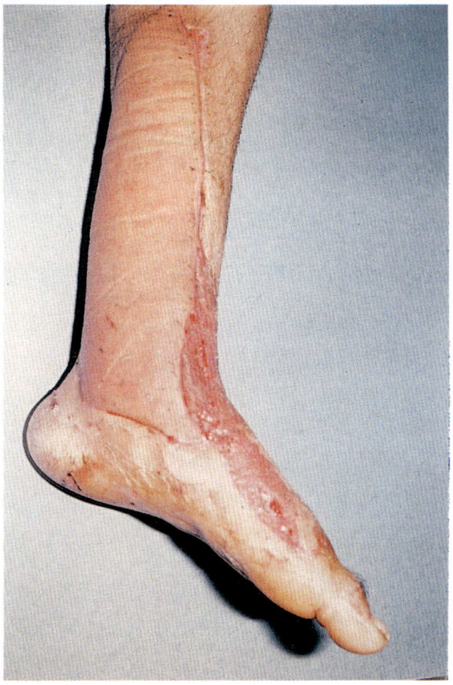

Fig. 22-13

Donor site scar following flap harvesting.

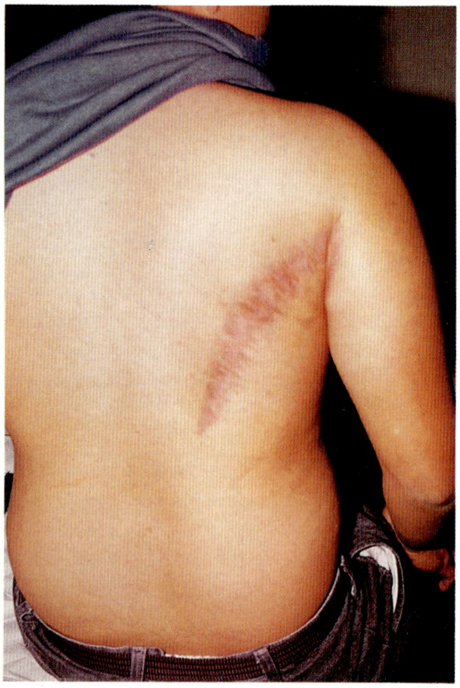

Fig. 22-14

Suggested Reading

Dos Santos LF. The vascular anatomy and dissection of the free scapular flap. *Plast Reconstr Surg.* 1984;73:599.

Swartz WM, Banis JC, et al. The osteocutaneous scapular flap for mandible and maxillary reconstruction. *Plast Reconstr Surg.* 1986;77:530.

Chapter 23

Gracilis Muscle and Myocutaneous Flaps

Jonathan W. Jones, MD

The gracilis muscle may be transplanted for reanimation of the face and restoration of upper and lower extremity muscle function. It is also an ideal choice for closing compound defects about the distal lower leg and foot. The donor site scar is inconspicuous and no functional losses have been recognized following harvesting of this muscle.

Case Examples

Case #1

A 14-year-old girl fractured her tibia in a motor scooter accident. Anterior compartment necrosis resulted following plating of the fracture and casting. A gracilis myocutaneous free flap restored ankle dorsiflextion.

Anterior compartment defect with exposed orthopedic hardware.

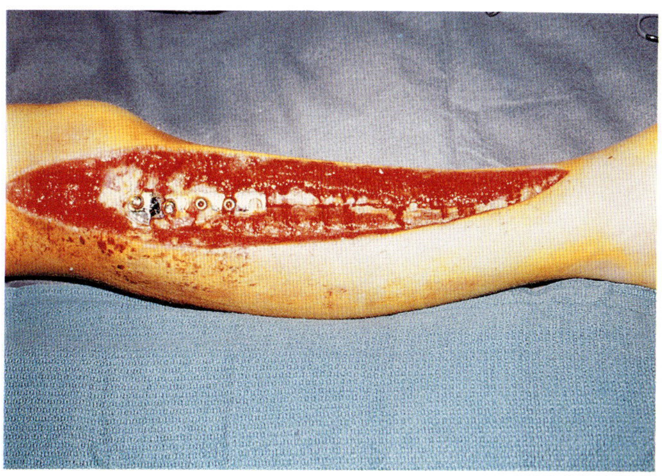

Fig. 23-1

Gracilis myocutaneous flap filling leg defect.

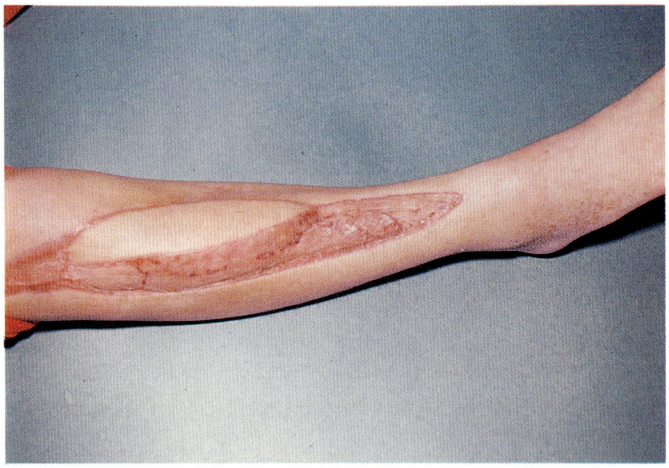

Fig. 23-2

Leg following scar revisions.

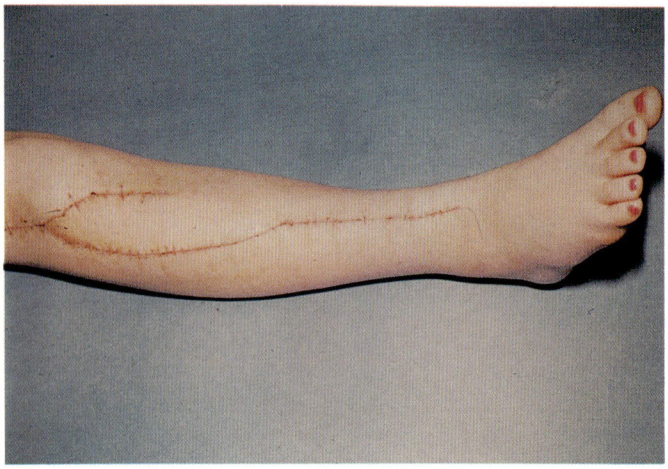

Fig. 23-3

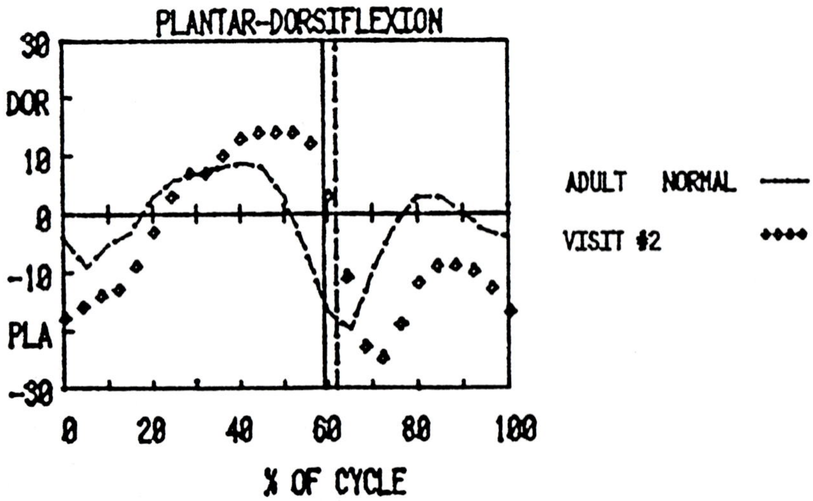

Fig. 23-4. Contractile activity of gracilis muscle during walking.

Case #2

A 15-year-old boy underwent resection of an osteosarcoma of the distal tibia. Immediate coverage was provided with gracilis free flap.

Tibia defect following osteosarcoma resection.

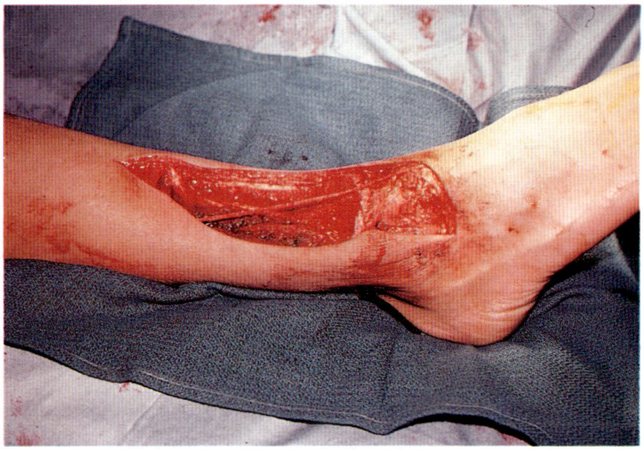

Fig. 23-5

Skin-grafted gracilis muscle.

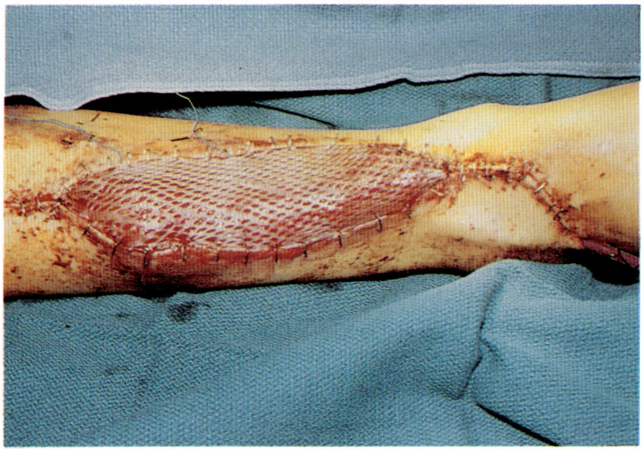

Fig. 23-6

Mature skin-grafted gracilis transplant.

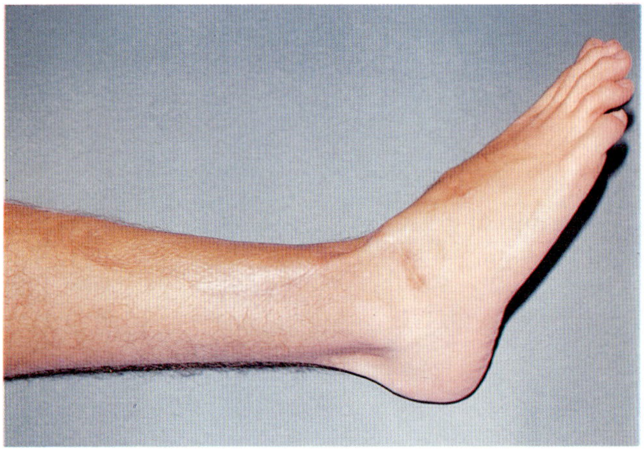

Fig. 23-7

Case #3

A 47-year-old woman sustained a severe crush injury to her right arm. The avulsed volar forearm muscles were replaced with a gracilis free flap. This enabled partial restoration of finger and thumb flexion. The obturator nerve to the gracilis was sutured to the median nerve. Sural nerve cable grafts were also interposed to restore protective sensation in the median distribution.

Arm crush injury defect.

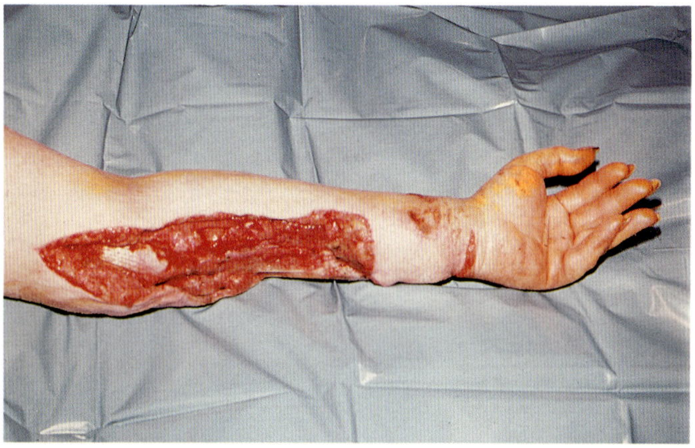

Fig. 23-8

Landmarks for gracilis dissection.

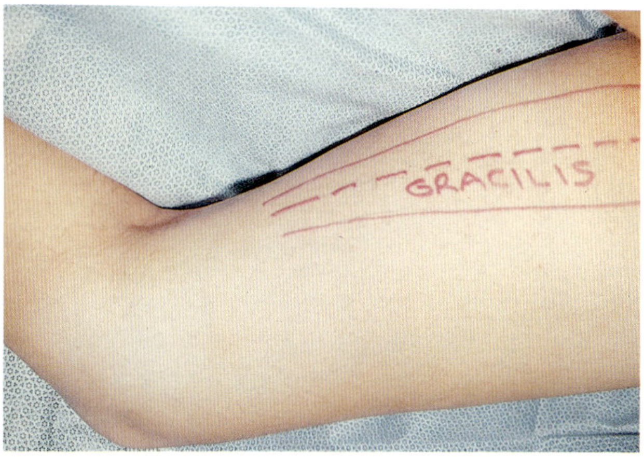

Fig. 23-9

Elevation of gracilis muscle, arrow at dominant pedicle.

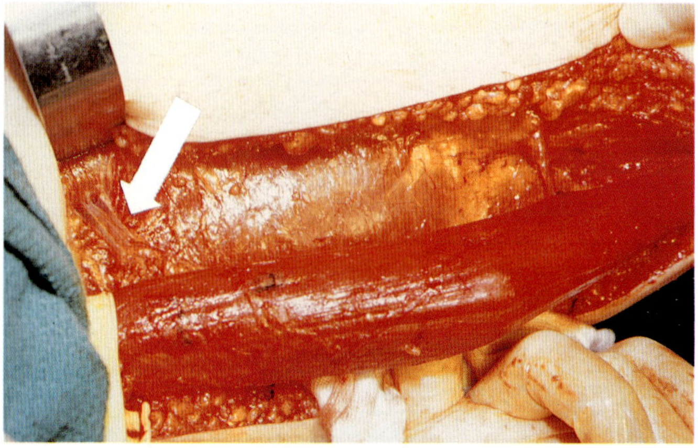

Fig. 23-10

Gracilis muscle transplanted to forearm.

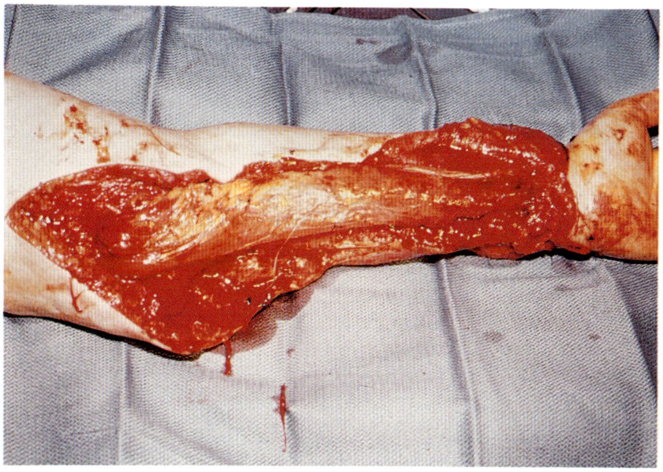

Fig. 23-11

Sural nerve graft replacing avulsed median nerve.

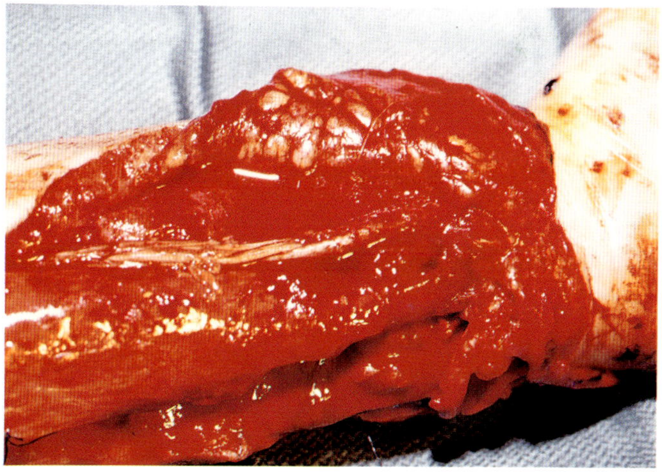

Fig. 23-12

Forearm with healed wounds.

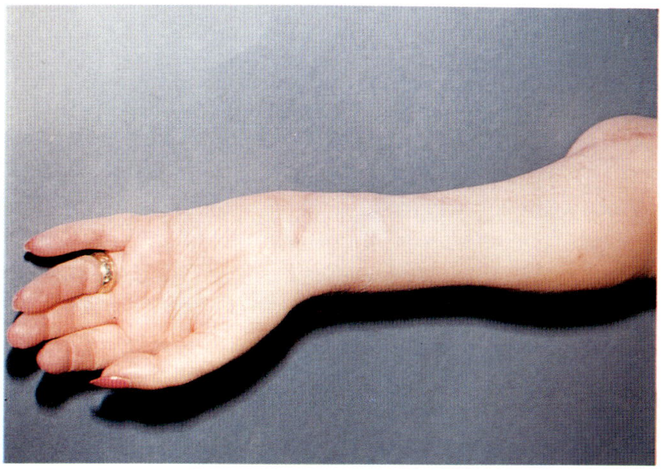

Fig. 23-13

Fingers at extension.

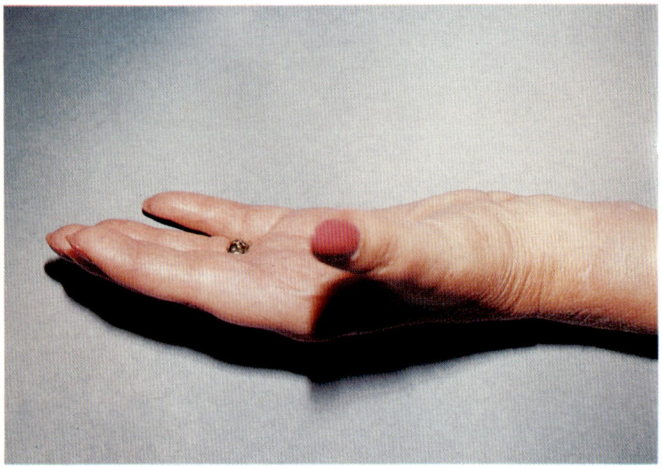

Fig. 23-14

Fingers flexed by gracilis transplant.

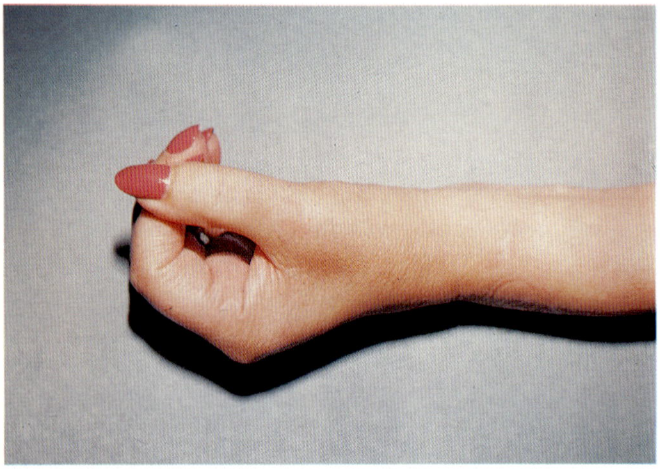

Fig. 23-15

Suggested Reading

Harii K, Ohmori K, Torii S. Free gracilis muscle transplantation with microneurovascular anastomosis for treatment of facial paralysis: a preliminary report. *Plast Reconstr Surg*. 1976;57:133-145.

Kobayashi S, Sekiguchi J, et al. (abst.) Functional free gracilis muscle to provide active dorsiflexion of the foot. *Reconstr Microsurg*. 1989;5,2:181.

Manktelow RT. *Microvascular Reconstruction*. Berlin: Springer-Verlag; 1986;37-44.

Chapter 24

The Lateral Arm Free Flap

Jonathan W. Jones, MD

Small, thin innervated skin paddles can be harvested from the lateral upper arm leaving a less conspicuous scar than the radial forearm free flap. Dissection of this flap is technically demanding and the pedicle is relatively short but in thin patients this flap can very effectively resurface hand, foot, and facial defects.

Case Examples

Case #1

An 18-year-old male sustained a degloving injury of his heel in a motorcycle accident. The skin grafted calcaneus repeatedly ulcerated despite the use of custom footwear. Transplantation of an innervated lateral arm fascia-cutaneous flap to the heel enabled the patient to discontinue using his cane, resume jogging, and participate in intercollegiate athletics.

Skin-grafted calcaneus with recurrent ulcerations.

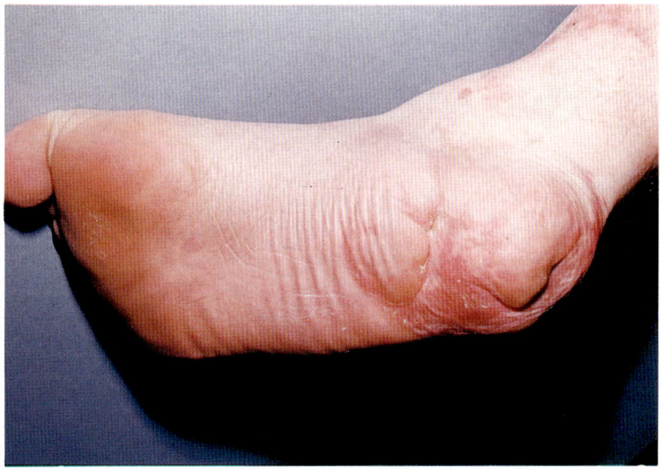

Fig. 24-1

Skin markings showing territory of lateral arm flap.

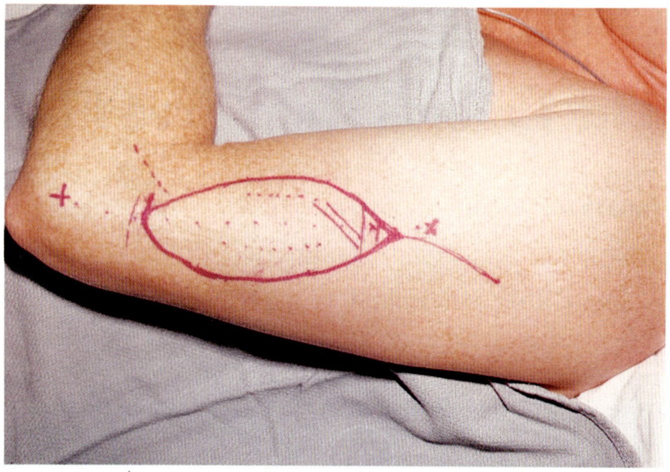

Fig. 24-2

Dissection of lateral arm flap.

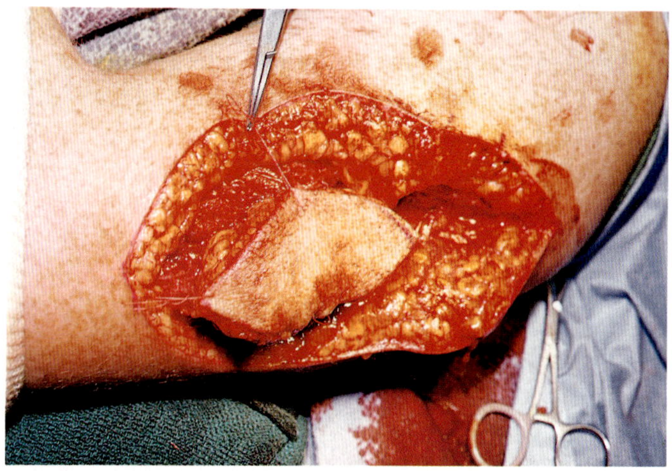

Fig. 24-3

Elevated flap with radial collateral vessels intact.

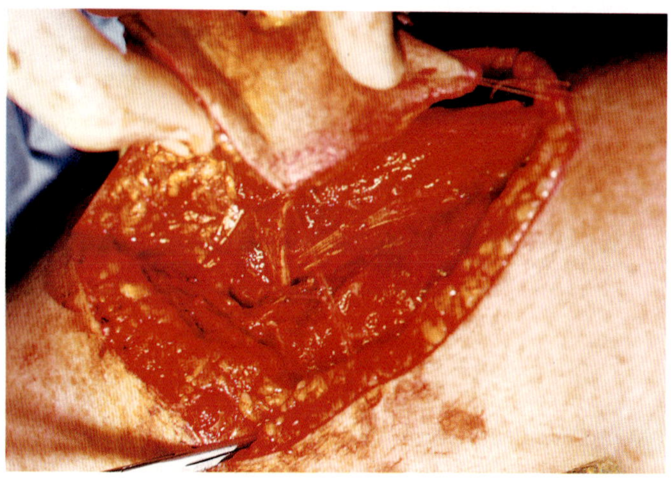

Fig. 24-4

Posterior tibial vessels exposed.

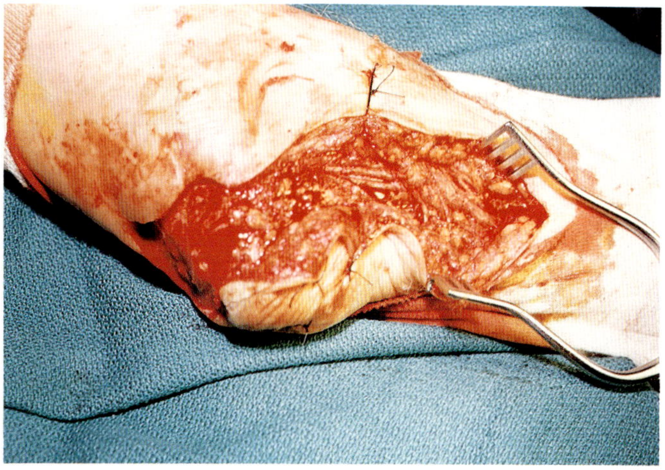

Fig. 24-5

Anastomosis of radial collateral artery and veins to posterior tibial vessels. Posterior cutaneus nerve of lateral arm flap sutured to sensory branch of posterior tibial nerve.

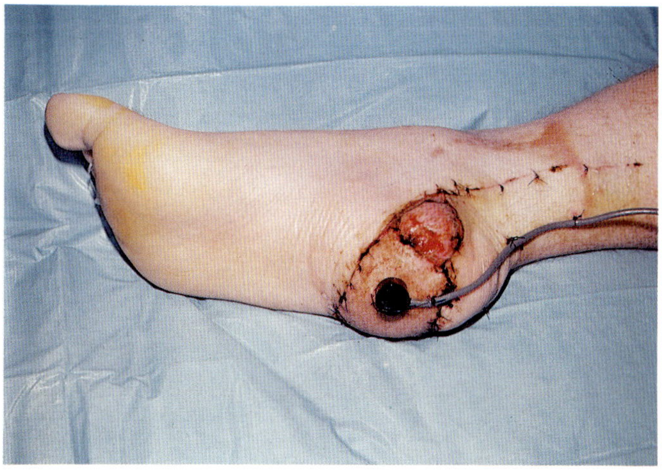

Fig. 24-6

Appearance of heel three years following transplant.

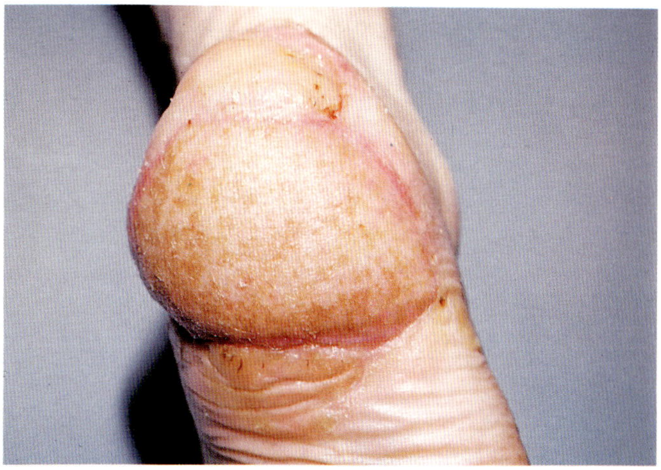

Fig. 24-7

Case #2

A 29-year-old male accidentally amputated his great toe with a hatchet while cutting wood. Transplantation of a lateral arm flap enabled preservation of the great toe metatarsal head.

Metatarsal head exposed.

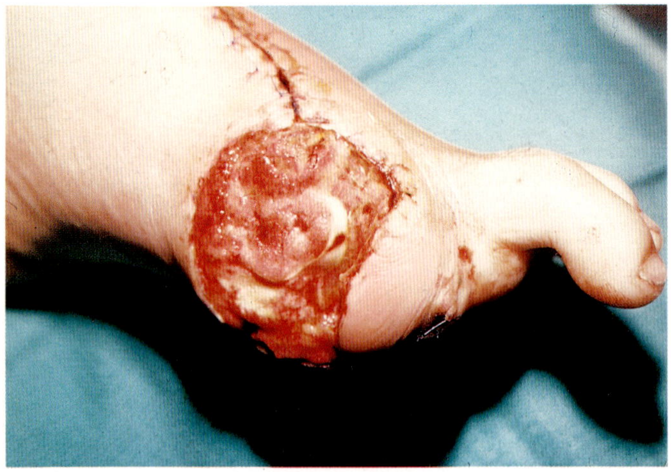

Fig. 24-8

Lateral arm donor site.

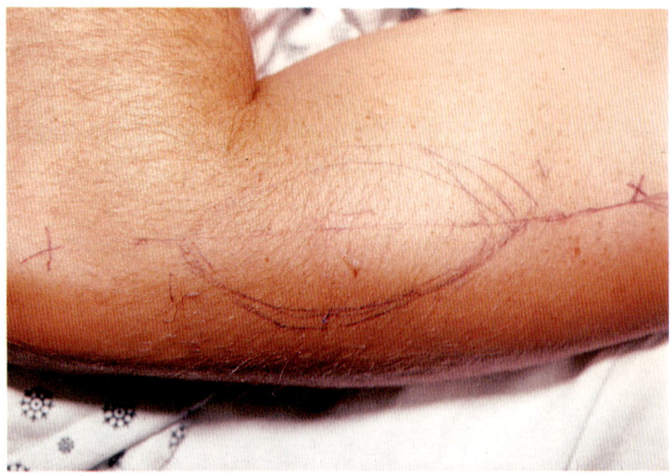

Fig. 24-9

Foot defect sealed with lateral arm flap.

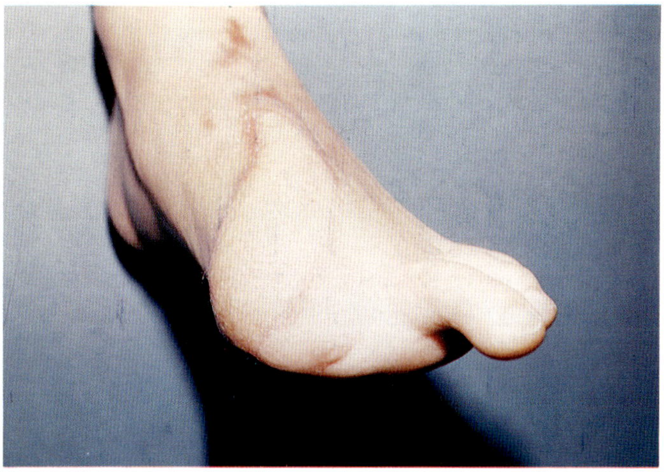

Fig. 24-10

Suggested Reading

Clemente CD. *Anatomy, A Regional Atlas of the Human Body*. Baltimore: Urban and Schwarzenberg; 1987; Fig. 58, 60.

Katsaros J, Schusterman M, Beppu M, Banis JC, Jr, Ockland RD. The lateral arm flap: anatomy and clinical applications. *Ann Plast Surg*. 1984;12:489-500.

Chapter 25

The Radial Forearm Free Flap

Jonathan W. Jones, MD

The radial forearm free flap is ideally suited for head and neck reconstruction. The long radial artery pedicle allows closure of posterior pharyngeal defects with anastamoses in the neck. The flap may be folded over to reconstruct full thickness defects of the cheek, nose, and lips.

Case Example

Case #1

A 34-year-old male with a multiply recurrent squamous cell carcinoma of the cheek required wide excision. A radial forearm flap containing the palmaris longus tendon provided oral lining and outer cover.

Recurrent squamous tumor of left lower lip.

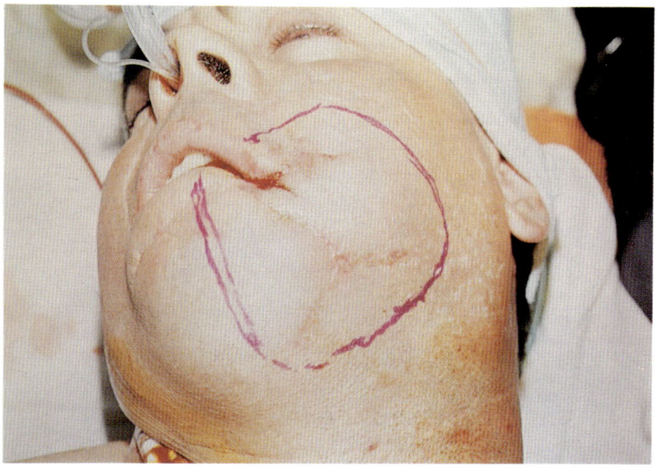

Fig. 25-1

Defect following tumor excision showing saggital resection of out portion of mandible.

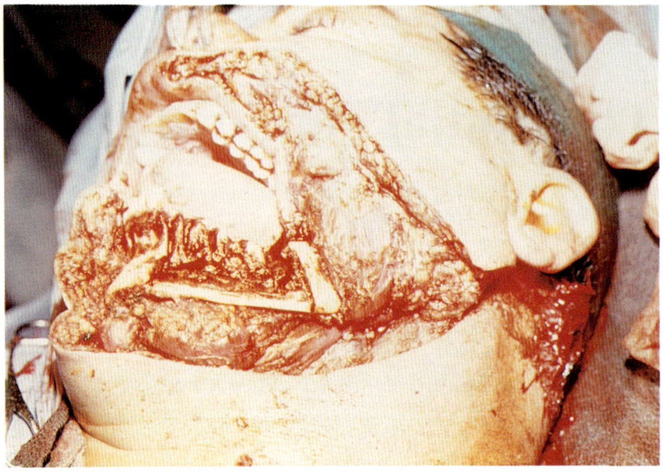

Fig. 25-2

Radial forearm flap outlined.

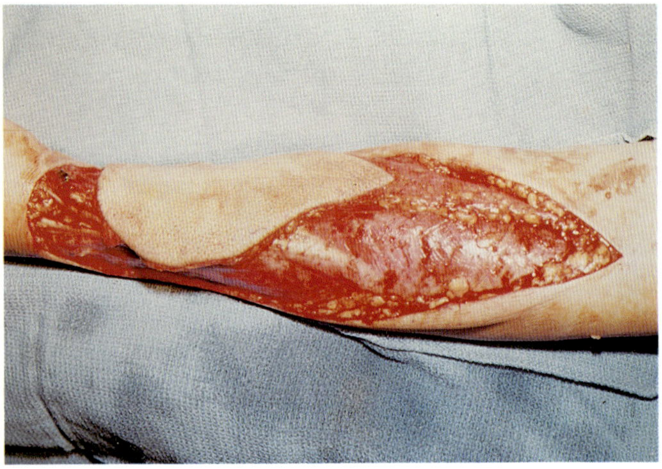

Fig. 25-3

Elevated flap perfused by radial artery, venae comitantes, and subcutaneous veins.

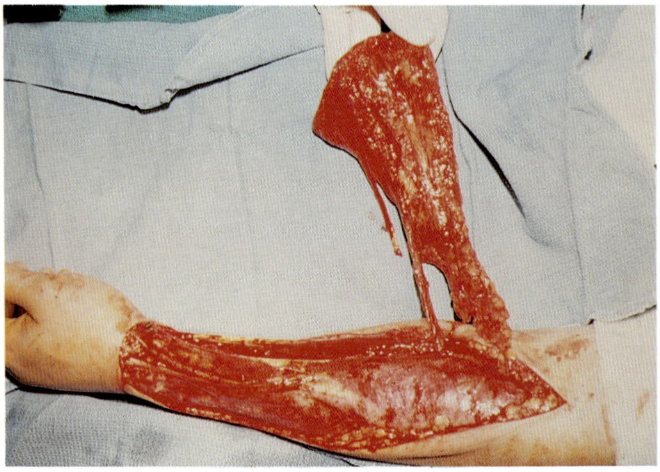

Fig. 25-4

Flap folded over palmaris longus tendon for simultaneous intraoral closure.

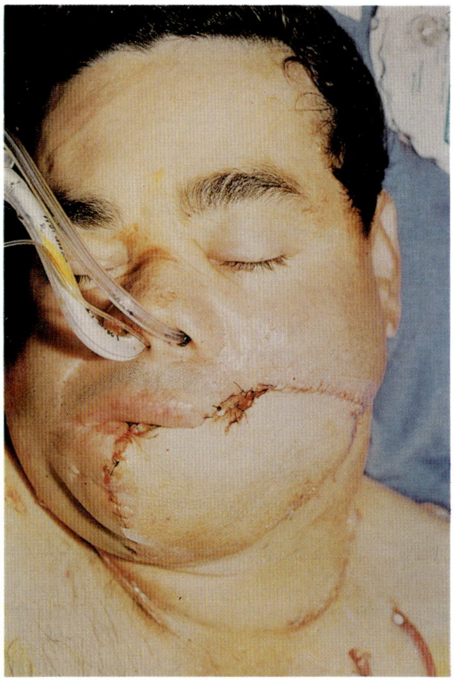

Fig. 25-5

Early postoperative result. Lower lip and commissure revisions planned.

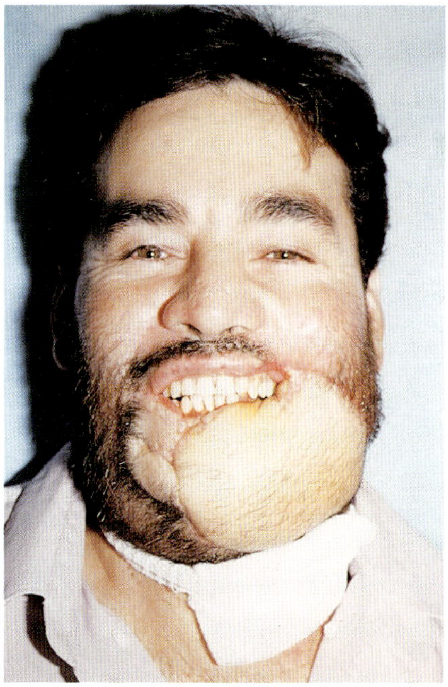

Fig. 25-6 A

Flap has an improved contour one year later following resolution of edema and minor revisions.

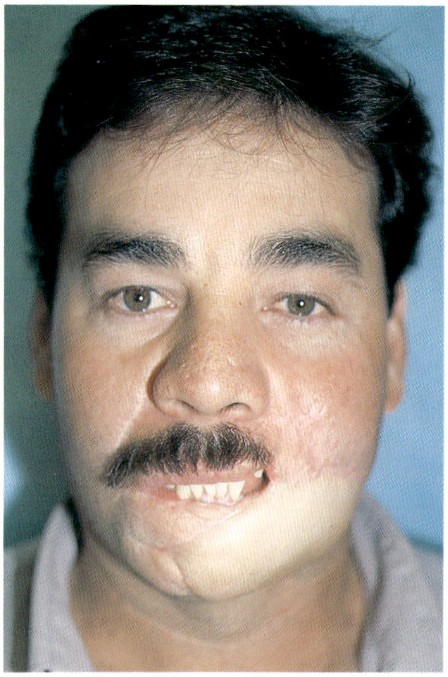

Fig. 25-6 B

Case #2

A 63-year-old woman with squamous carcinoma of the foot required resurfacing following tumor excision. A radial forearm flap provided durable closure.

Plantar ulcerations with foci of squamous carcinoma.

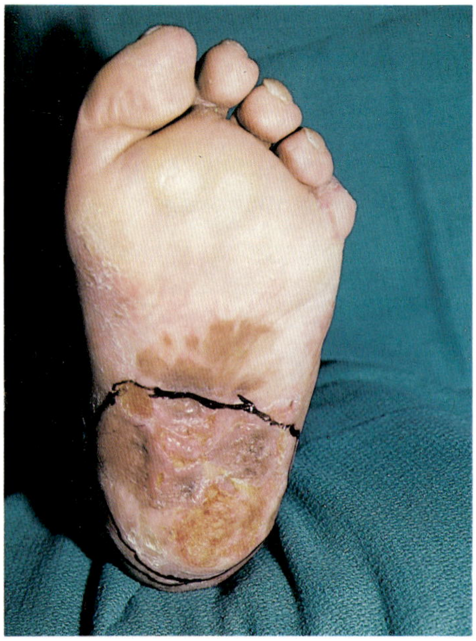

Fig. 25-7

Forearm donor site.

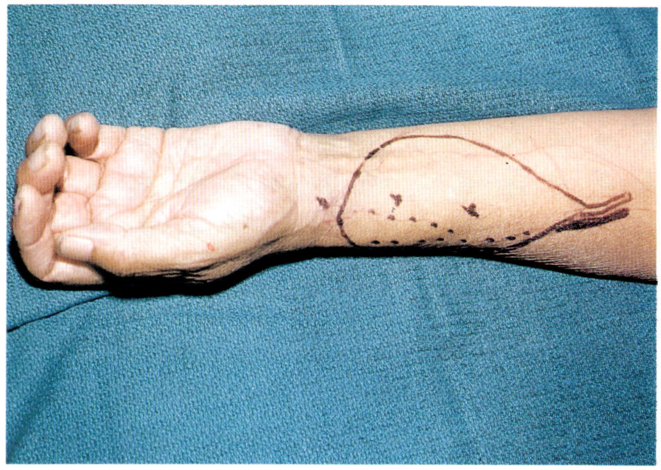

Fig. 25-8

Flap, five years later.

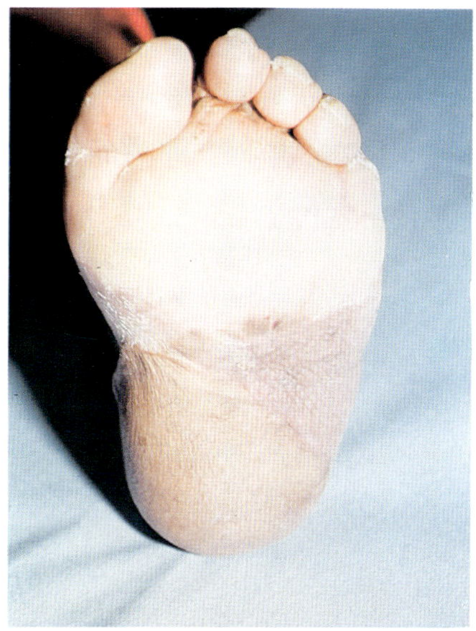

Fig. 25-9

Donor site scar.

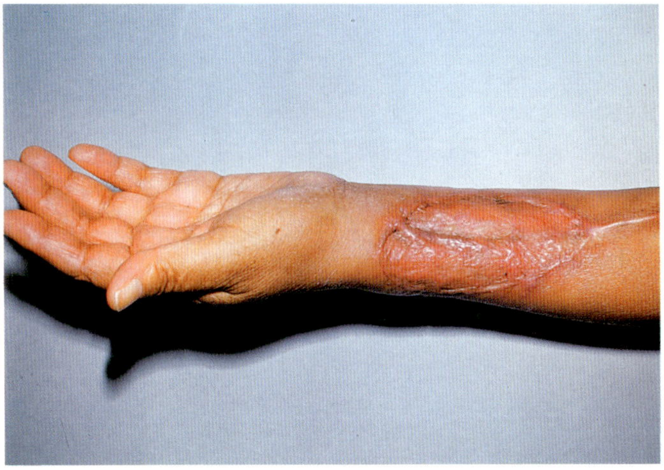

Fig. 25-10

Custom sandals allow ambulation without cane.

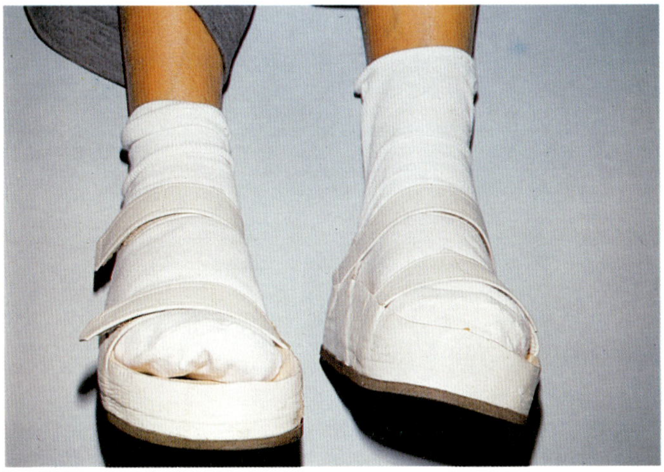

Fig. 25-11

Suggested Reading

Song R, Gao Y, Song Y, et al. The forearm flap. *Clin Plast Surg*. 1982;9:21-26.

Soutar DS, Scheilier LR, Tanner NS, McGregor IA. The radial forearm flap: a versatile method for intraoral reconstruction. *Br J Plast Surg*. 1983;36:1.

Chapter 26

Rectus Abdominus Muscle and Myocutaneous Flaps

Jonathan W. Jones, MD

Shortly following the introduction of the transverse rectus abdominus myocutaneous flap for breast reconstruction, extensive studies were undertaken to determine the blood supply of the rectus abdominus muscle. The entire rectus muscle may be transplanted on the inferior epigastric pedicle. Alternatively, a large transverse lower abdominal skin paddle may be taken with only enough muscle to allow preservation of cutaneous perforators.

Case Examples

Case #1

A 2-year-old child was run over by an automobile and sustained an extensive degloving injury of the ankle. Bone, tendon, and joint exposure resulted. The inferior epigastric artery and venae comitantes of the rectus myocutaneous flap were anastamosed to the dorsalis pedis vessels.

Foot avulsion defect in three-year-old child.

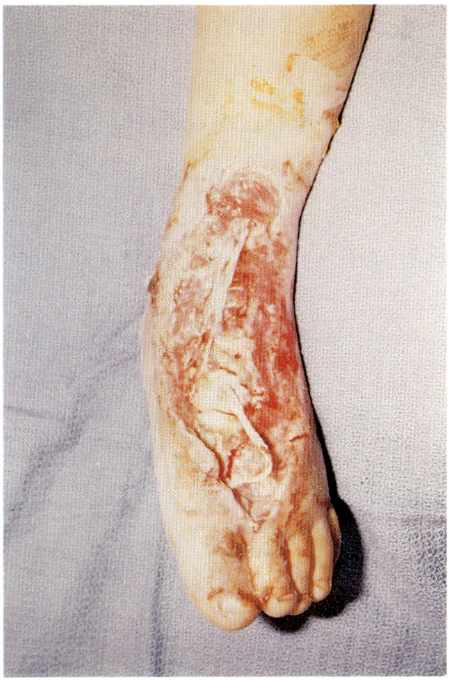

Fig. 26-1

Outline of skin paddle.

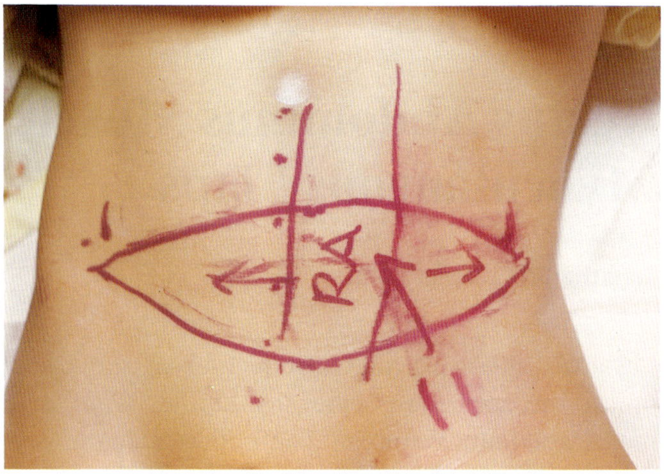

Fig. 26-2

Circumscription of flap.

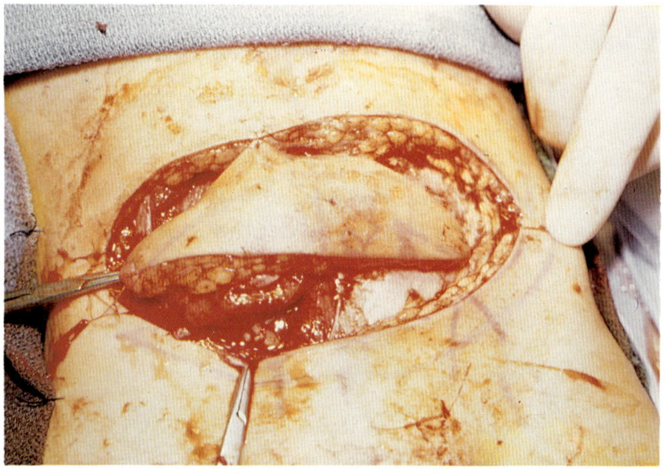

Fig. 26-3

Rectus abdominus myocutaneous flap elevated.

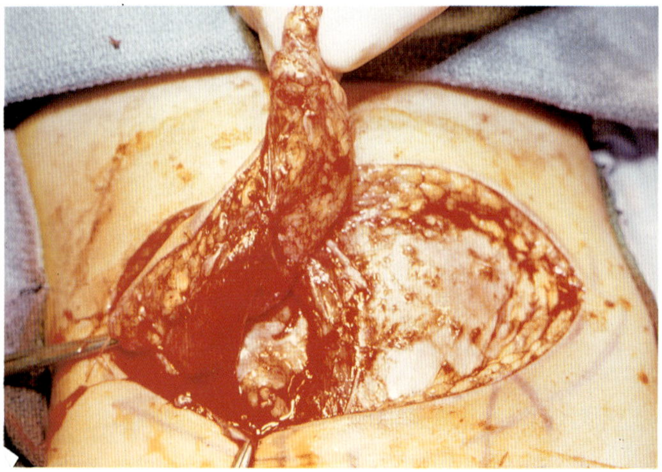

Fig. 26-4

Rectus flap transplanted to ankle.

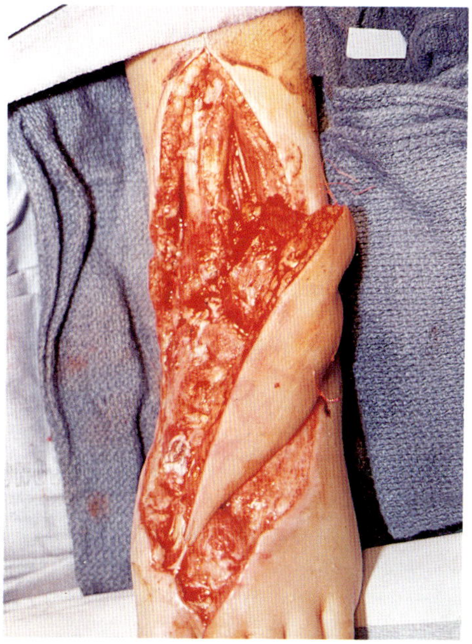

Fig. 26-5

Anterior tibial vessels exposed.

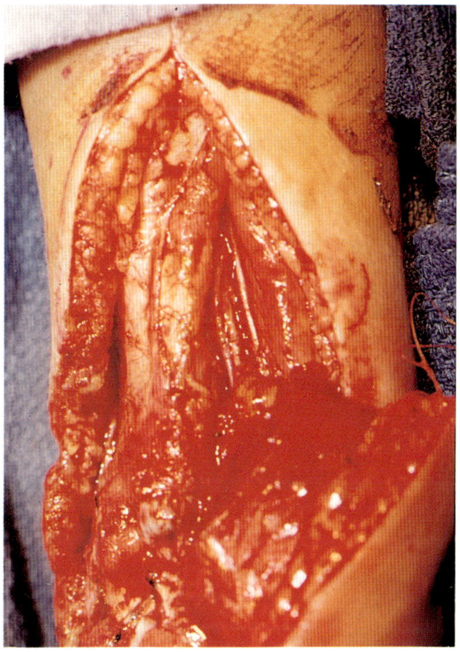

Fig. 26-6

Anastamosis of inferior epigastric vessels to anterior tibial vessels.

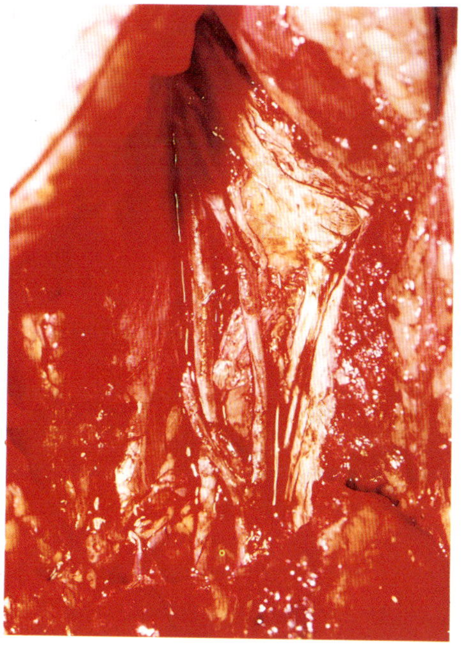

Fig. 26-7

Early postoperative appearance showing skin graft at margin.

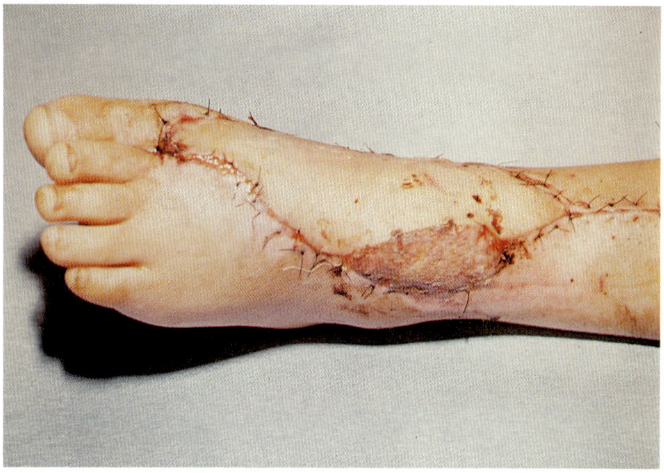

Fig. 26-8

Late postoperative appearance.

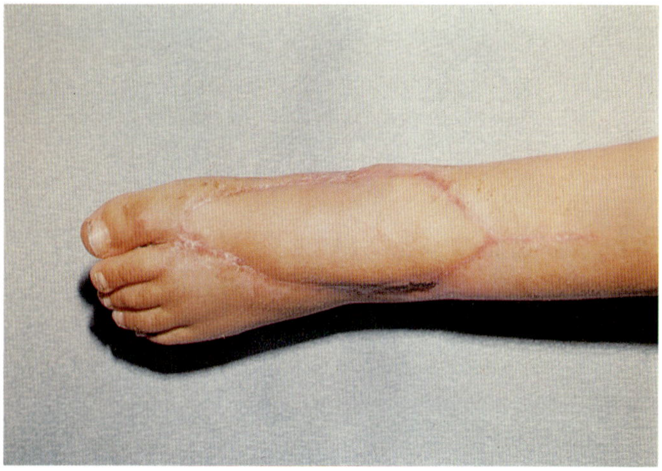

Fig. 26-9

Case #2

A 22-year-old man sustained extensive injuries in a motorcycle accident. The rectus abdominus muscle was transplanted to the lower leg and antbiotic impregnated methylmethacrylate beads were placed in the bone defect. These beads were subsequently removed and replaced with a free fibula graft.

Tibia defect following motorcycle accident.

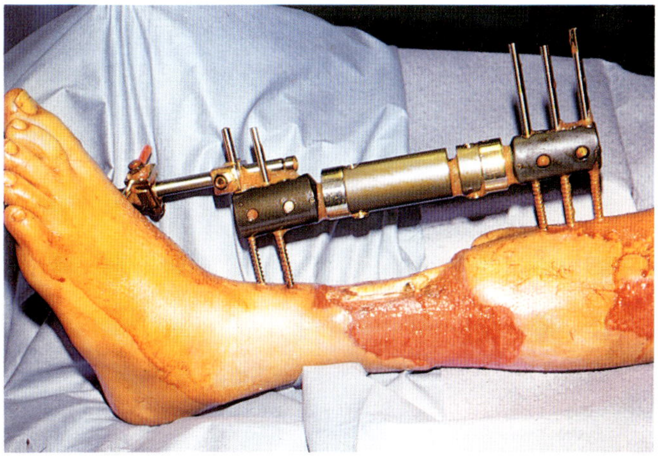

Fig. 26-10

Anterior view of leg wound.

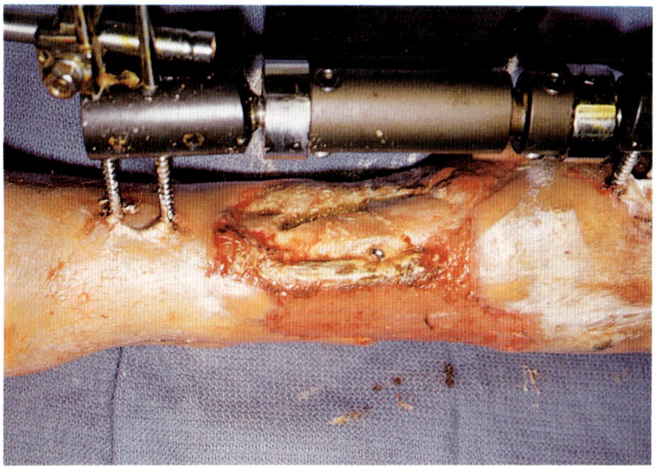

Fig. 26-11

Rectus flap transplanted to cover bone.

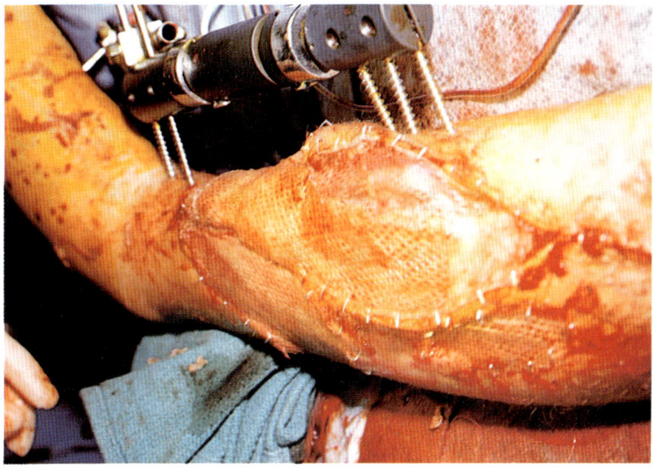

Fig. 26-12

Early appearance of flap.

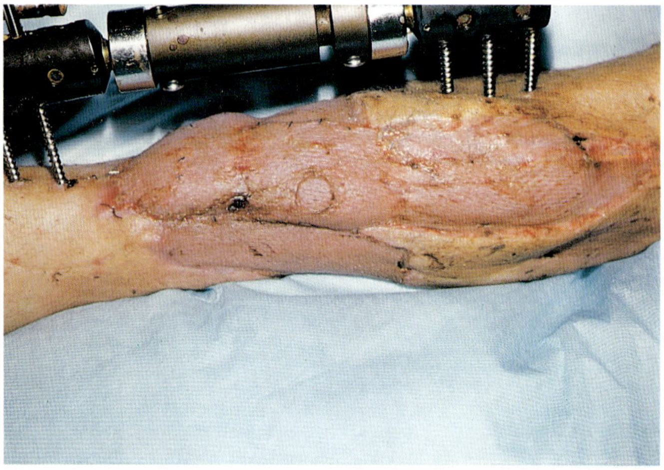

Fig. 26-13

Medial view of rectus flap providing stable coverage of tibia fracture.

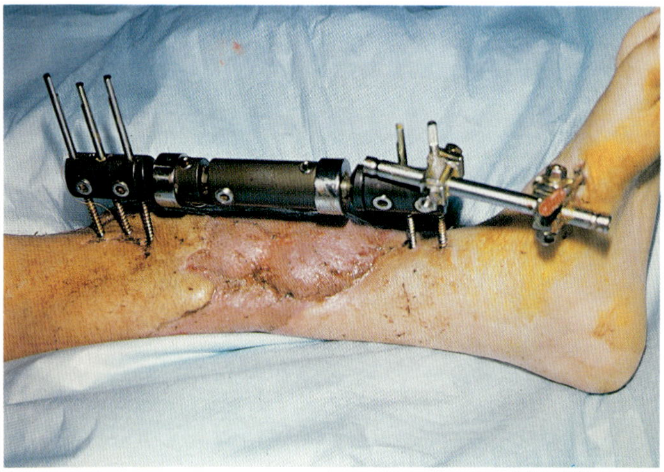

Fig. 26-14

Suggested Reading

Bunkis J, Walton RW, Mathes SJ. The rectus abdominus free flap for lower extremity reconstruction. *Ann Plast Surg*. 1983;11,5:373-380.

Grotting JC, Urist M, Maddox WA, Vasconez LO. Conventional tran flap versus free microsurgical tram flap for immediate breast reconstruction. *Plast Reconstr Surg*. 1989;83,5:828-841.

Koshima I, Soeda S. Inferior epigastric artery skin flaps without rectus abdominus muscle. *Br J Plast Surg*. 1989;42:645-648.

Chapter 27

The Latissimus Dorsi

Jonathan W. Jones, MD

The subscapular artery splits to form the circumflex scapular and thoracodorsal arteries; the latter supplies the proximal 80% of the latissimus dorsi muscle. Often, the thoracodorsal artery only has one significant accompanying vein but the 3 mm diameter of the artery and vein enable reliably patent anastamoses.

The latissimus dorsi muscle is ideal for closure of circumferential defects of the legs and massive cranial defects.

Case Examples

Case #1

A 39-year-old male sustained 12,000 volt electrical injuries. Bone and tendon exposure resulted following debridement of necrotic tissues. Stable coverage was provided with a latissimus dorsi muscle.

Electrical burn of ankle.

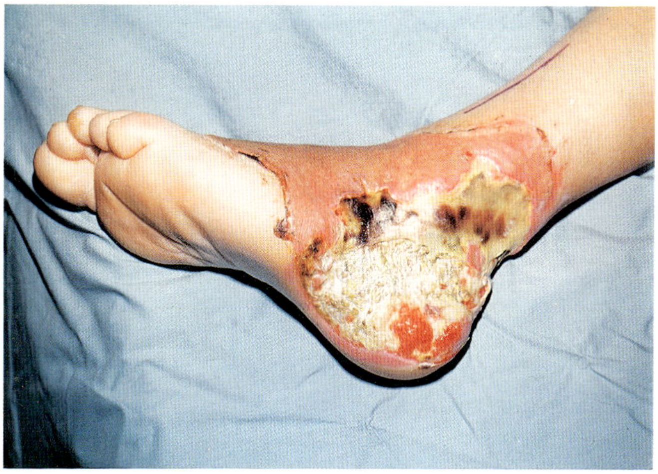

Fig. 27-1

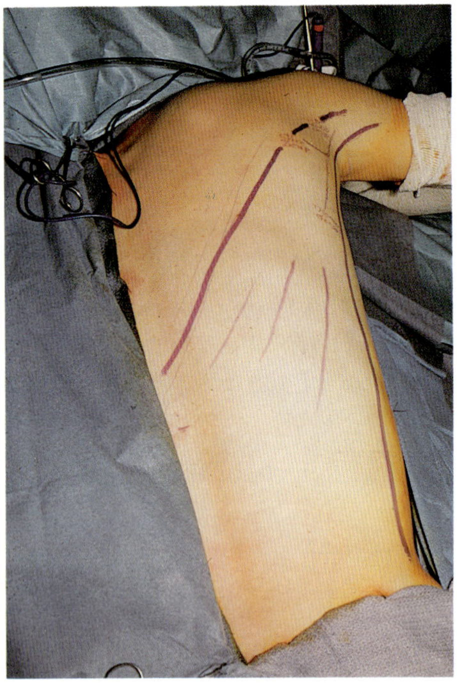

Fig. 27-2

Latissimus dorsi surface landmarks.

Elevation of latissimus dorsi muscle via oblique back incision.

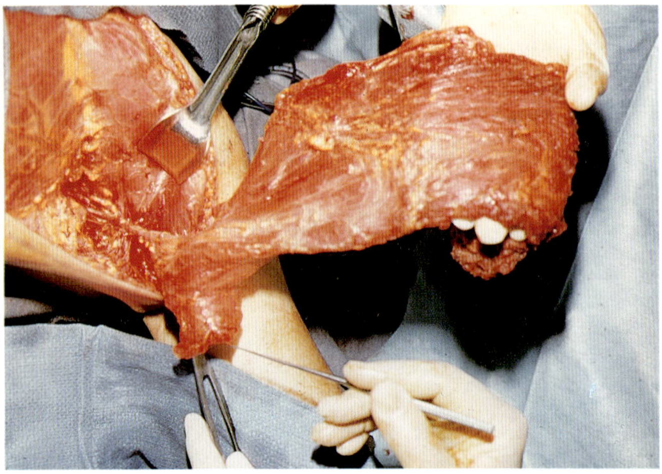

Fig. 27-3

Muscle transplanted to medial ankle defect.

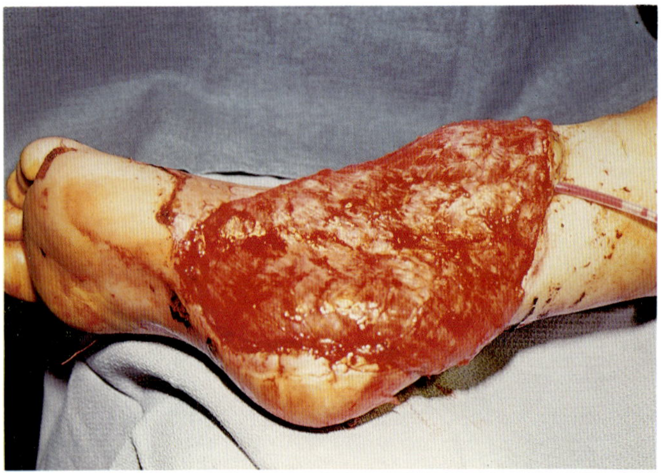

Fig. 27-4

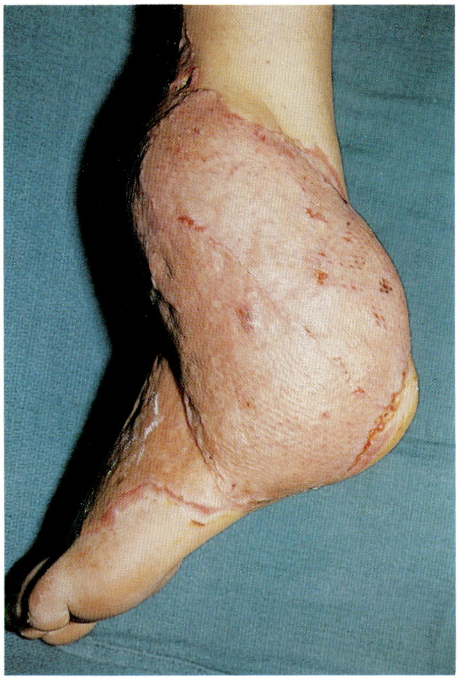

Fig. 27-5

Early postoperative appearance of flap.

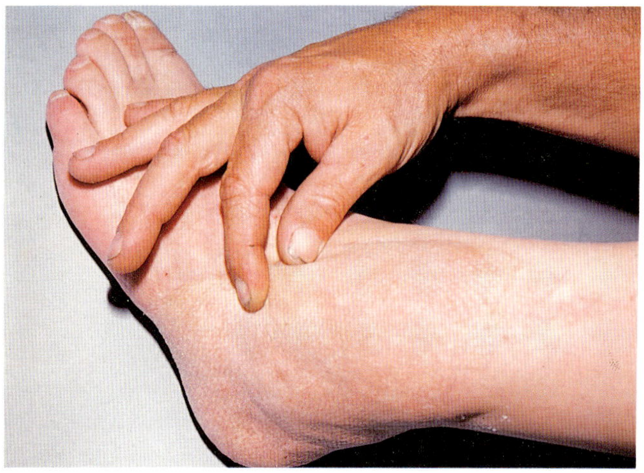

Fig. 27-6

Previously bulky flap may be pinched between fingertips.

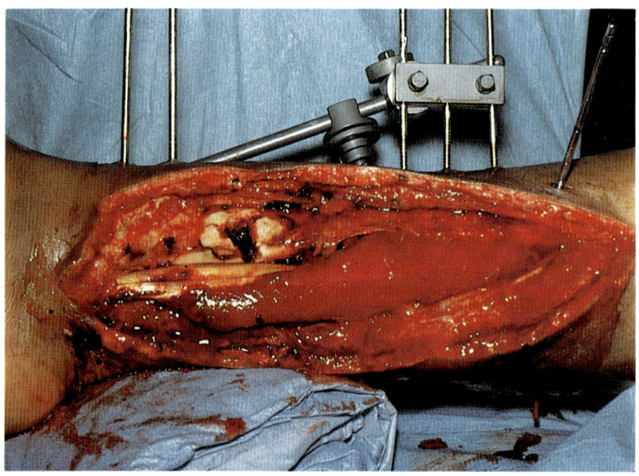

Fig. 27-7

Typical motorcycle injury to lower third of leg.

Elevation of latissimus dorsi muscle.

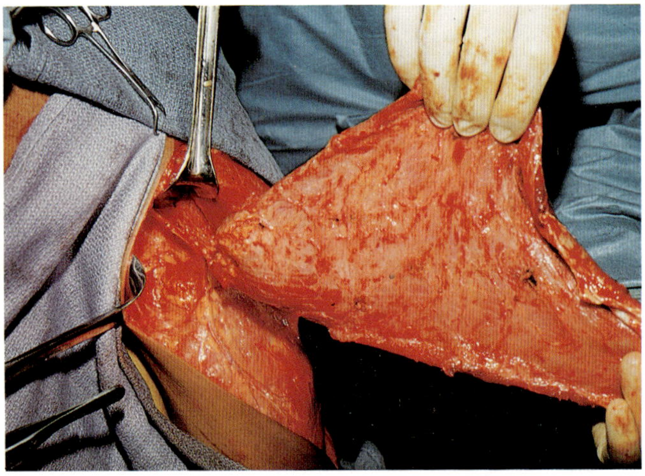

Fig. 27-8

Thoracodorsal vessels to latissimus dorsi muscle.

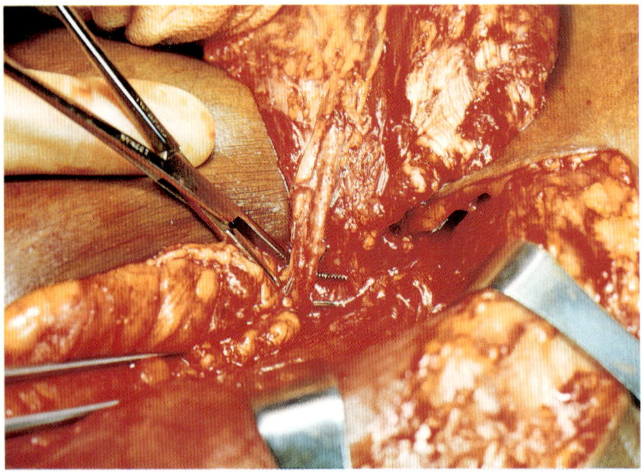

Fig. 27-9

Lower leg injuries sealed with latissimus dorsi flap.

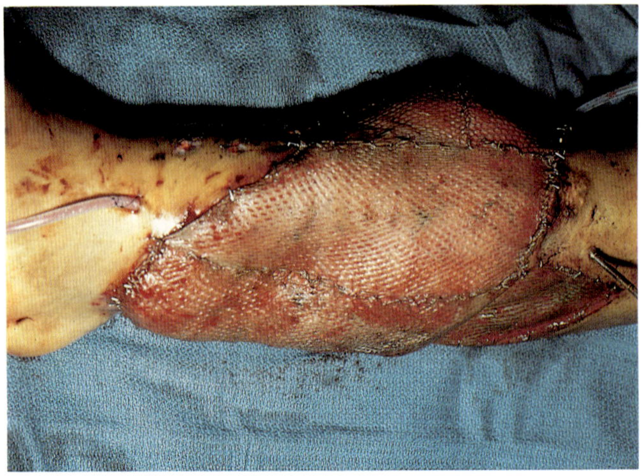

Fig. 27-10

Leg defect closed with transplanted latissimus flap and skin graft.

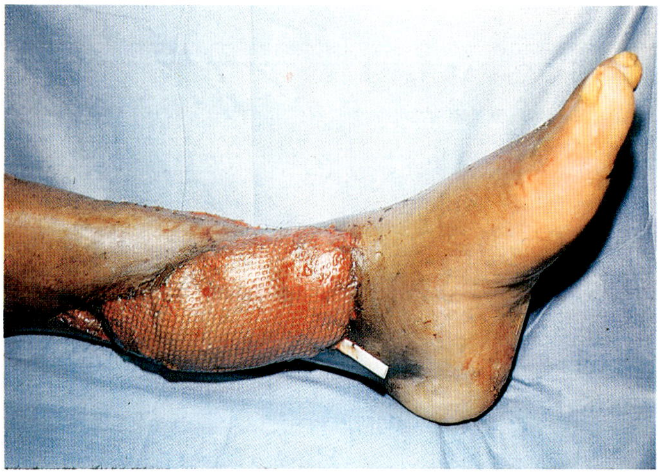

Fig. 27-11

Case #2

An 81-year-old male underwent resection of a massive squamous cell tumor. Both the latissimus dorsi muscle and a parascapular fasciacutaneous flap were transplanted to cover the defect. The common subscapular vessels were anastamosed to the superficial temporal vessels.

Cranial defect following tumor resection. Fascia patch replaces dura defect.

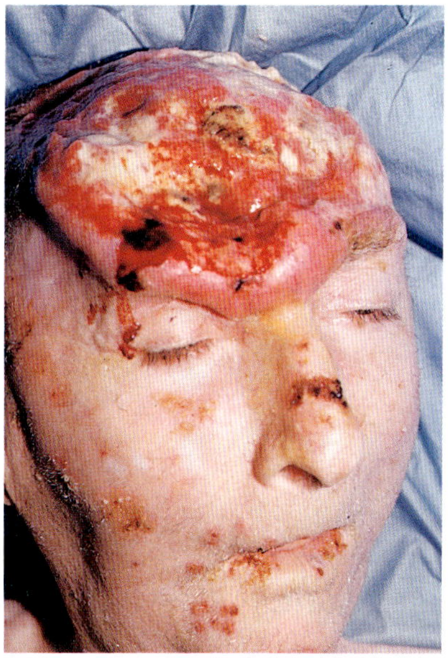

Fig. 27-12

Anastamosis of thoracodorsal to superficial temporal vessels.

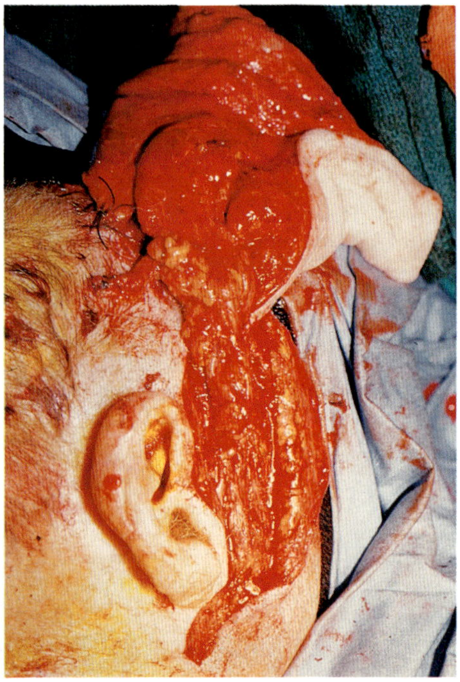

Fig. 27-13

Latissimus and parascapular flaps transplanted to cranium.

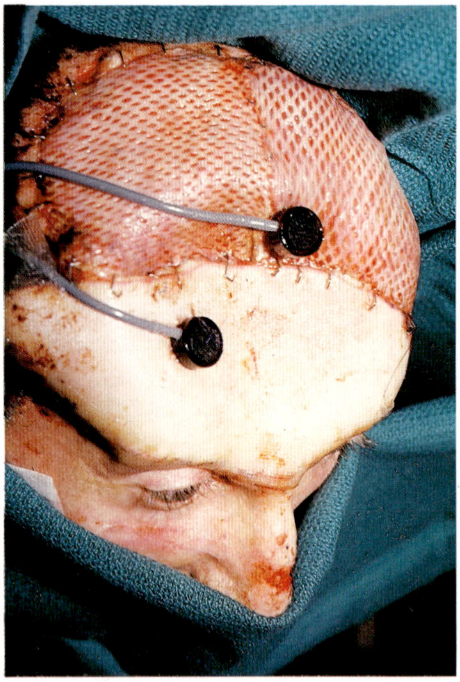

Fig. 27-14

Suggested Reading

Batchelor AGG, Sully L. A multiple territory free tissue transfer for reconstruction of a large scalp defect. *Br J Plast Surg*. 1984;37:76.

Mau JW, Jr, Lukash FN, Gallieo GG, III. Latissimus dorsi free muscle flap in lower extremity reconstruction. *Plast Reconstr Surg*. 1981;65:603-607.

Roswell AR, Davies DM, Eisenberg N, Taylor GI. The anatomy of the subscapular thoracodorsal arterial system: study of 100 cadaver dissections. *Br J Plast Surg*. 1984;37:574.

Chapter 28

Adjunctive Measures

Milbhor D'Silva, MD
Sun Lee, MD

Anatomy

Diagrams and photographs only yield two-dimensional representations of three-dimensional structures. Therefore, dissections should be performed in the anatomy laboratory before any new flap is attempted. Microsurgical skills must similarly be mastered in a laboratory setting.

Organization

The responsible surgeon should provide the operating room personnel with a list of instruments required, a description of table orientation and patient positioning needs, and staffing information such as when two nursing teams will be required for concurrent donor and recipient site surgery.

Anesthesia

The anesthesiologist is a key member of the reconstructive team. Administration of regional and/or general anesthetics, good hydration, maintenance of body temperature, and provision of sympathetic blocks will help ensure the success of the procedure. Continuous scaline, axillary, and epidural sympathetic blocks may be maintained two to three days postoperatively.

When anastamoses are performed on the trunk, the anesthesiologist may also need to coordinate ventillation of the patient with the surgeon.

Exposure of Recipient Vessels

Exposure of recipient vessels in a traumatized limb can often be the most time-consuming and challenging part of the flap transfer procedure. When possible, enough side branches should be ligated so as to allow elevation of the vessels out of the wound on small neurosurgical pledgets. Most surgeons have experienced the frustration of trying to perform an anastamosis in the depths of a wound that is filling up with blood; here the assistant must deftly control suction, irrigation and intermittent application of opthalmologic sponge "spears" to soak up blood.

Order of Vessel Repair

If anastamoses are expiditiously performed, it makes no difference which vessels are repaired first. Usually, the deepest structure is repaired first. After an artery and vein have been repaired, the temporary occlusion clips are removed, and the flap is allowed to perfuse. Lastly, the second vein is repaired. I prefer not to repair just the artery and allow the vein to bleed for several minutes as is favored in some centers; the one exception might be in the replantation of severed limbs where one does not want a large volume of acidotic blood to re-enter circulation.

Anastamosis Technique

Technique for small vessel anastamosis are reviewed elsewhere in this text. The posterior wall technique was used for all tissue transfers listed in chapters 31-39. For vessels over 2 mm in diameter, 9-0 nylon on a taper needle was generally used; 10.0 nylon was used for anastamoses of small vessels.

End-to-side arterial anastamoses are performed whenever possible. The ideal areteriortomy instrument has yet to be developed. For very large vein grafts which are to be anastamosed to the popliteal vein, an aortic punch yields an excellent hole.[1] For very small vessels only a small slit is required. Many texts describe how an oblique arteriotomy may be made by lifting a portion of the vessel and cutting out an ellipse with curved scissors. This is often difficult to perform in fibrotic vessels as fragmentation of the media may result. Instead, a longitudinal arteriotomy is first made with a blade and small half-ellipses of the full thickness of the vessel wall are next excised. The single oblique cut method reported by Hidalgo[2] is a simpler method yet.

A variation of the posterior wall technique with the first suture placed at the mid-point of one side wall may be used for the end-to-side repair. A running suture placed with standard vascular surgery technique is often preferable to interrupt sutures when the media is friable.

Vascular Spasm

If brisque pulsatile bleeding is not noted at the recipient site arteriotomy or cut-end of the vessel, the transplant will not succeed. Often the artery must be trimmed back more and more proximally until good bleeding is noted. Vein grafts may then be required. Gentle hydrostatic dilation of artery with nitroglycerine (10 micrograms/cc) will often correct arterial spasm. Venous spasm is very rarely noted; if good vein dilation is not apparent following anastamosis, then vein spasm may be suspected. Here, too, gentle hydrostatic dilation of the vein with nitroglycerine solution will often correct this problem. Our laboratory studies show 100% anastamosis patency with and without rat femoral artery and vein dilation, contradicting other suggestions that vessel dilation might adversely affect anastamosis patency.

Vein Grafts

Purple dye is painted on the proximal end of the in-situ vein graft. The "purple is proximal" convention avoids confusion between members of the surgical team and consequent incorrect vein orientation.

The proximal vein graft anastamosis is performed first and a temporary occlusion clamp is then placed at the end of the vein graft. Arterial pulsations will dilate, stretch and unkink the graft; then the distal anastamosis is performed.

A saphenous vein graft with a large "y" tributary may be used to both perfuse the flap and improve blood flow to the extremity.

Artery Versus Vein Confusion

Occasionally an artery will be accidentally anastamosed to a vein. This problem can be avoided by marking the vessels in some way before division of the donor pedicle. With testicular translocations, the spermatic artery must be marked with a small suture before the pedicle is divided since it is nearly impossible to differentiate between the cut ends of the 0.4 mm diameter artery and veins.

Dragged-In Adventitia

Heparinized saline from a 3 cc syringe with a 27 gauge needle may be used to balloon out the adventitia and enable easier distal adventitia trimming. If adventitia is dragged into the lumen with a suture, then the ends of the vessel should be trimmed and the anastamosis redone.

Anticoagulation

Harri's exellent free flap success rate without anticoagulation[3] argues against the need for anticoagulants. Other replantation studies show improved success rates with anticoagulation. When intraoperative thromboses occur despite well-performed anastamosis, then heparin may be started at the time of anastamosis revision. We often give 2,000 to 5,000 units of heparin intravenously before pedicle division and give Dextran 40 at 10 to 20 cc/hr for the subsequent 48 hours.

Wound Closure

Care must be taken to avoid kinking or compressing the pedicle at the time of wound closure. Small skin grafts may be required at the flap margins. Dressings are loosely applied and the flap recipient site is elevated.

Monitoring

Flaps are visually inspected for color and briskness of capillary refill. Toe to hand transplants and digital replants are also monitored with pulse oximetry. Surface infrared reflective photoplethysmograph probes are used for most free flaps. Doppler monitoring is employed to monitor buried vascularized bone grafts and deepithelialized flaps.

Discharge

Patients who have undergone digital replantation, and those who have undergone transfer of flaps to the upper extremities or head and neck, are discharged on the fifth postoperative day. Those who have undergone flap transfers to the lower extremities maintain elevation of these regions for nine days and thereafter gradually resume crutch walking.

References

1. Harris GD, Finseth F, Buncke HJ. Posterior wall first microvascular anastamotic technique. *Br J Plast Surg*. 1981;34:47-49.
2. Shaw NW, Hidalgo DA. *Microsurgery in Trauma*. Mt. Kisko, NY: Futura Publishing Co.; 1987;47.
3. Harii K. *Microvascular Tissue Transfer: Fundamental Techniques and Clinical Applications*. Tokyo: Igaku-Shoin; 1983.

Section IV

Gynecologic Microsurgery

Chapter 29

Introduction and Patient Preparation

Raphael B. Durfee, MD

INTRODUCTION

Surgery with the use of magnification is a recent addition to Gynecologic surgery; it was first introduced formally in 1975 at a special conference in the United States. Preliminary work had been done for several years at clinics in Sweden, France, England and British Columbia in Canada. These techniques have had a deep influence on the practice of Gynecologic microsurgery in general. Among these are the use of lactated Ringer's solution to keep the abdominal wound, cavity, and organs wet at all times; fine point bipolar cautery for better hemostasis; highly defined accurate apposition of tissues using sutures of small caliber made of synthetic, nonreactive materials; and a change in the material used for packing the bowel out of the pelvic field of operation.

There are many changes in the approach to the patient, including much improved informed consent, pre-operative management, and operating room practices. There must be a detailed consultation with the patient and her mate, especially with regard to their past histories. If the operation contemplated is tubal ligation reversal, the surgeon must have all available records and knowledge of what was done and the postoperative course. Complete knowledge of the different types of sterilization procedures available and in use for women must be an essential part of the surgeon's education.

Modern diagnostic methods are explained at the consultation, along with a description of surgical methods employed. Risks are to be detailed, together with chances for success. Indications for a given operation are presented. Preoperative methods are reviewed and intraoperative care is described, including the use of photography and the application of the laser as indicated. What may be expected postoperatively is outlined, and all questions are to be answered clearly in simple language and in detail. Informed consent forms are read, understood and signed, including permission for photography and the use of video monitors. There must be no lack of knowledge on the part of the patient, nor must there be any excessive anticipation of perfect success. These are expensive elective operations and should not be undertaken lightly.

A complete medical history should be obtained which includes all operative reports, delivery records, x-rays, ultra sound reports, special study findings, and any pathology reports. Preoperative laboratory studies are done and a preoperative consultation with an anesthesiologist is scheduled. If fertility is the objective of the surgery, the male partner must be proven to be fertile and capable of normal intercourse; the woman must have demonstrable, unequivocal evidence of regular ovulation; and there must be no other impediments to conception except the immediate condition under consideration.

A complete physical examination which includes a detailed complete pelvic evaluation should be conducted. Any abnormal findings in the pelvis must be investigated. At the conclusion of the workup, if there are any changes in the contemplated surgery, they should be explained, together with the reasons for doing so. For example, it may be necessary to use a laparoscopic examination in the surgery just prior to the laparotomy to verify or rule out certain suspected abnormalities or to determine just exactly what previous surgery has been done. Both partners need to know that there may be changes in the proposed surgery based upon pathology seen at laparoscopy, including cancellation of the laparotomy. In such cases, the partner should be notified at once. Cancellation of the procedure can result from laparoscopy findings such as: unsolvable problems of post infection adhesions related to P.I.D., endometriosis, or postoperative adhesions due to other pelvic surgery. A suggestion should be made at this time to include operative placement of the ovaries to a maximum point for later retrieval of an ovum for I.V.F. (In Vitro Fertilization). Any other conditions found in the pelvis should be managed according to the best surgical practice, including what may be necessary to preserve the health and future of the woman even with sacrifice of fertility.

The surgeon involved in microsurgery should be calm, rested, and with very little scheduled for the rest of the day. There should be no demands upon him/her by obstetric problems or any other emergency requests. The entire team must be clearly integrated for the procedure and all instruments and equipment readied for the operation. The surgeon should check all instruments and all sutures, etc., including the function of the microscope to be sure that all of the ancillary aspects of the operation are in order. The surgeon and his assistants should be seated and comfortable throughout the surgery.

The patient is admitted early on the morning of the surgery N.P.O. midnight, with the only other request being that she bathe the evening before with a mild antiseptic soap and use no skin oils or creams. No preoperative enema is given, a vaginal wash is optional but in our opinion unnecessary. No preoperative hair removal is advised.

Anesthesia is entirely in the control of the specialist. We only request an IV administration of 20 mg of Decadron and an antibiotic of choice prior to the skin incision. The skin is prepared with iodinized solutions and soaps unless contraindicated and pubic hair has been previously immediately removed by careful dry shaving; special care is taken to be sure that the skin is not cut nor the hair follicles traumatized. Draping is according to usual surgical practice. An inlying Foley catheter is placed in the bladder. There are those who prefer to place an acorn catheter or H.U.I. intrauterine elevator at this point, and others who prefer to pack the vagina so as to elevate the uterus in the pelvis. We do not believe in this manipulation because of the possibility of introducing pathogenic bacteria into the uterus and operative areas from the cervix or vagina.

The abdomen is opened in the usual manner: scalpel incision in the skin, usually transverse. The fat layer and the abdominal fascia are opened with bipolar cutting and coagulation cautery; no ligatures are ordinarily used. The peritoneum is opened transversely with a scalpel and extended with fine blunt-tipped scissors. A specially adapted O'Connor-O'Sullivan retractor is placed in the wound. We do not use any drapes for the wound edges; if these edges are kept moist throughout the operation, the tissues are in much better condition than if they are covered with any materials.

The operations are carried out and a photograph is taken of the preoperative appearance and the postoperative immediate result. When necessary, 70% Dextran solution is placed in the peritoneal cavity, but this is not routine; a liter or more of lactated Ringer's solution may be used at this point if desired but is not mandatory. No other intra-peritoneal medications are used. The plastic packs are removed and the peritoneum is closed, usually with #3-0 synthetic suture such as Dexon or Vicryl. The abdominal incision is closed in the usual manner with a continuous suture of the same material in the fascia and no sutures in the fat layer unless it is unusually thick, in which case interrupted sutures of similar fine material are used. We prefer to close the skin with a continuous subcuticular suture of #3-0 synthetic as above. Usually we cover the incisional area with a fine application of a collodian material and do not use an abdominal bandage of any other kind. This closure reduces incisional pain and seals the wound against outside contamination and is much more effective than any other cover.

Postoperative, the patient is kept as comfortable as possible. Much of this is accomplished by the expert anesthesiologist who uses several medications and devices to accomplish the desired effect. We suggest continuation of the I.V. Decadron 20 mg every six hours I.V. for four to six doses, after which the dose is reduced by oral administration over the next four days from 20 mg to 10 mg the third day, 5 mg the fourth day, 2 mg 2x daily for the fifth day. This prevents any undue withdrawal problems with the steroid. In the absence of any reason to continue, the antibiotic is stopped at two doses.

This regimen produces an optimum of postoperative recovery. Almost no narcotic pain relievers are needed, ambulation is very rapid, the patient has no nausea, is hungry, has excellent immediate bowel function, and needs no bladder catheter. The patient usually goes home in the afternoon of the second post-operative day, almost entirely pain free, with restoration of all her normal body functions.

In sixteen years we have had no wound or intra-abdominal infections, no wound breakdowns, no hematomas, no seromas, no skin separations. No sutures have to be removed and the wound heals with a hair-line scar.

Details of all aspects of these operations follow.

Indications for Microsurgery

The indications for microsurgery are increasing. The primary indications are:

Tubal Ligation Reversal

Extensive knowledge of different kinds of tubal ligation is very important. Most reversals are tubal anastomoses or neo-salpingostomy and fimbrial release. Some involve lysis of adhesions.

Tubal Pathology

Many of these are perisalpingeal or intrasalpingeal. The severity of either is a vital factor in predicting favorable results of surgery. Intra-tubal disease is more ominous from the standpoint of possible ectopic pregnancy later.

1. Pelvic inflammatory disease, which is common, is not usually reversible in any but the mild to very moderate cases with minimal damage to the mucosa, minor hydrosalpinx and minimal external adhesions.
2. Endometriosis, which also has become common, has been recently managed by combined micro and laser surgery.
3. Salpingitis isthmica nodosa appears to be increasing in numbers and severity. Patent tubes can be obtained if the uterine interstitial portion is normal. Otherwise, tubouterine implantation or I.V.F. must be considered.
4. Peritubular adhesions. There has been marked improvement in the management of this problem by the use of combined microsurgery and the laser.
5. Cornual polyps respond to treatment by application of surgical procedures through the hysteroscope. Work has been done with tubaloscopy which may prove to be very beneficial both therapeutically as well as diagnostically.
6. Previous surgery for ectopic pregnancy has responded to conservative laparoscopic management with preservation of tubal tissue which lends itself to microsurgical procedures. Early diagnostic methods have increased the salvation of otherwise destroyed tubal tissues because the pregnancy is early and rarely ruptures the tubal wall.
7. Rare and minor conditions such as accessory tubal tissues and multiple fimbria or tubal ostia; congenital abnormalities, and phimosis of the fimbria, partial absence of tubal tissue, tubal duplication, and total tubal absence. Some of these do not lend themselves to repair.
8. Other pelvic conditions such as generalized pelvic adhesions from several sources; ovarian diseases ranging from simple cysts to endometriomas, polycystic disease of several types, rare benign tumors, rare congenital anomaly; and uterine anomalies, myomata, adenomyosis, endometriotic uterine cul-de-sac adhesions.

Contraindications for Microsurgery

1. Active infection, including tuberculosis.
2. Extensive adhesions with a frozen pelvis and/or intestinal involvement.
3. Massive bilateral hydrosalpinx with total ovarian masses.
4. Normal pelvis or very minor disease.
5. Absent tubes or ovaries, bilateral.
6. Any absolute contraindication to pregnancy.
7. Severe antifertility factors, e.g. anovulation.
8. Insufficient tubal tissue, under 4 cm length.
9. Age over 40 years.

10. Severe endometrial cavity adhesions or disease.
11. Two or more previous surgical failures.
12. The presence of any emergency situation.
13. Ambivalent personality or severe psychoneurosis.

Microsurgery in Gynecology

The following is a list of most microsurgical procedures:

1. Tubal surgery, most commonly tubal ligation reversals.
   Lysis of extra and peritubular adhesions.
   Tubal anastomosis:
   Isthmus-cornua (interstitial).
   Isthmus-isthmus.
   Isthmus-ampulla.
   Isthmus-fimbria.
   Different anastomosis on each side.
2. Ovarian surgery.
   Lysis of extra and periovarian adhesions.
   Dissection, coagulation, laser of endometriosis externa.
   Excision of ovarian cysts (all kinds possible).
   Wedge resection.
   Ovarian reconstruction.
   Ovarian suspension.
   Ovarian transplantation.
3. Treatment of endometriotic lesions, not ovarian (pelvic).
4. Uterine surgery combined macro and micro.
   Myomectomy.
   Excision of uterine horn.
   Adhesion lysis.
   Uterine unification operations.
   Reperitonization.
5. Retroperitoneal dissection and repair as indicated.

Female Sterilization

It is difficult to reverse tubal ligation procedures in women without knowledge of what these operations are, how they are done, and what pathology may exist in the pelvis after such techniques.

Tubal ligation may be done by laparotomy, minilaparotomy, colpotomy, culdoscopy, hysteroscopy, laparoscopy, at cesarean section or any abdominal operation.

Direct operations are single or double ligation with or without incision or resection: Madlener, Pomeroy, Aldridge, Irving, Parkland, Watson, Kroner fimbriectomy, Oxford and other European methods, and Uchida, which may be the best.

Indirect operations are: electrofulguration by laparoscopy, Fallope ring and clip applications (unipolar and bipolar), ligation and fimbriectomy, hysteroscopic cauterization of the internal tubal os, fulguration of the interstitial area, transuterine silastic plugs, and P block.

Other operations are: cornual resection, total salpingectomy, bilateral ovariectomy, total hysterectomy—vaginal and abdominal, and cesarean hysterectomy.

Successful fimbrial release.

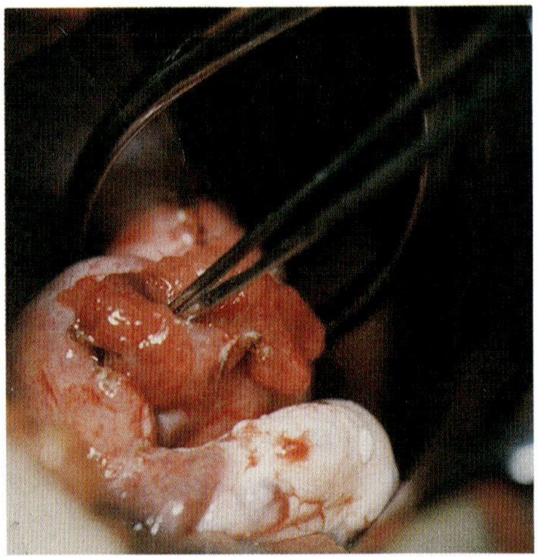

Fig. 29-1

Normal Fallopian tube. It is important to know where and how much blood supply exists.

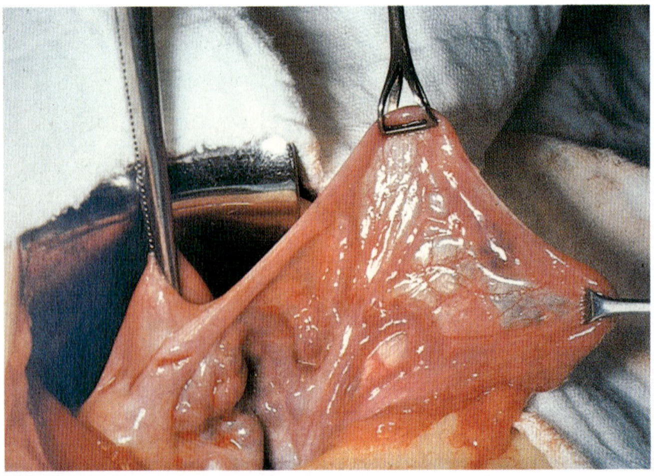

Fig. 29-2

Female sterilization tubal ligation procedures

Pomeroy, Step 1. It reduces the failure rate a great deal to use the largest size plain catgut available to produce the greatest initial reaction.

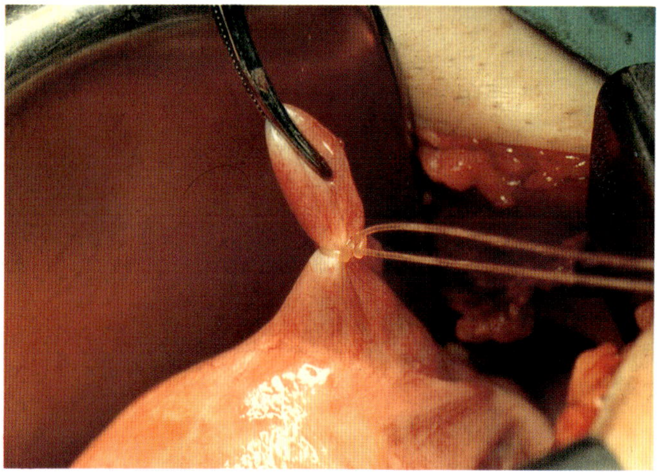

Fig. 29-3

Pomeroy, Step 2.

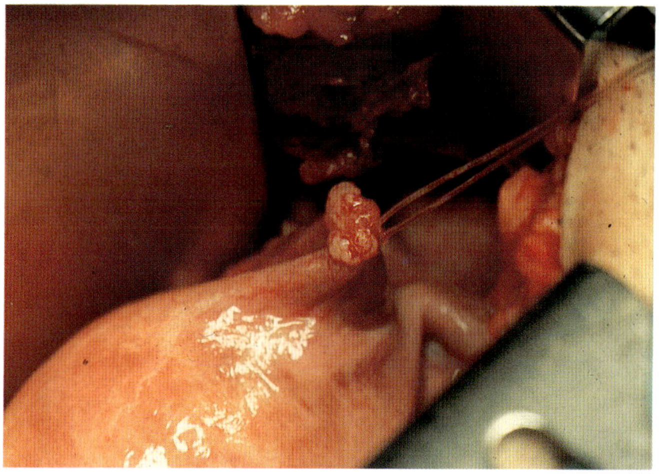

Fig. 29-4

Madlener, both steps. Crush and tie without cutting. Never use permanent ligature (Figs. 29-5 and 29-6 reprinted with permission from Knight[1]).

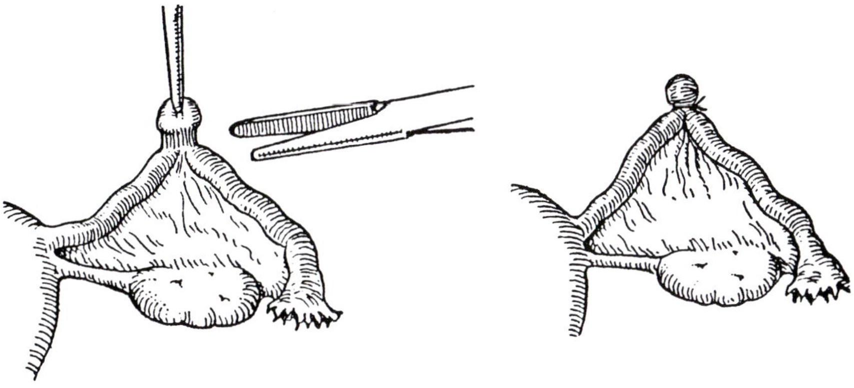

Fig. 29-5

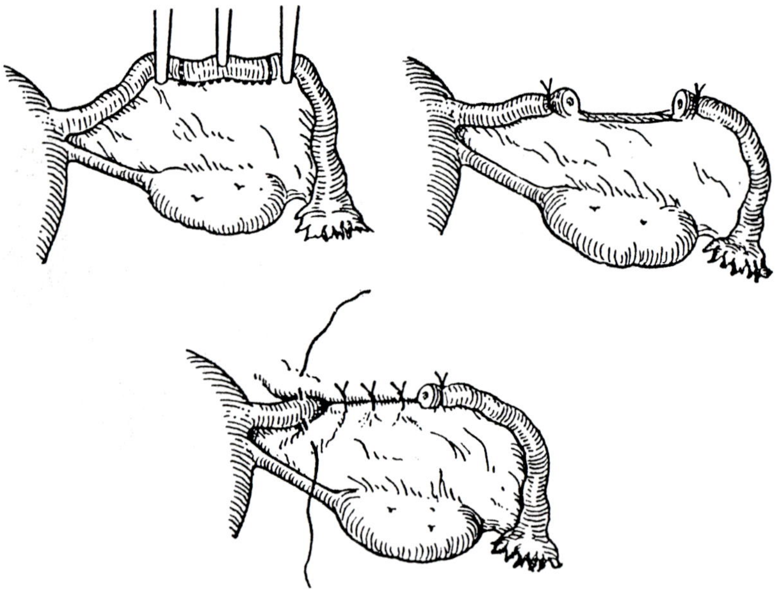

Fig. 29-6

Watson, segment resection and ligation.

Parkland, ligate each side.

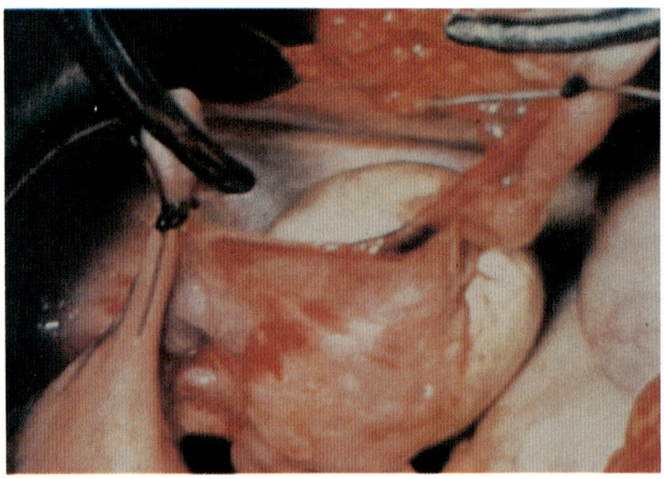

Fig. 29-7

Kroner fimbriectomy, never ligate with permanent ligature. Excision point at arrow (Figs. 29-8 through 29-16 reprinted with permission from Pernoll[2]).

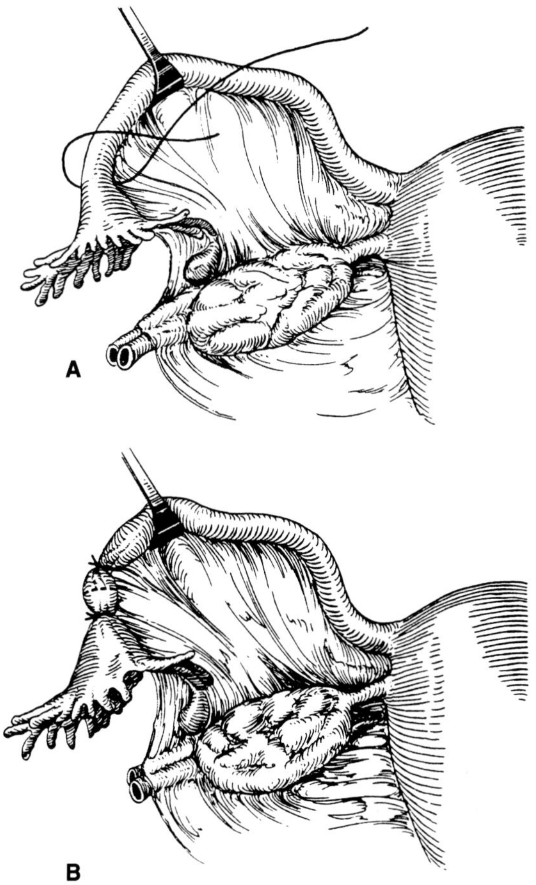

Fig. 29-8

Irving, Step 1.

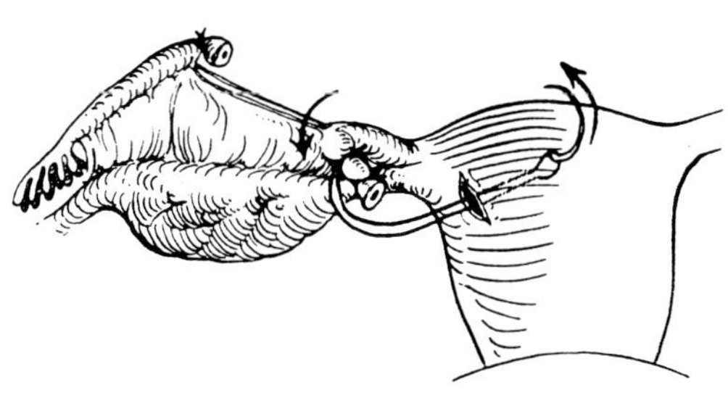

Fig. 29-9

Irving, Step 2.

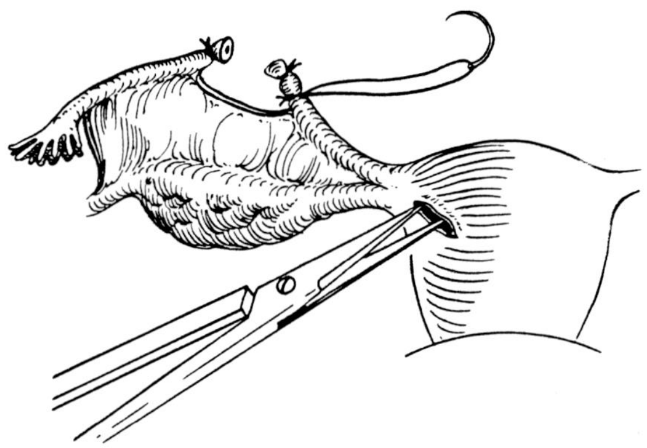

Fig. 29-10

Irving, Step 3.

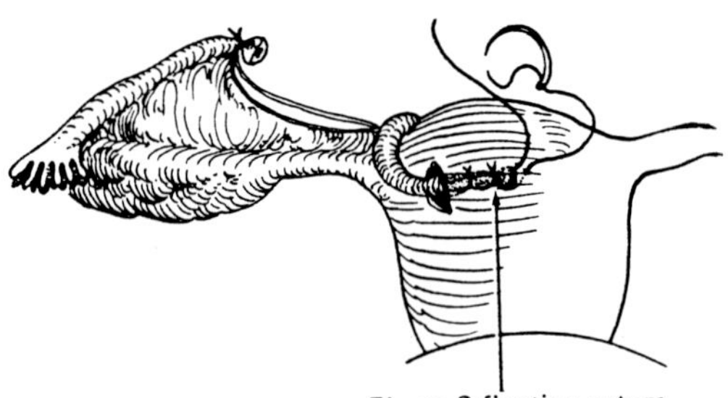

Fig. 29-11

Irving, Step 4. This procedure has one advantage, proximal tubal tissue is intact. There may be bleeding from the uterine wall implantation site. Tubal length may be lost.

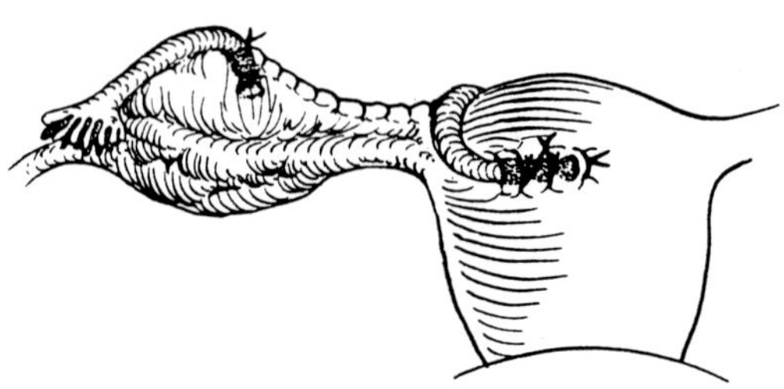

Fig. 29-12

Uchida, Step 1. Inject serosal with saline solution. Then incise superiorly to muscle. Injection reduces blood loss.

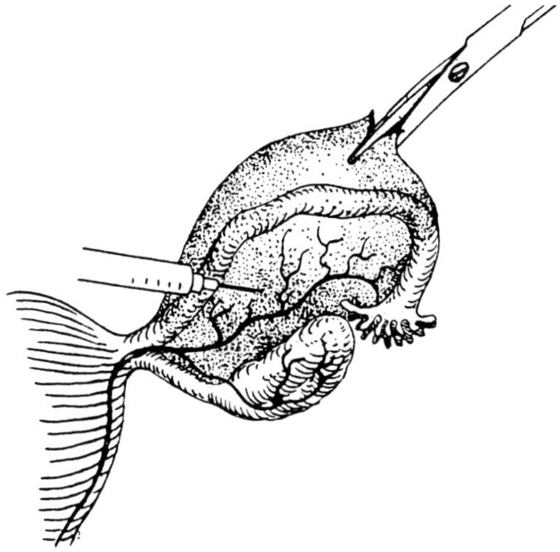

Fig. 29-13

Uchida, Step 2. Muscle and mucosa emerge from the incised area. No blood loss.

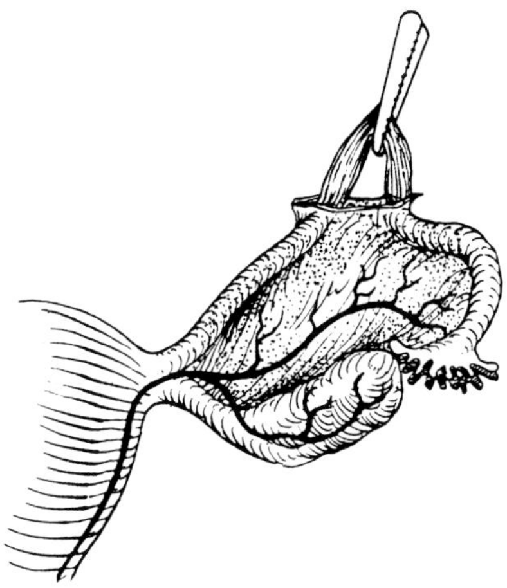

Fig. 29-14

Uchida, Step 3. Fimbriated end is untouched, while the proximal end at the uterus is stripped of serosa. This can usually be done without damage to blood vessels.

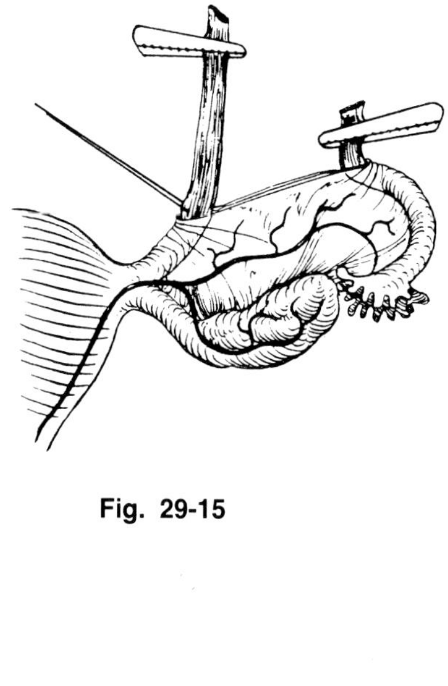

Fig. 29-15

Uchida, Step 4. About 5 cm of muscular tube is cut away; the end is buried automatically in serosa. Fimbriated end and serosal opening are closed and tied together. A modification is to excise all the distal tube. Uchida's procedure has proven to be probably the best procedure, with minimal failure rate and minimal complications. It must be done correctly. DO NOT suture the mucosal incision.

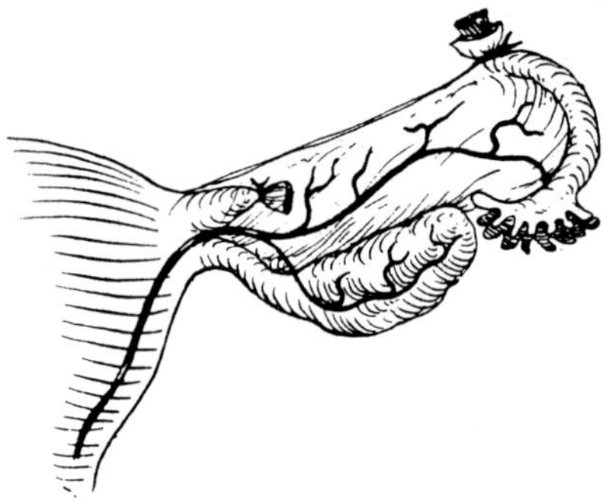

Fig. 29-16

Cornual resection. The cornua is excised to the endometrium, wound is closed with permanent suture, tube is ligated with catgut (Reprinted with permission from Knight[1]).

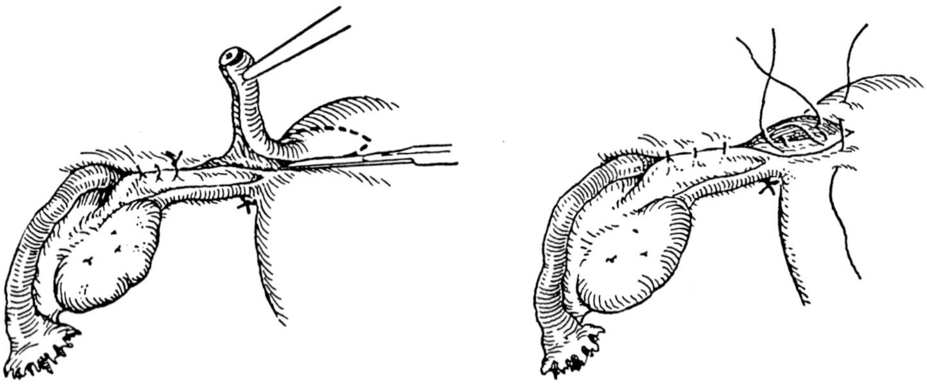

Fig. 29-17

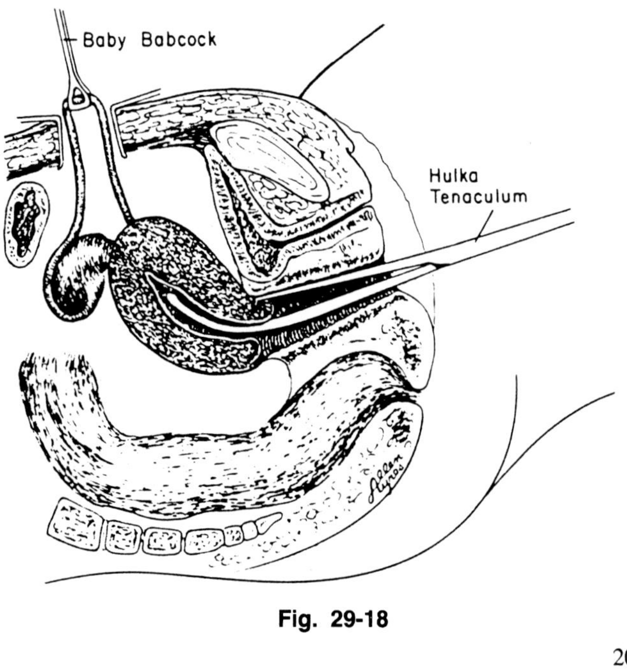

Fig. 29-18

Minilaparotomy (Reprinted with permission from Penfield[3]). Any procedure can be done this way. Hasson canula may be used, see Ch. 30, Figs. 30-38.

Tubal sterilization procedures

Posterior colpotomy incision. Inserts: upper left, Pomeroy; center, clip; lower right, Fallope ring. Black and white, fimbriectomy (Line art reprinted with permission from Mattingly[4]).

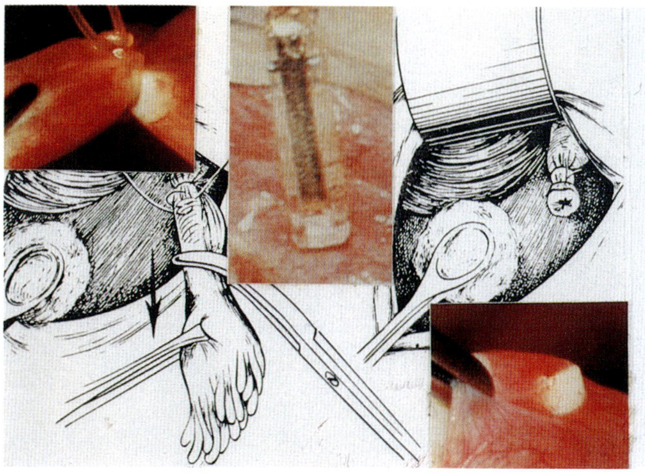

Fig. 29-19

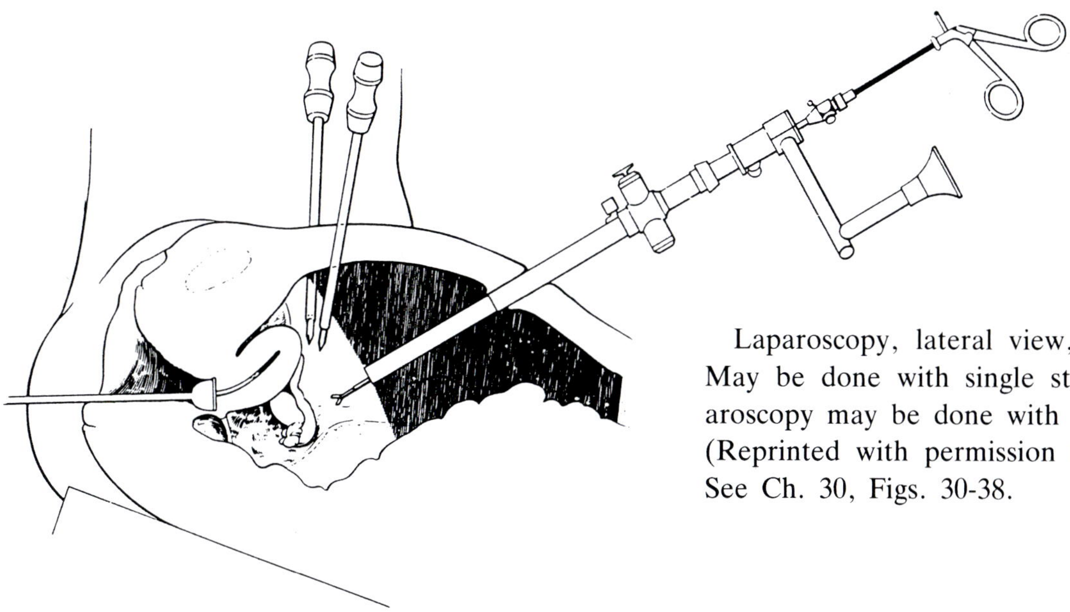

Laparoscopy, lateral view, double stick. May be done with single stick, open laparoscopy may be done with Hasson canula (Reprinted with permission from Patton[5]). See Ch. 30, Figs. 30-38.

Fig. 29-20

Bipolar electrocoagulation by laparoscopy. Burn is greater with unipolar current (Figs. 29-21 through 29-23 reprinted with permission fro Phillips[6]).

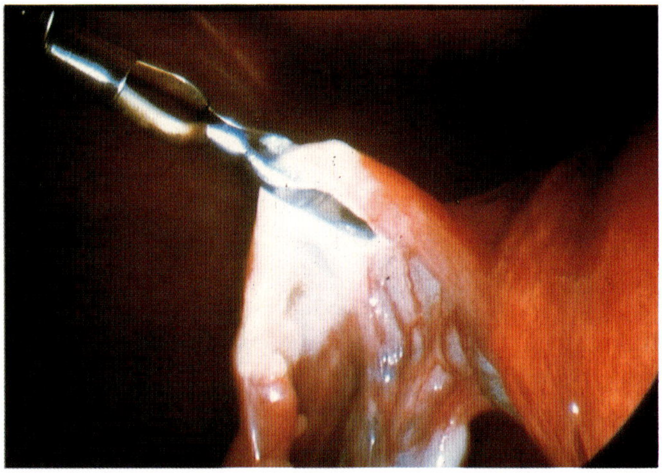

Fig. 29-21

Thermal coagulation with cut. This insures tubal separation.

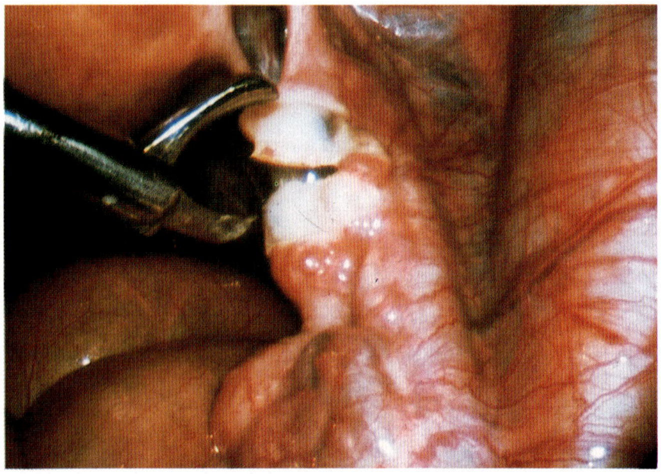

Fig. 29-22

Clip application by single stick laparoscopy.

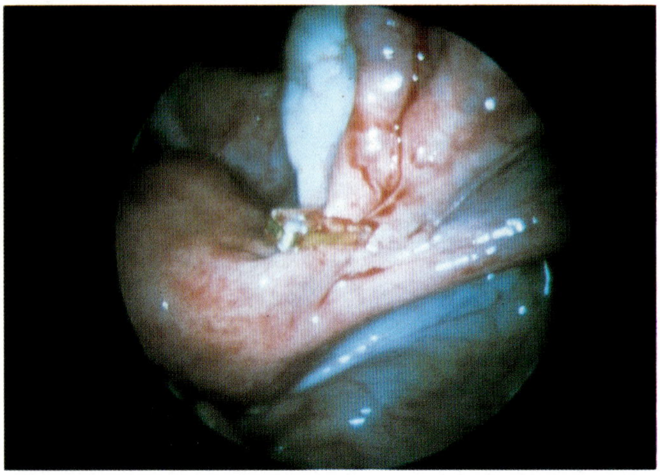

Fig. 29-23

Fallope ring application by same approach. Insert shows application with loaded ring.

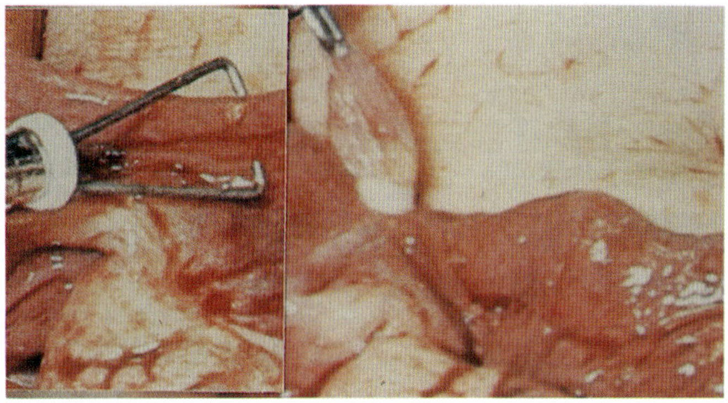

Fig. 29-24

Patient Preparation

The patient has been anesthetized, an inlying catheter has been placed in bladder, the pubic hair has been dry shaved. Immediate preoperative dry shaving prevents trauma to the skin and cuts the hair very close; this reduces bacterial growth in the follicle. The skin preparation is with an iodine soap followed by Betadine solution specially made for skin and which releases nascent iodine. In this patient, the white triangle on the lower abdomen is the mark of a swim suit, with the adjacent skin suntanned.

Lateral view prior to skin preparation.

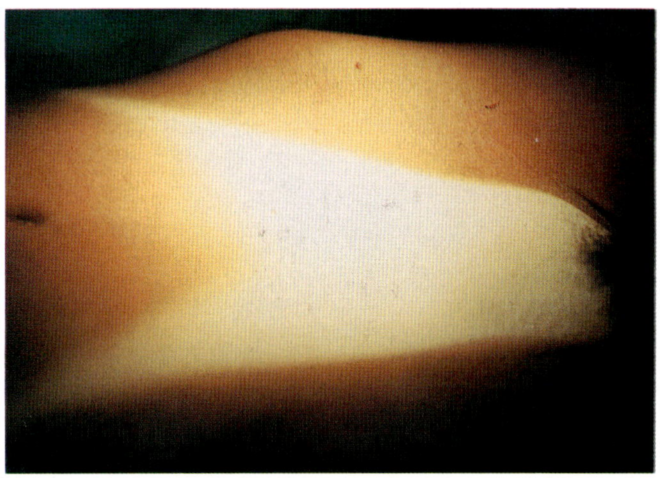

Fig. 29-25

Same, front view.

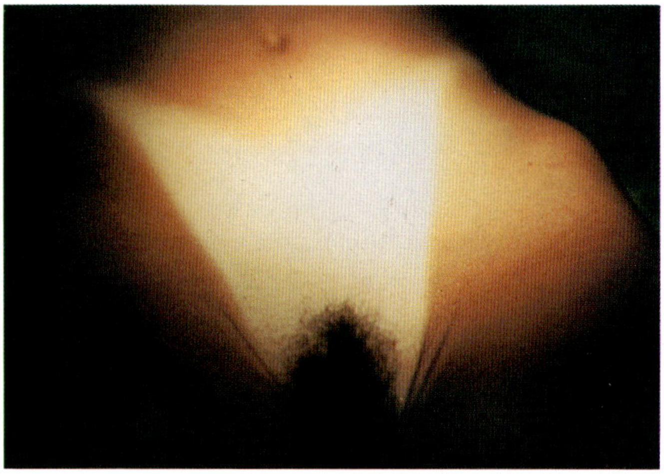

Fig. 29-26

Inlying catheter from another case with an adherent plastic drape.

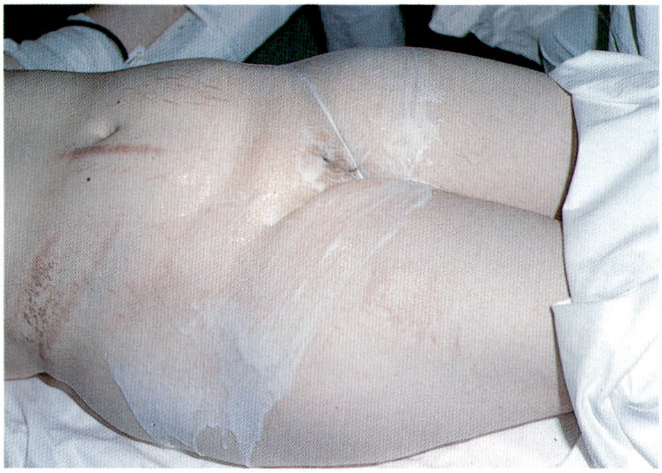

Fig. 29-27

Antiseptic soap wash.

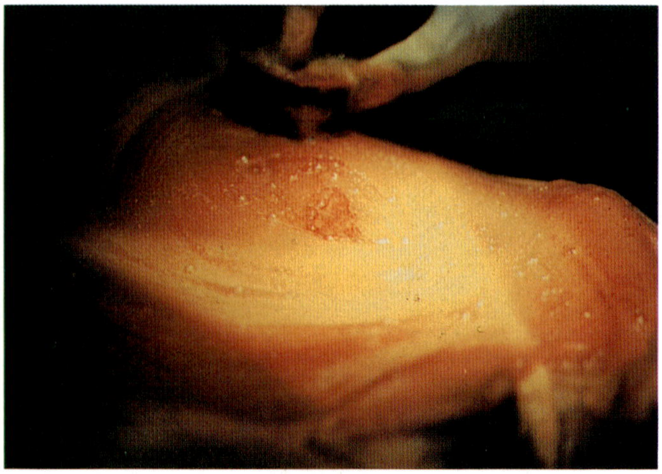

Fig. 29-28

Wash extends to breast line for transverse incision, to the neck for midline incision.

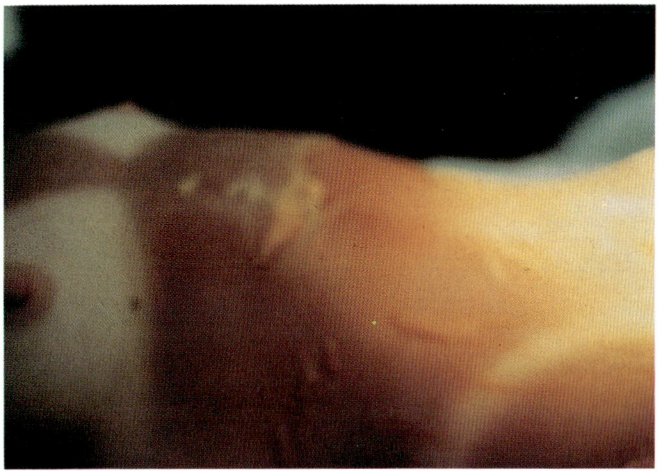

Fig. 29-29

Soap has been removed. Betadine solution applied, and dried.

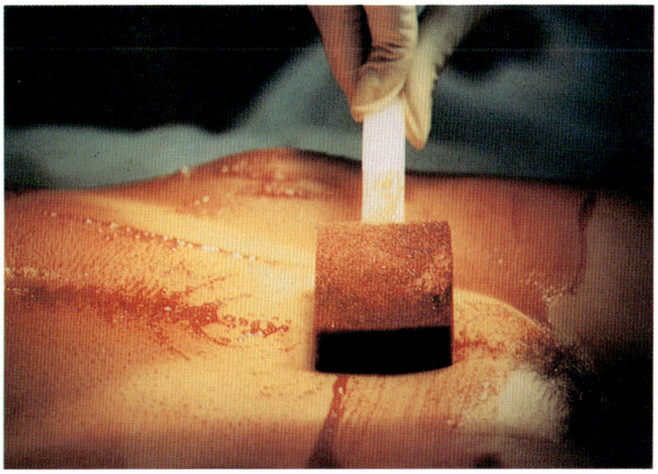

Fig. 29-30

Draping

Sterile towel draping.

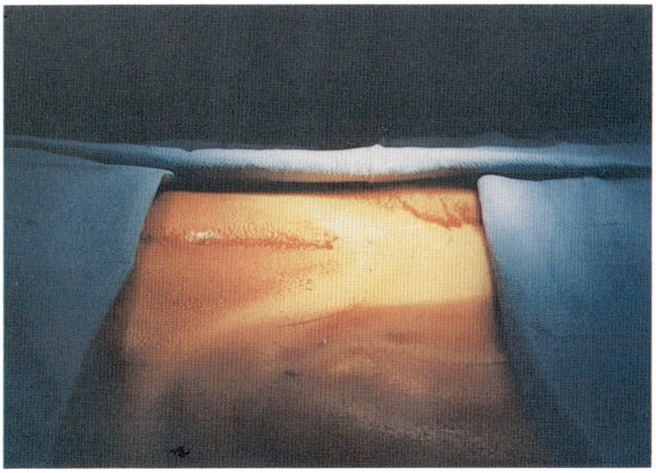

Fig. 29-31

Towels in place.

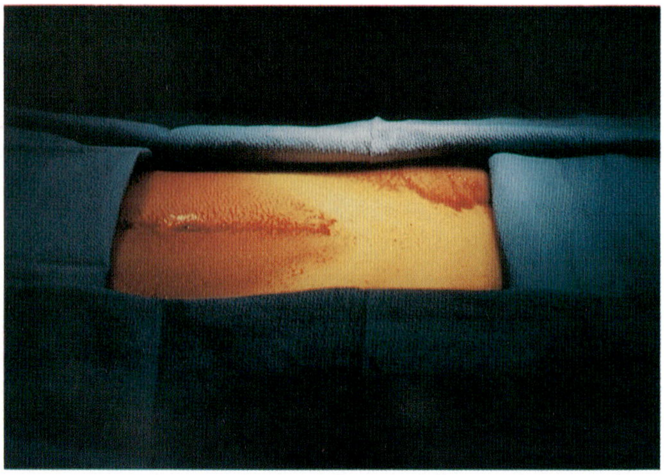

Fig. 29-32

Towels clipped in place.

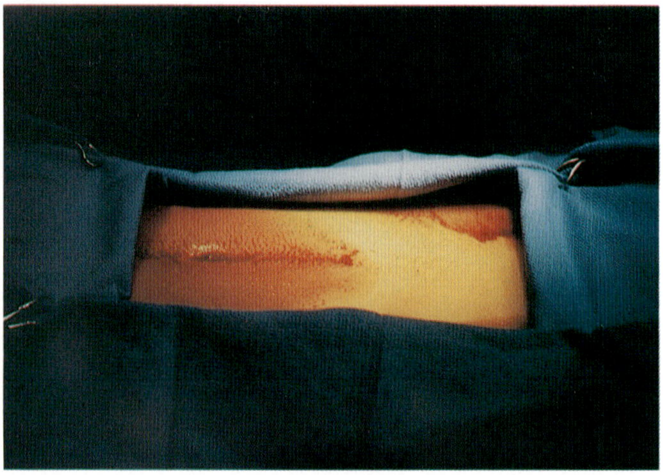

Fig. 29-33

Waterproof paper drape.

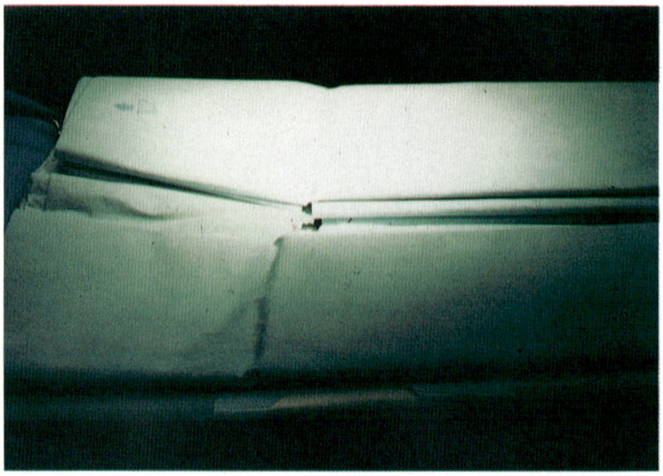

Fig. 29-34

Operating Room Set-up

Ready for incision.

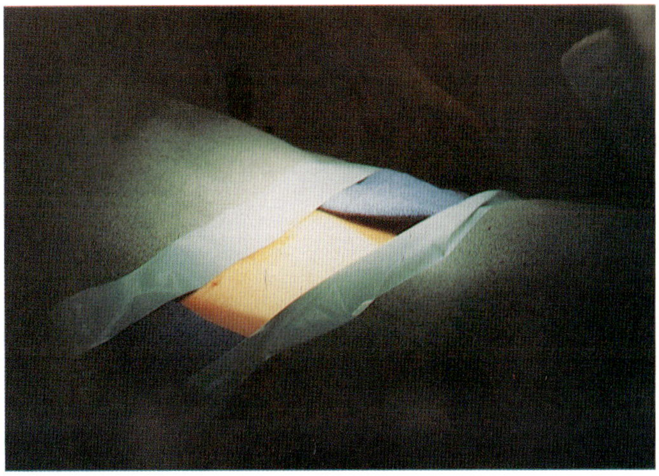

Fig. 29-35

Special plastic drape may be used.

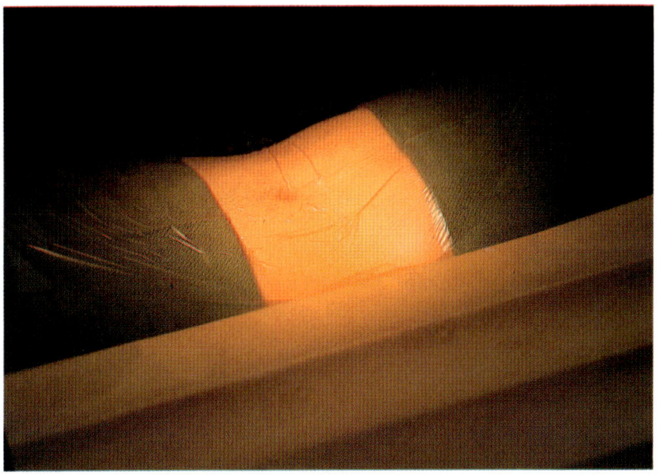

Fig. 29-36

Mayo stand without micro instruments.

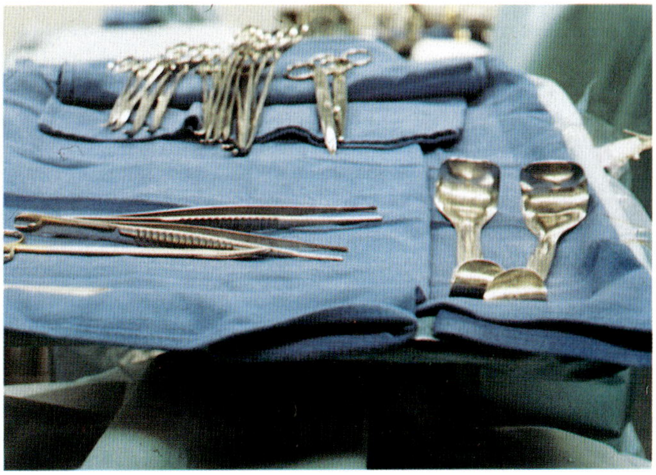

Fig. 29-37

Back table with standard retractors and instruments.

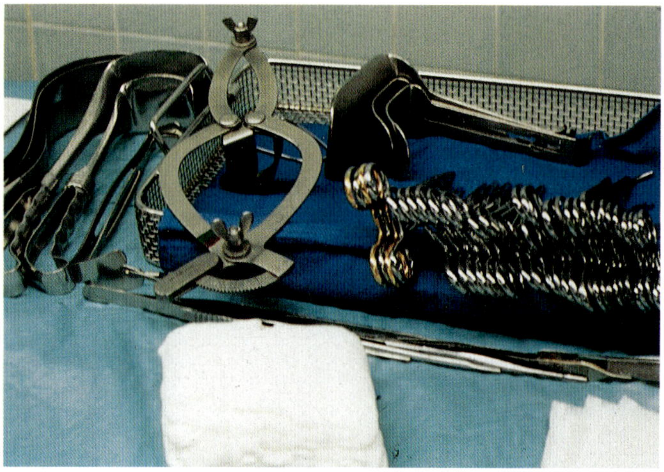

Fig. 29-38

Hand controlled electro-cautery, also has micro tip.

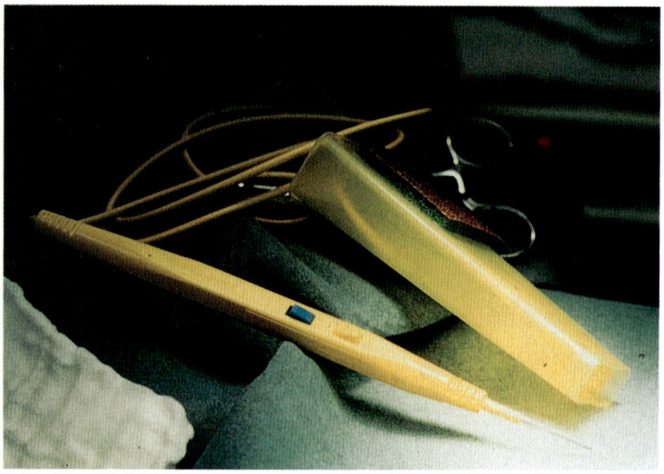

Fig. 29-39

References

1. Knight R. Tubal sterilization. *Am J Obstet Gynecol.* 1946;51:201-209.
2. Pernoll M, Benson R. *Current Obstetric and Gynecologic Diagnosis and Treatment.* East Norwalk, Ct: Appleton-Lange; 1989.
3. Penfield JA. Minilaparotomy for female sterilization. *Obstet Gynecol.* 1979;54:184-188.
4. Mattingly RF, Thompson JD. *Telinde's Operative Gynecology.* 6th ed. Philadelphia, Penn: JB Lippicott Company; 1985.
5. Patton G, Kistner R. *Atlas of Infertility Surgery.* 2nd ed. Boston, Mass: Little, Brown and Company; 1984.
6. Phillips J. Instructional slides from: *Endoscopy in Gynecology.* Published by A.A.G.L., Downey, Calif; 1985.

Chapter 30

Microscopes, Instruments, Devices And Pelvic Packs

Raphael B. Durfee, MD

MICROSCOPES

Any number of operating microscopes are available. They are free standing and mobile, fixed in the ceiling and swing, attached to an operating table and can be removed. They come in many shapes and sizes and can be very complicated or remarkably simple. A choice of what to procure is a very individual matter and must be adapted to each particular environment. They must be dual binocular with changeable magnification lenses. The use of a sterile plastic drape is also an individual matter. Gas sterilized plastic bag covers for the operator's arms and hands are cheap, easily sterilized, available in any grocery store, and allow for great adaptation for everything from focusing to photography without and changes of expensive operating gloves. Each microscope must be cleaned on a daily basis to remove any dust particles or accumulated dirt. The surgeons and nurses must be aware that the microscope is not sterile, and should there be the slightest suspicion that an instrument or anything else in the sterile field has come into contact with it, the item must immediately be removed. There is no room for argument about this matter, just do it. The surgeons should sit directly across from each other on comfortable stools with easy access to the eyepieces; all preliminary adjustments of the microscope and everything else is done before scrubbing the hands and arms. Since the majority of operating tables have a central pedestal, the table needs to be properly adapted as shown in the operating room photographs.

INSTRUMENTS

It is almost a necessity for each surgeon to have his/her own set of microinstruments. These should be selected with great care and should be very diverse and versatile so that everything that could possibly be needed for the surgery is ready. Everyone has a feel for certain equipment as to weight, size and fit to the hand. Sets are available by several instrument makers and should be contained in labeled steel cases suitable for sterilizing. These are specially made to protect and carry everything. Never allow anyone to clean and prepare these sets who is not aware of their fragility and value; one careless move can ruin the finest set of microinstruments. A similar attitude must be maintained in the operating room; all instruments must be passed from the scrub nurse to the surgeon by direct hand to hand contact; no instrument should be allowed to rest on the table, because if it falls to the floor the chances are it is ruined. They must be protected from rust, demagnetized from time to time, constantly checked under magnification for hooks and defects, and discarded if not always perfect. Each operator should accumulate all of the things he or she wishes, to provide the most complete armamentarium.

DEVICES

Various special devices are available for intra-abdominal microsurgery and most of these become an individual choice; many are included here by illustration. There are very few unnecessary items in this category for those who perform several diverse kinds of microsurgery. Special headlamps are preferred by some operators, but this is impractical except with loupes. Many prefer loupes adapted to each person's eyes and these have an advantage as to mobility of the head; for some, however, this is a disadvantage because it is difficult to fixate the head for any prolonged length of time. Loupes are excellent in situations in which there is a great deal of combined, micro, macro, and laser manipulations.

PELVIC ORGAN MANIPULATION

Divergence of opinion is greater in this area than anywhere else in Gynecologic microsurgery. The problem is to raise the uterus up into the wound, stabilize it and bring the adnexal tissues into the field. Some surgeons use vaginal packing or a Valchek or acorn cannula to raise and anteflex the uterus. This can also be done with a HUI. We prefer to leave the cervix and vagina untouched and use a Buxton or Shirodkar clamp to lift the uterus and obstruct the canal at the end of the internal cervical os. This prevents any possibility of introducing pathogenic bacteria from the cervix or vagina.

Microscopes

Zeiss operating microscope with photographic controls.

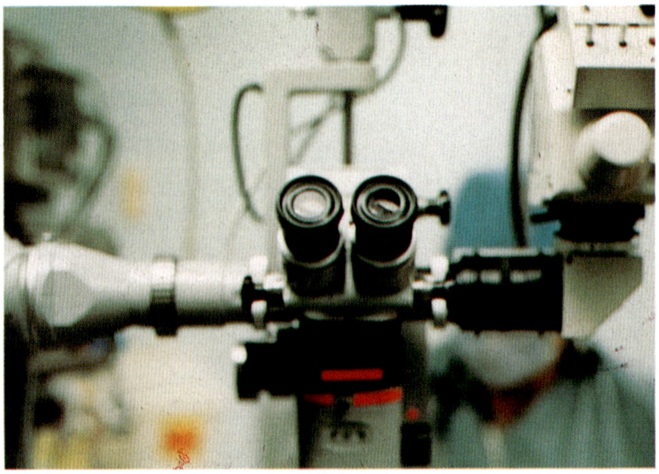

Fig. 30-1

Basic Zeiss microscope, mobile.

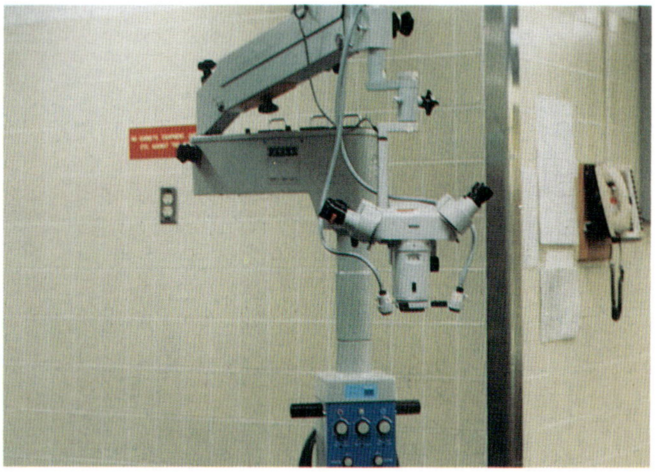

Fig. 30-2

Laser control with Zeiss microscope; CO_2 Laser.

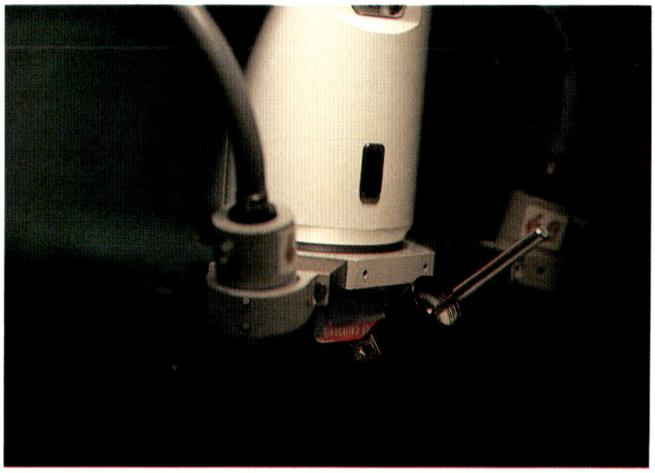

Fig. 30-3

Ceiling mounted Zeiss microscope, not practical, reduced mobility.

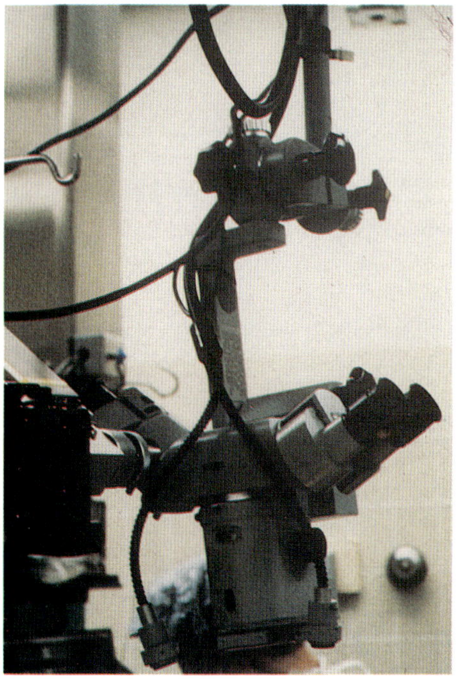

Fig. 30-4

Undraped Zeiss microscope; surgeons seated facing each other; retractor in place; plastic hand and arm drapes for focusing, movement, photography. These can be changed without changing gloves.

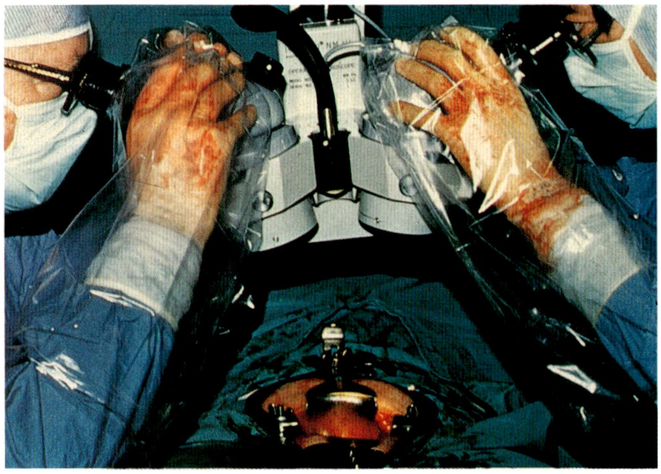

Fig. 30-5

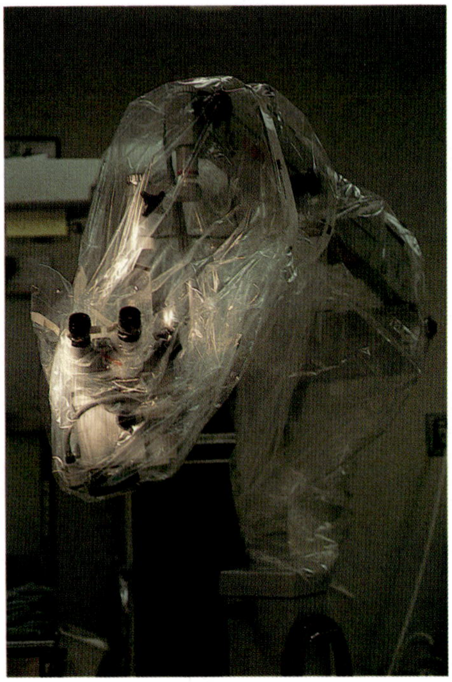

Fig. 30-6

Draped Zeiss microscope used by many; however, it is hard to apply and may be contaminated by a surgeon's head, etc. Not really necessary or practical.

Elmed OPX 500 RC AM-MI reversible operating table.

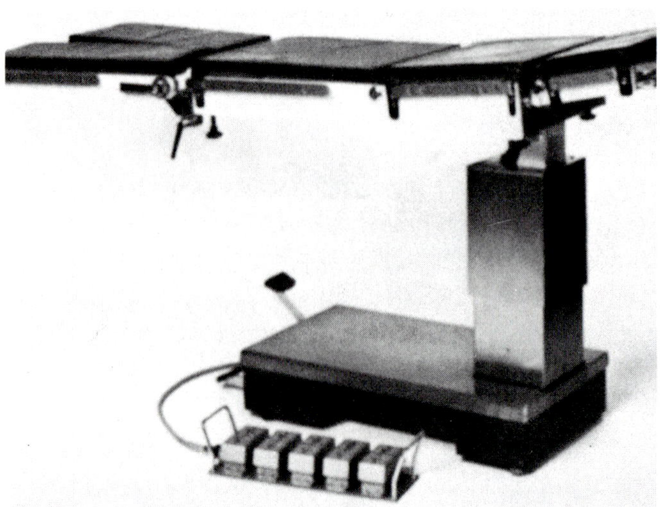

Fig. 30-7

Steel extender for any standard table (Figs. 30-8 through 3-10 courtesy of Good Samaritan Hospital, Portland, Oregon).

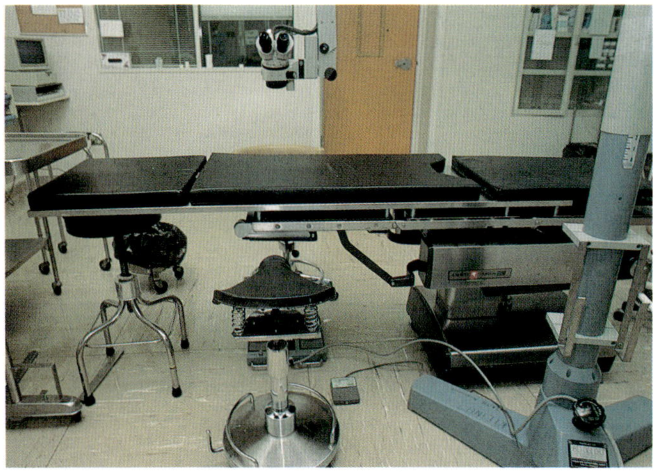

Fig. 30-8

Same extender with operating room set-up. Note stools, control pedals for microscope.

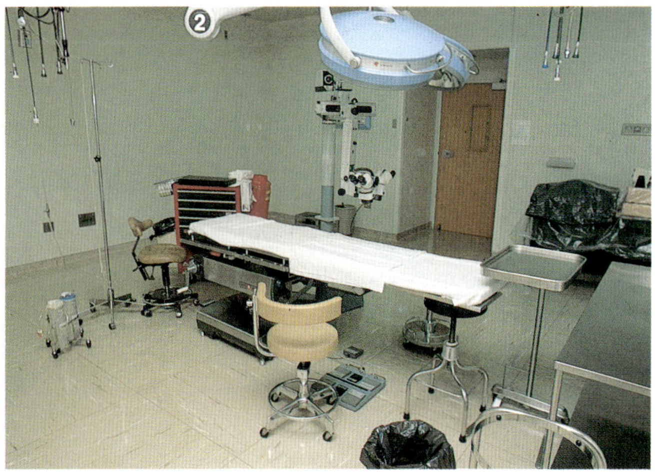

Fig. 30-9

Another view.

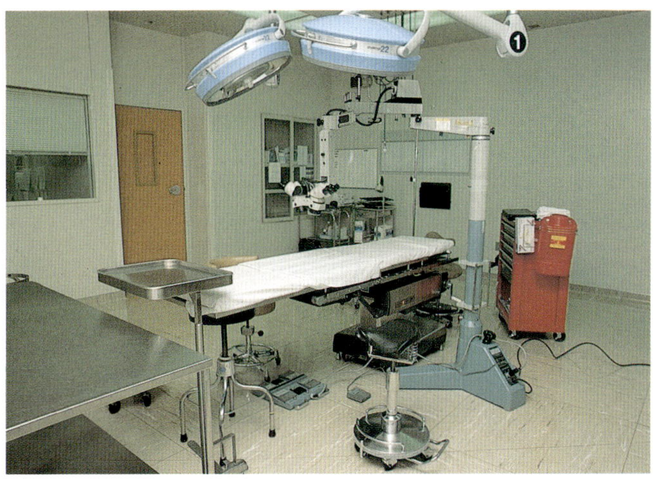

Fig. 30-10

Initial step in packing the pelvis with plastic drape to elevate the pelvic organs into the wound.

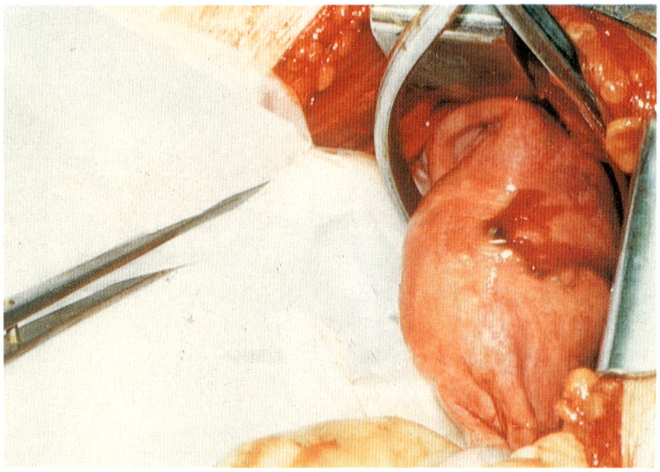

Fig. 30-11

Material fills the deep pelvis and cul-de-sac; no gauze sponges are ever used for packs, only for protection when using the laser.
Note: The draping material shown here is used in eye surgery; it is abundant, fairly heavy, easy to use. If not available, almost any plastic material can be used; bowel bags are especially good and are almost always in the operating suite.

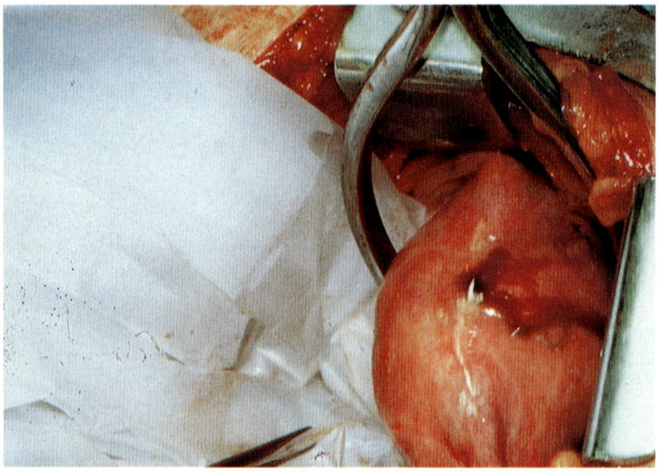

Fig. 30-12

Excess material is trimmed.

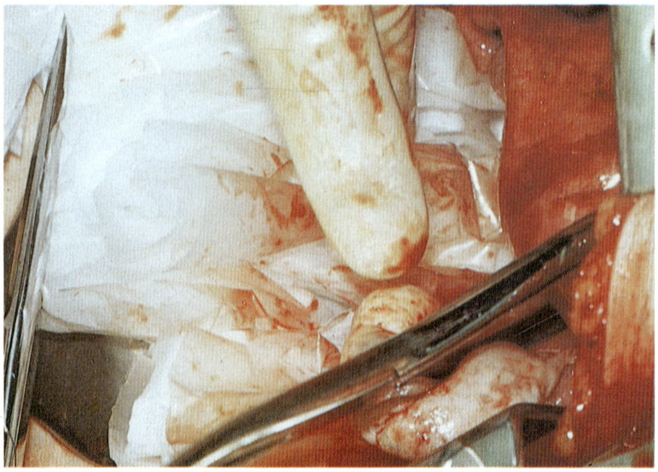

Fig. 30-13

Some plastic may be placed in the anterior space if needed.

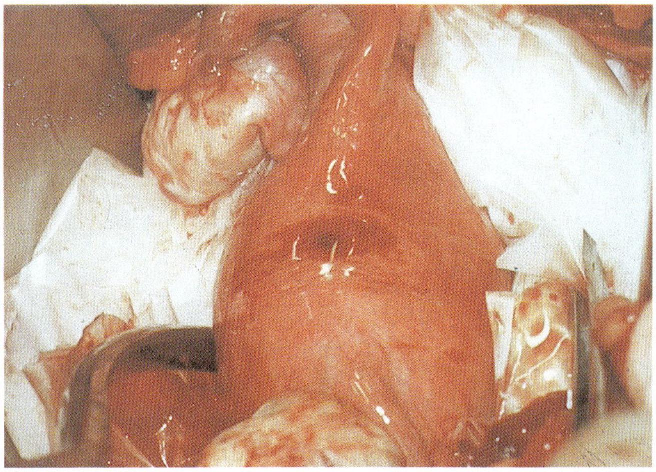

Fig. 30-14

Place a wound protector if desired.

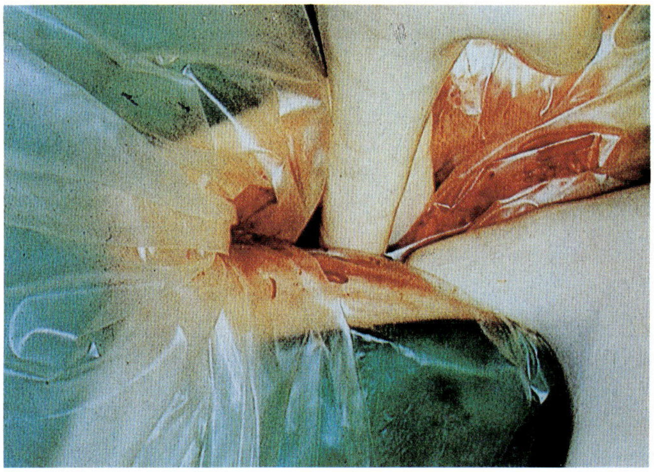

Fig. 30-15

The Kirschner retractor in place.

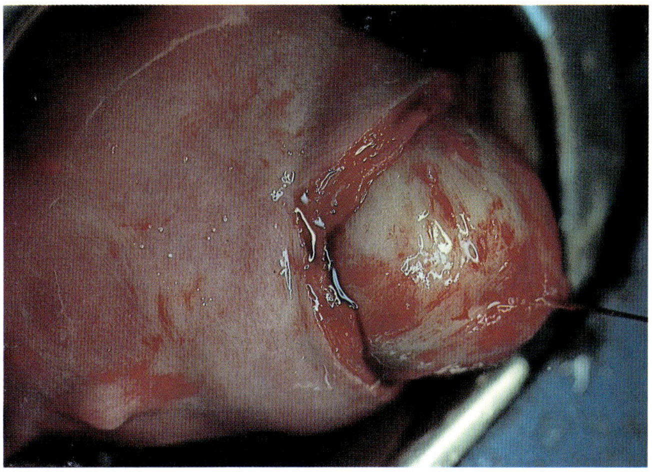

Fig. 30-16

A modified O'Conner-O'Sullivan retractor in place.

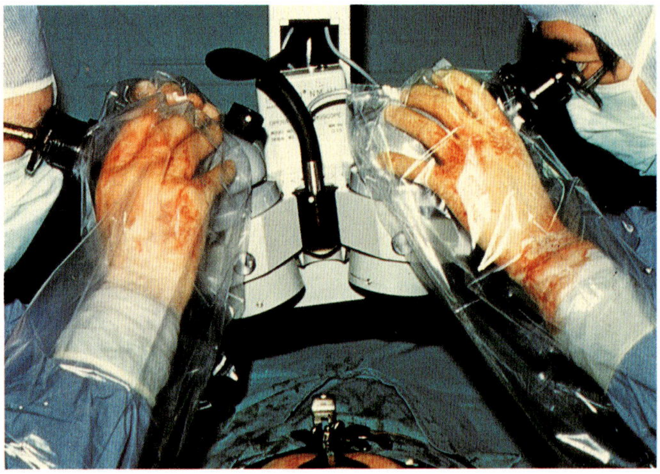

Fig. 30-17

Pelvic organs on plastic laparotomy pads.

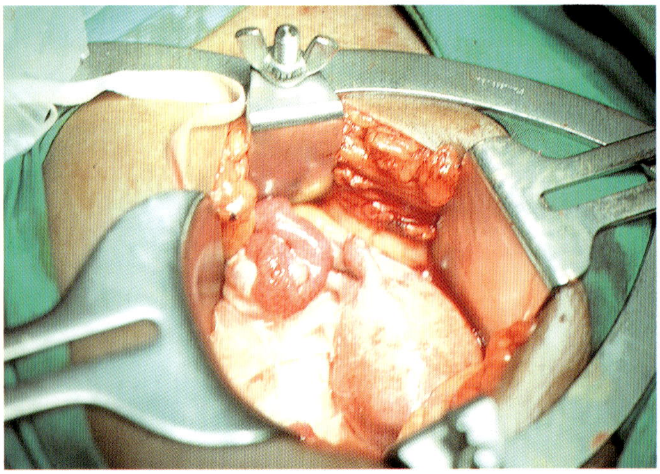

Fig. 30-18

Modified O'Connor-O'Sullivan retractor with all blades.

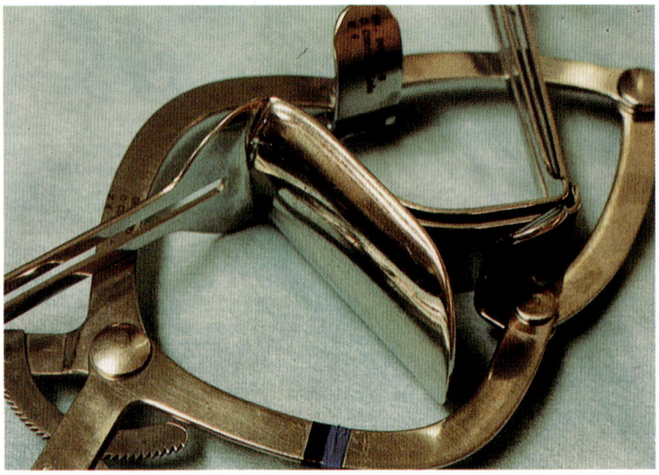

Fig. 30-19

Kirschner retractor (Elmed).

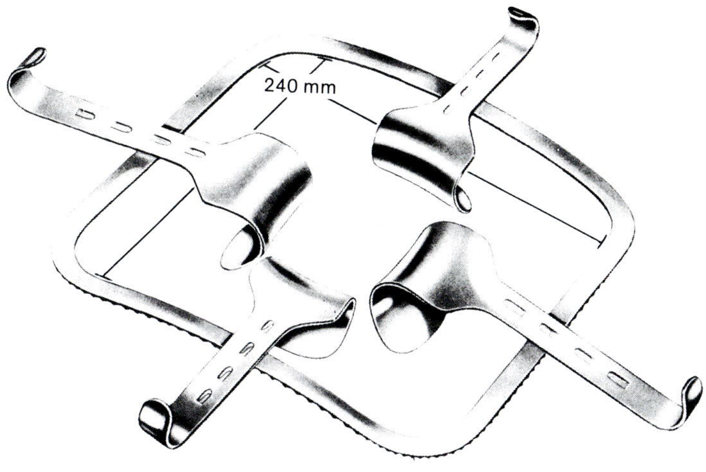

Fig. 30-20

Slight curved, short, lateral blades for O'Connor retractor with wing nut.

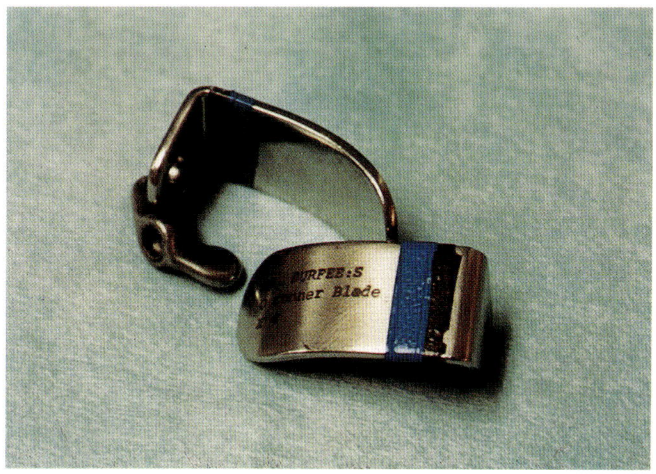

Fig. 30-21

Same, mounted.

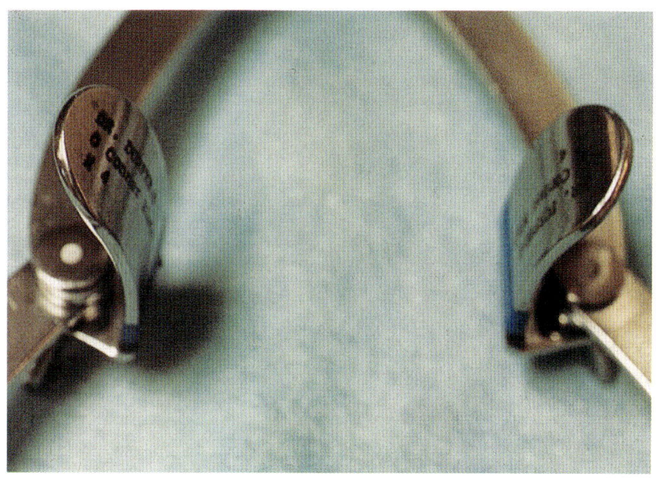

Fig. 30-22

Micro irrigator (Elmed).

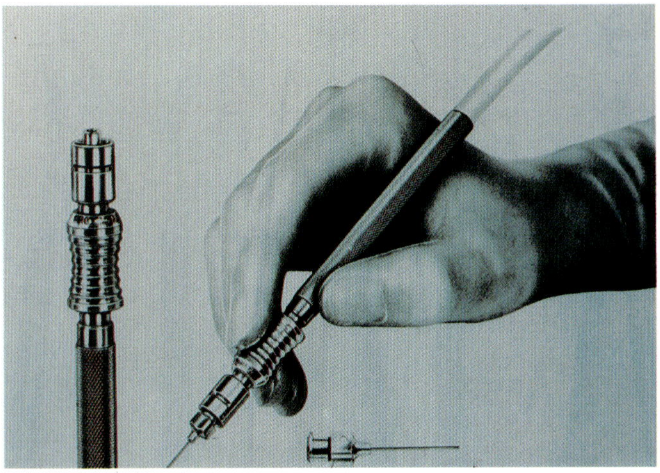

Fig. 30-23

Suction irrigator (Elmed).

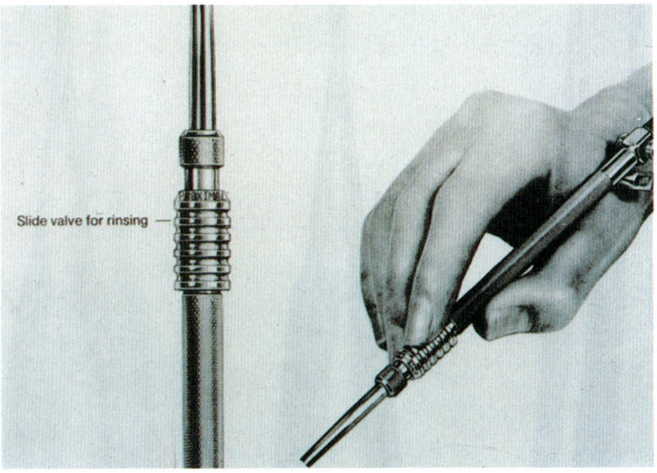

Fig. 30-24

60 ml syringe with intracath tip for irrigating.

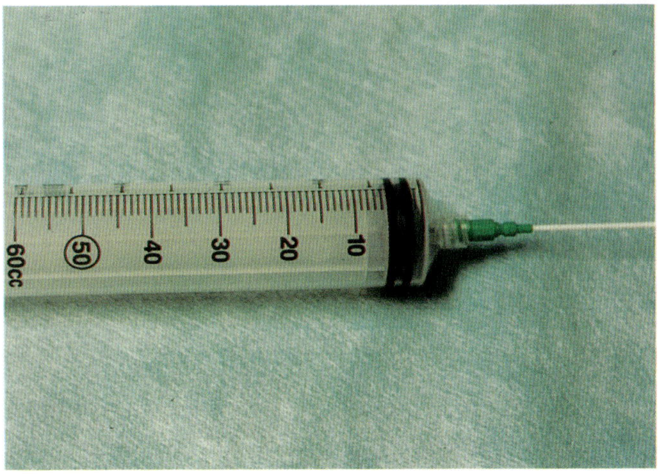

Fig. 30-25

IV apparatus for irrigating (Baxter).

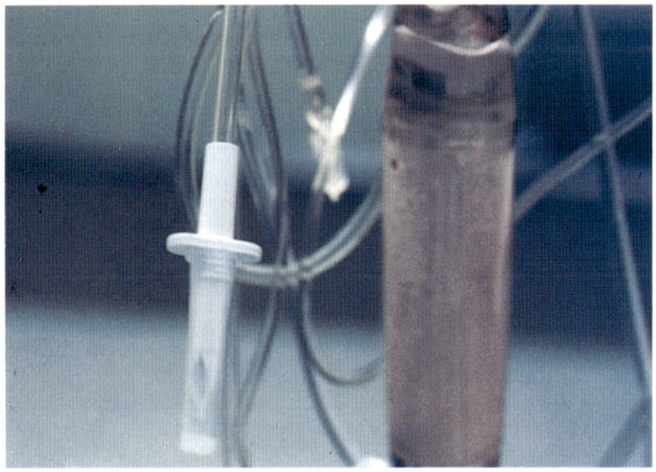

Fig. 30-26

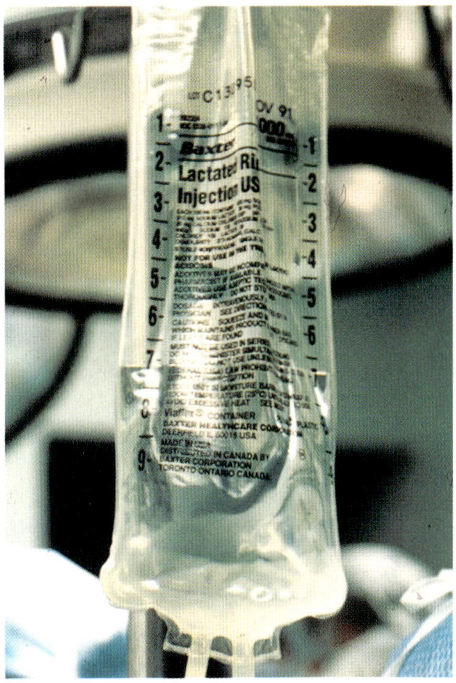

Fig. 30-27

One liter lactated Ringer's solution with heparin (5000 μ) for irrigation (Baxter).

Buxton clamp occludes internal cervical os from outside.

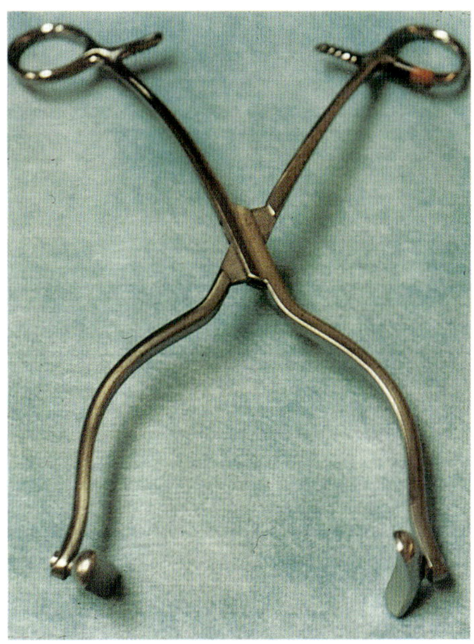

Fig. 30-28

Buxton clamp, note movable tips.

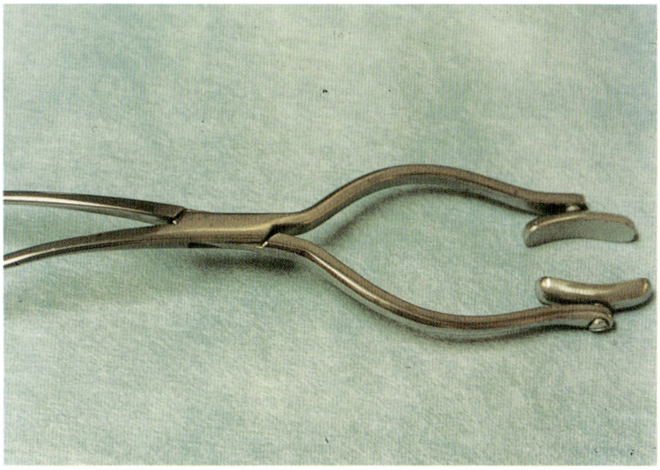

Fig. 30-29

Steel autoclave and transport case for microsurgical instruments.

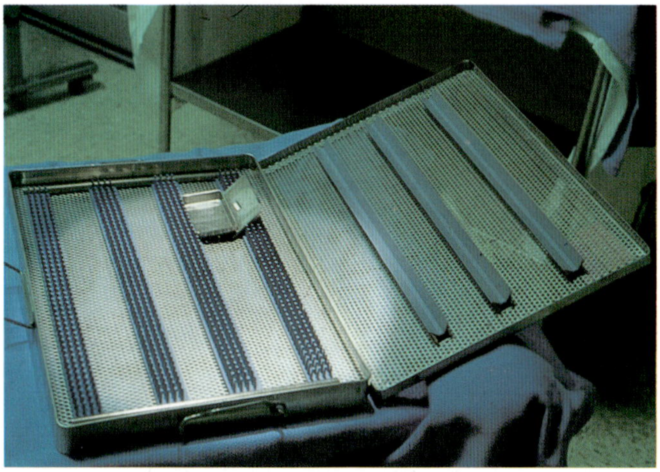

Fig. 30-30

Enlarged picture of needles for comparison; 6-0 at the left, 4-0 center, 2-0 right.

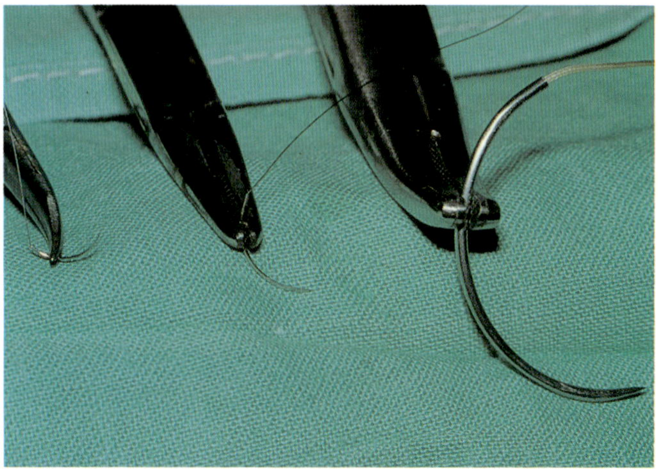

Fig. 30-31

A list of the basic instruments for Gynecologic microsurgery. There are many other variations and additions not listed here.

Fine-tipped forceps (2 or 3)
Fine-toothed forceps (1)
Platform-tying forceps (2)
Ring-tipped forceps (2)
Needle-holder (3 different)
Scissors, sharp, straight (1)
Scissors, small sharp tissue (1)
Scissors, angled iris (1)
Scissors, suture cutting (1)
Probe with handle (1)
Lacrimal probes (4)
Stangel tubes (3)
Teflon angled rods (4)
Buxton or Shirodkar clamp (1)
Cork-boring set
Tube holder (2)
Tube holding clips (3)
Gomel knife holder (1)
Gomel curved steel blades (6)
Gomel irrigation device (1)

Needle holders are a matter of personal preference. Vickers Brown right- and left-handed, hold needles very well; Castroviejo holder, locking, nice handling for tiny needles; Winston or Codman plastic holder, for slightly larger needles.

Sutures range from 5-0 to 10-0 and may be Vicryl, Dexon, PBS, or nylon. 2-0 blue nylon used for stents.

Lacrimal probes.

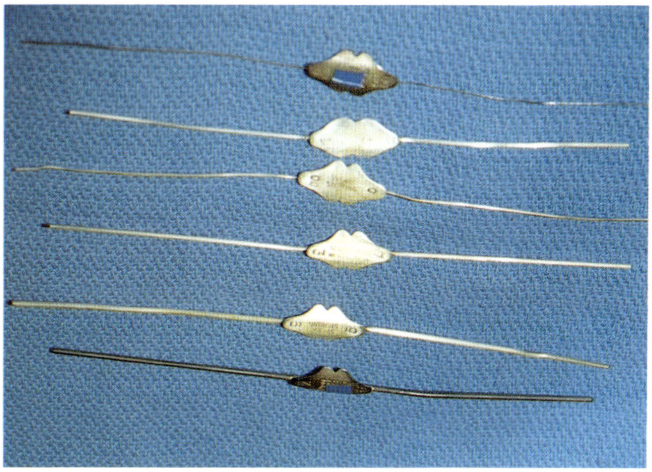

Fig. 30-32

Straight-handle probe.

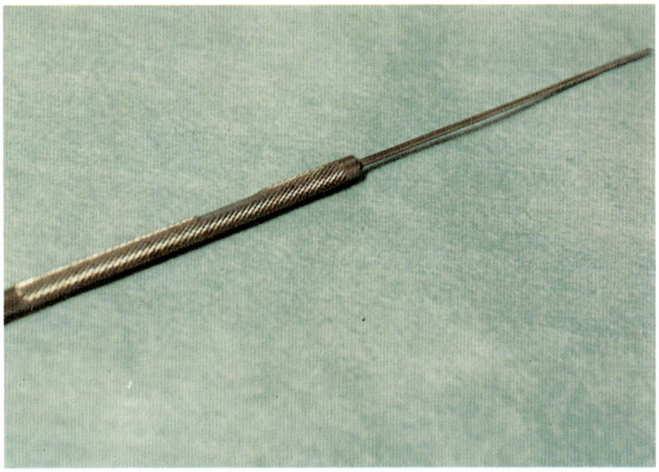

Fig. 30-33

18 intracath for uterine fundal injection and for irrigation with syringe.

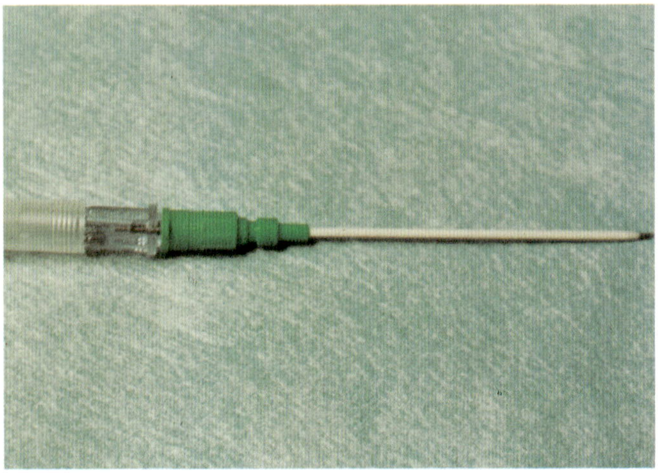

Fig. 30-34

Stangel tubal lavage tubes.

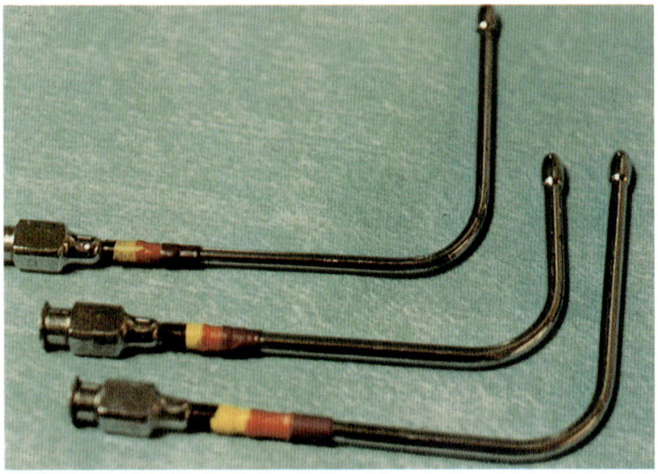

Fig. 30-35

Long-handled tube holder.

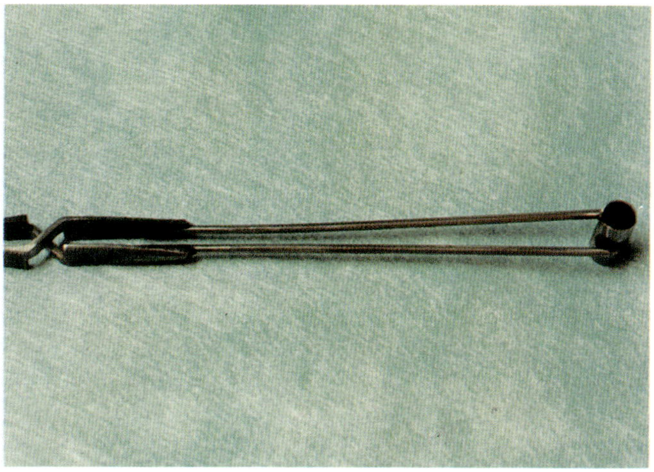

Fig. 30-36

Tubal clip holders.

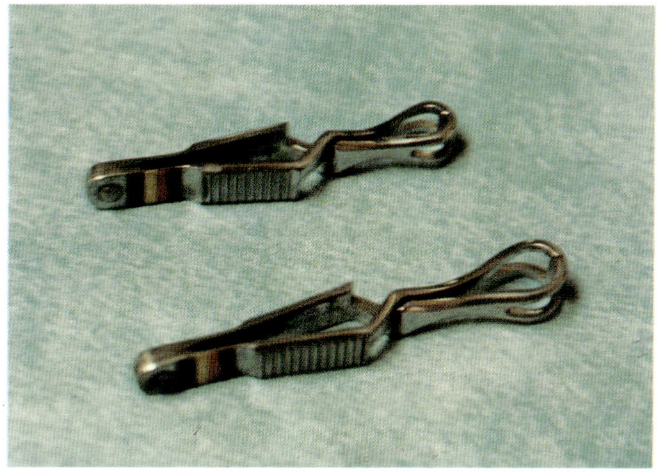

Fig. 30-37

Glass rods for adhesion lysis or use with a laser.

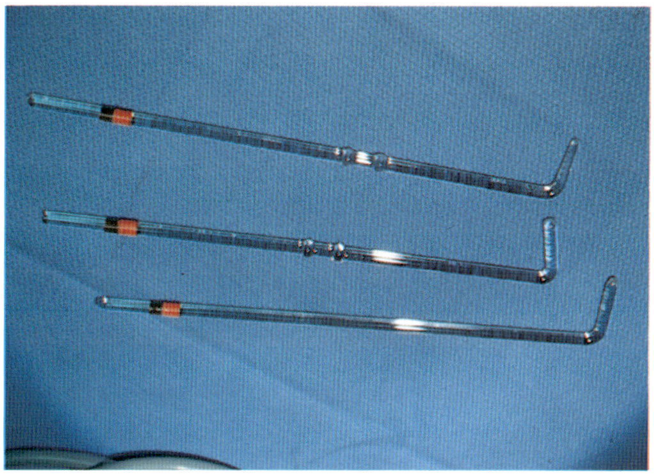

Fig. 30-38

Cork borer for tubal implants.

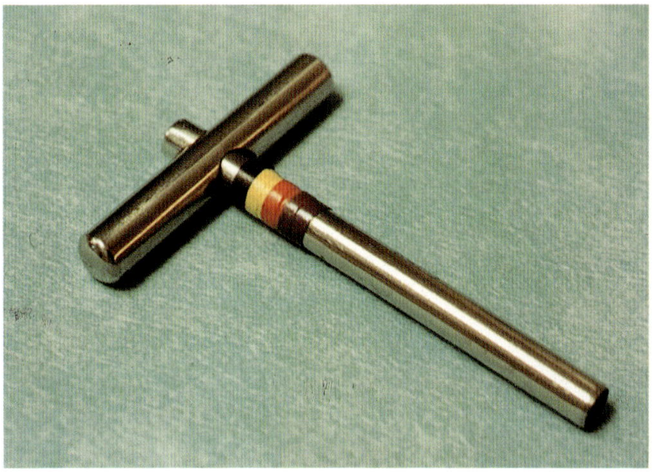

Fig. 30-39

Microtying forceps (Elmed).

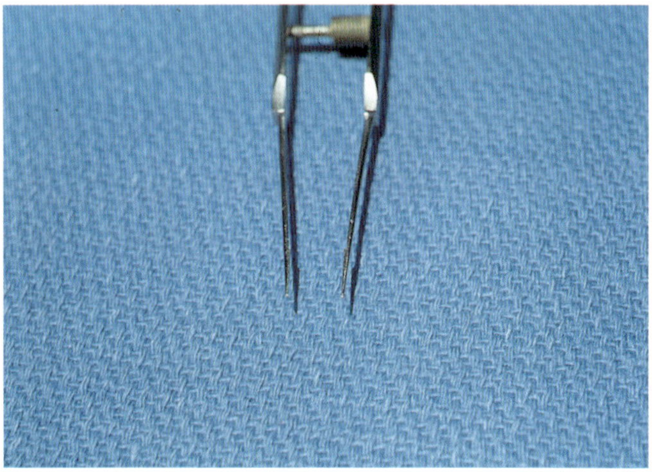

Fig. 30-40

Standard, curved tip nonlocking needle holder.

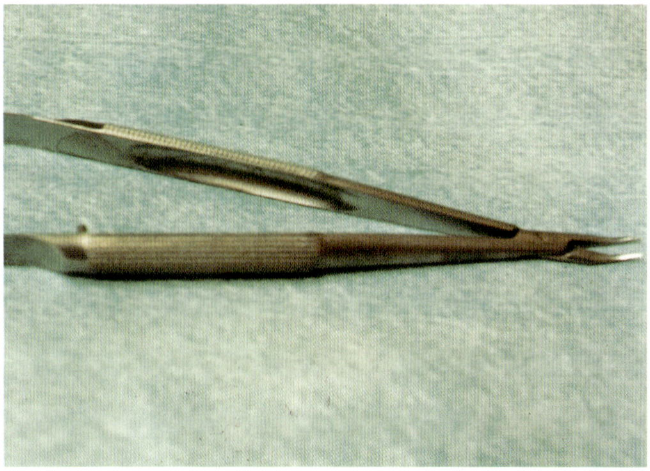

Fig. 30-41

Carbon dioxide laser with its base.

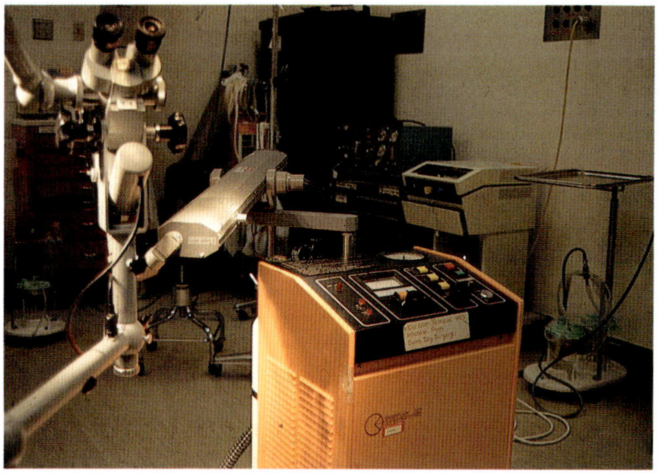

Fig. 30-42

Mobile base for laser.

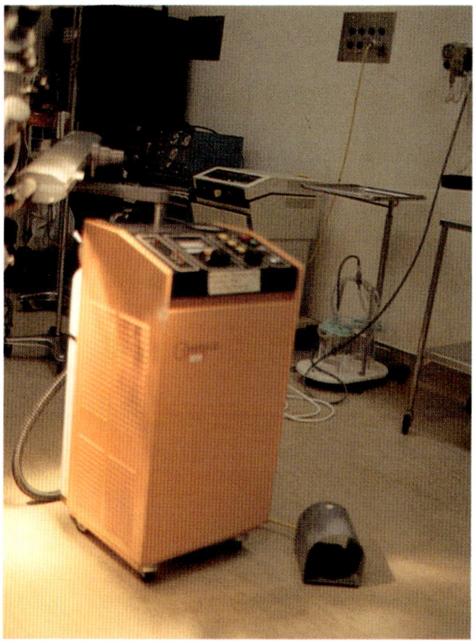

Fig. 30-43

Nonlocking straight needle holder.

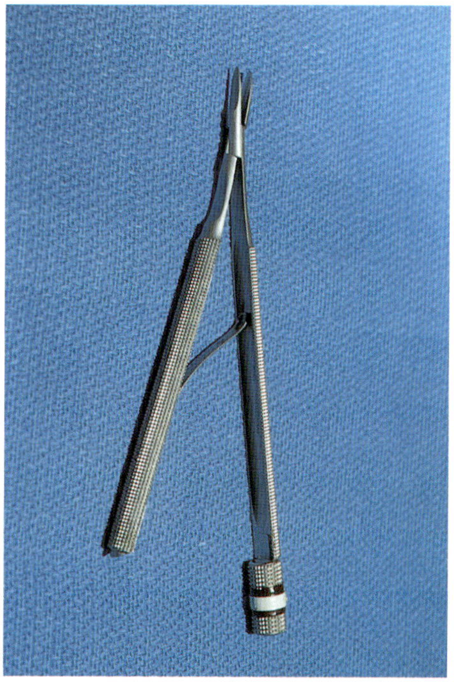

Fig. 30-44

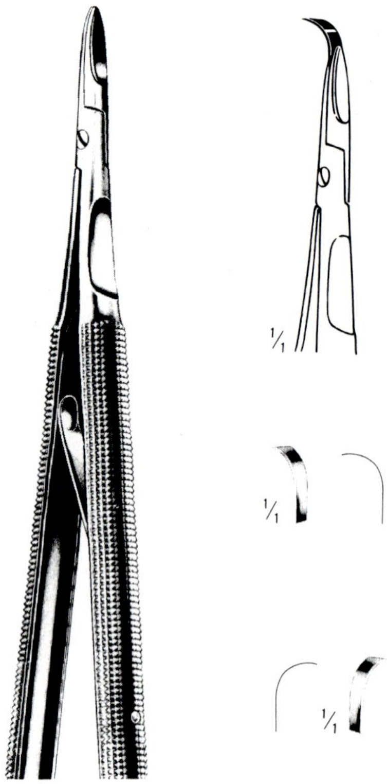

Fig. 30-45

Steel blade holder (Gomel) (Reprinted with permission from Elmed[1]).

Flat, sharp, iris scissors.

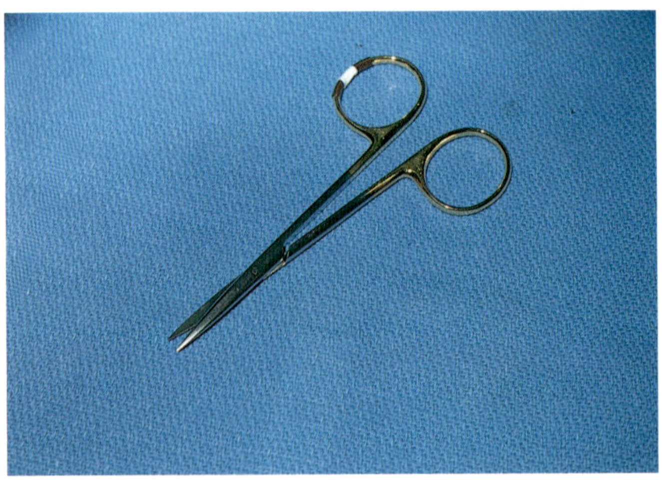

Fig. 30-46

All of these instruments are from the Elmed catalogue. Those designed by certain persons are given credit. Other manufacturers have equally fine tools; a list is included at the end of the chapter. Figs. 30-45 through 30-47 are all by Gomel. The inserts show mostly the handle end of the instrument. Gomel's steel blades are shown this way. Everyone should own a personal instrument set.

Flat and curved microscissors.

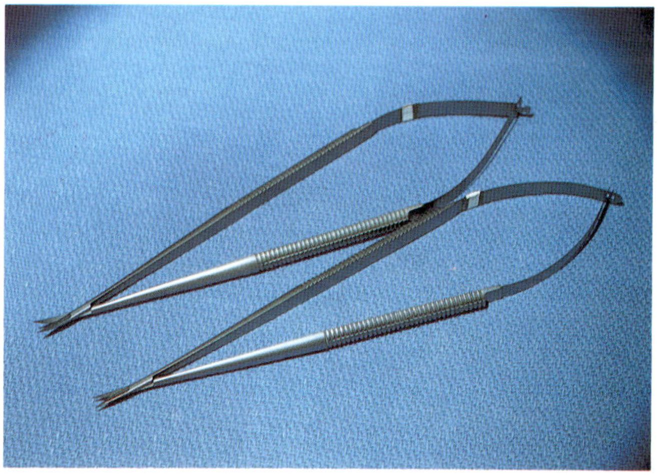

Fig. 30-47 A

Flat and curved tips.

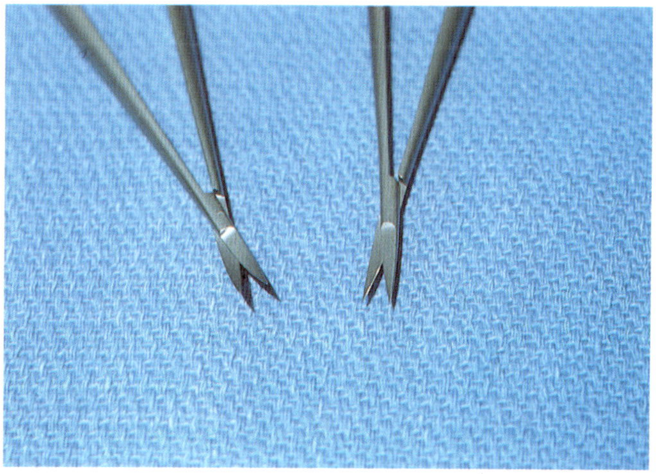

Fig. 30-47 B

Straight tissue-holding forceps.

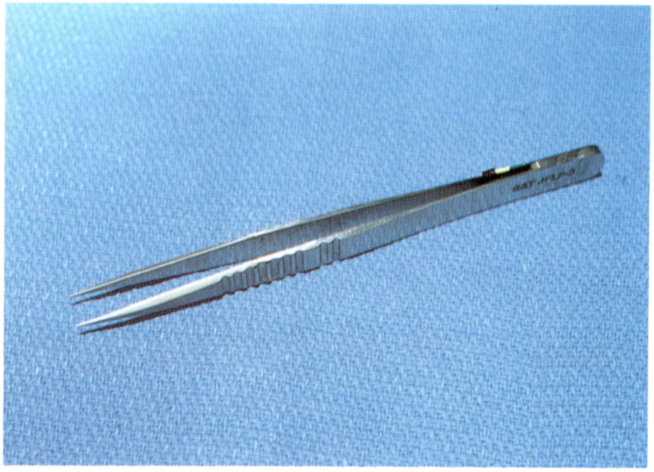

Fig. 30-48

Bipolar microcoagulator.

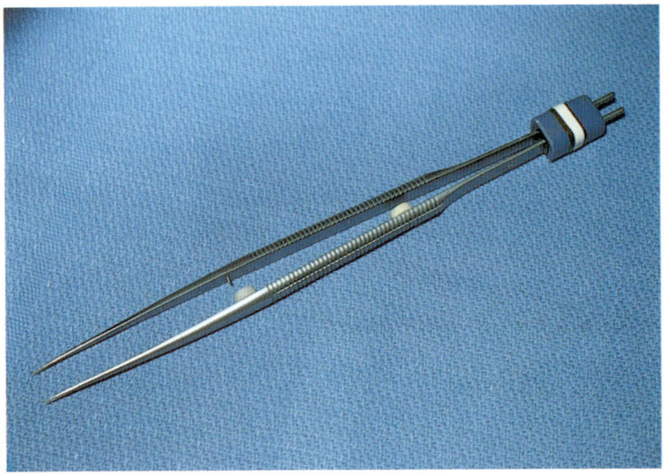

Fig. 30-49

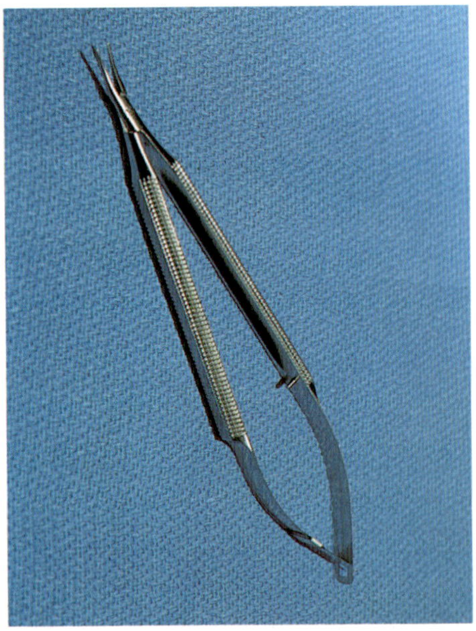

Fig. 30-50

Curved microneedle holder.

Long handle straight microneedle holder.

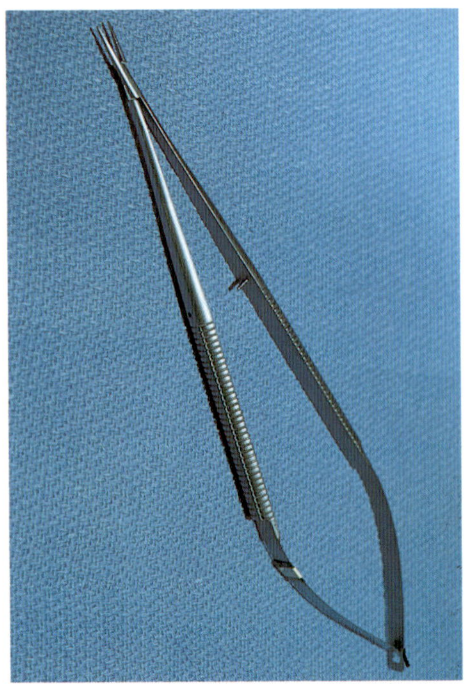

Fig. 30-51

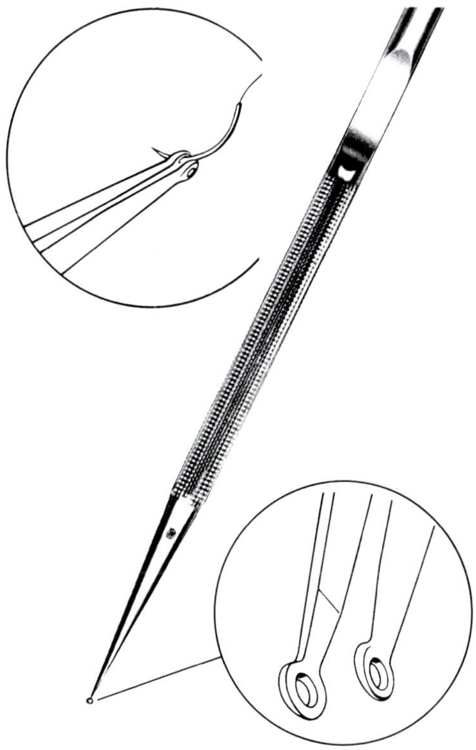

Fig. 30-52

Ring-end grasping forceps, can be used for microneedles (Reprinted with permission from Elmed[1]).

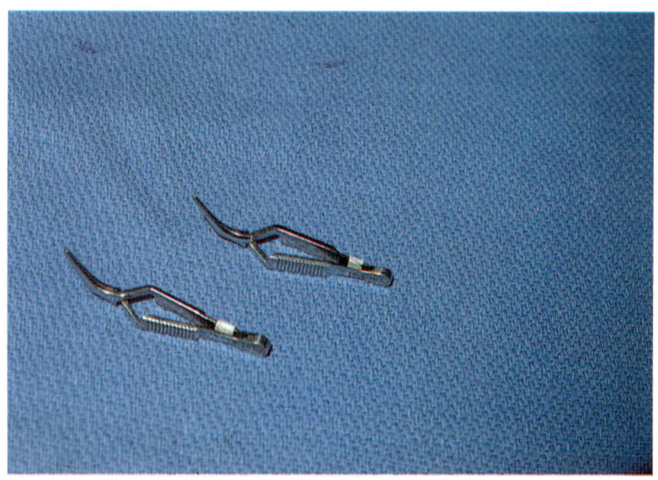

Fig. 30-53

Fine-tip self-closing tissue clips.

Size-graded straight probes.

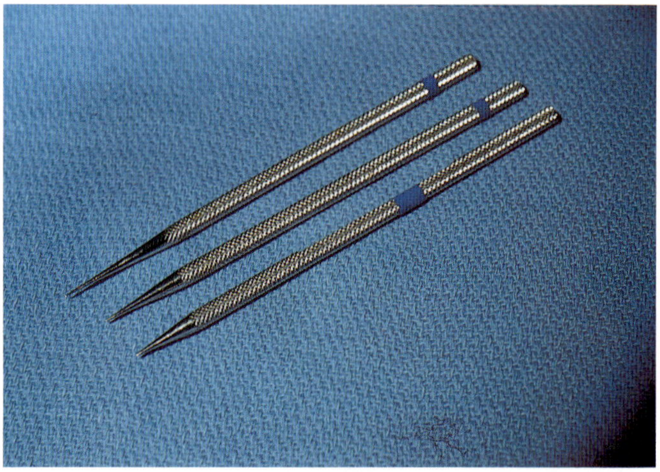

Fig. 30-54

Curved, long handle probe.

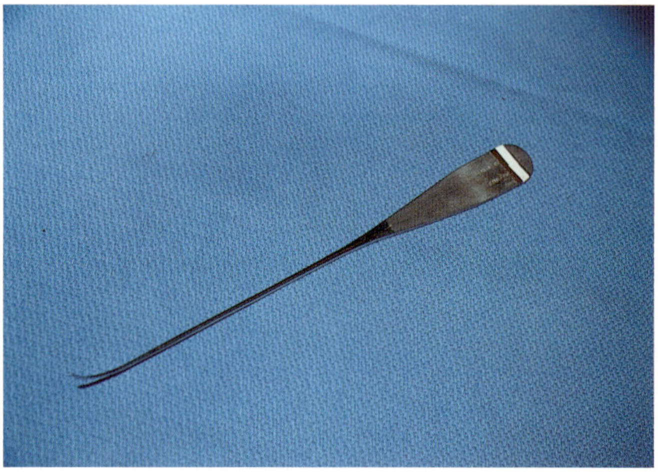

Fig. 30-55

References

1. Elmed Catalogue. Elmed Incorporated, 60 West Fay Avenue, Addison, Illinois

Chapter 31

Diagnostic Procedures and Surgical Findings

Raphael B. Durfee, MD

DIAGNOSTIC PROCEDURES

Many diagnostic procedures are now available to facilitate selection of patients for microsurgery, with or without the laser. Culdoscopy has been replaced by laparoscopy and hysteroscopy, but its value remains for use in areas where these expensive and sophisticated instruments are not available. Hysterosalpingography (HSG) is still very useful in certain cases and may be combined with ultrasonography in some investigations of infertility. HSG is of great assistance in determining postsurgical tubal patency. Laparoscopy and hysteroscopy are invaluable diagnostic modalities and are worth a thousand pelvic examinations.

Included in this review are a few surprises in pelvic findings that otherwise might not have been suspected. When invasive diagnostic procedures are not advisable, ultrasound methods can be very informative. Recent advances in the field of tubaloscopy will provide much more information and allow for observation of changes in tubal mucosal tissues and conditions of the interstitial portion of the fallopian tube, none of which are well known at present.

A few pathologic or unusual conditions found at surgery would not have been a surprise if a more complete or detailed diagnostic approach had been made. Prior knowledge of the condition of the pelvic organs permits a more comprehensive plan for specific therapy; e.g., any one of several conditions in which the use of the laser would be essential. This means that a laser machine should be in the operating room ready for use at any time. In most surgeries this requires previous planning, for the number of lasers available is limited.

Classic pelvic examination (Kelly[1]).

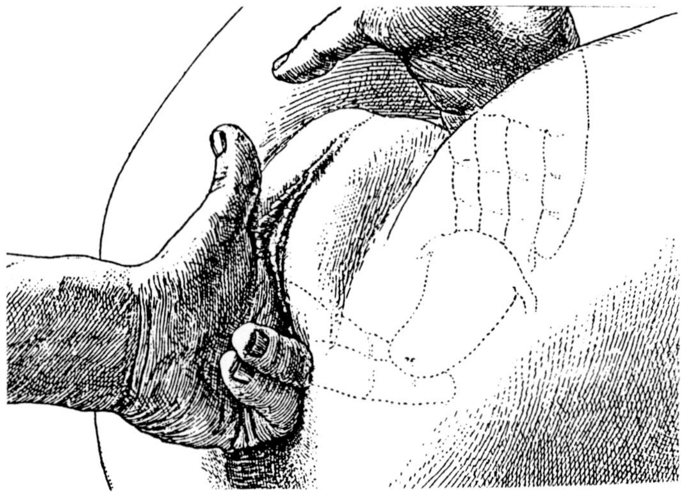

Fig. 31-1

Knee-chest position for culdocentesis (Kelly[1]).

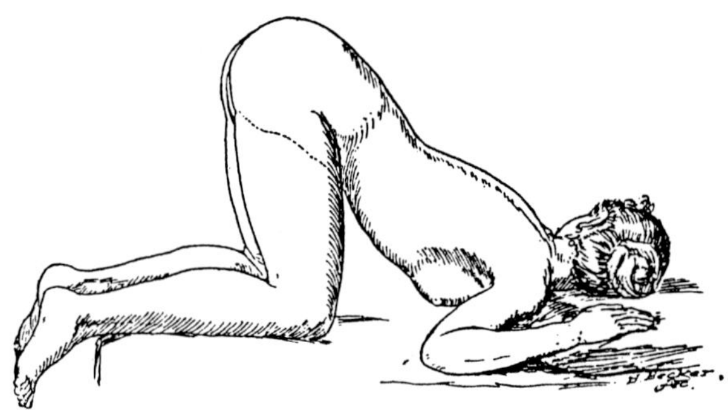

Fig. 31-2

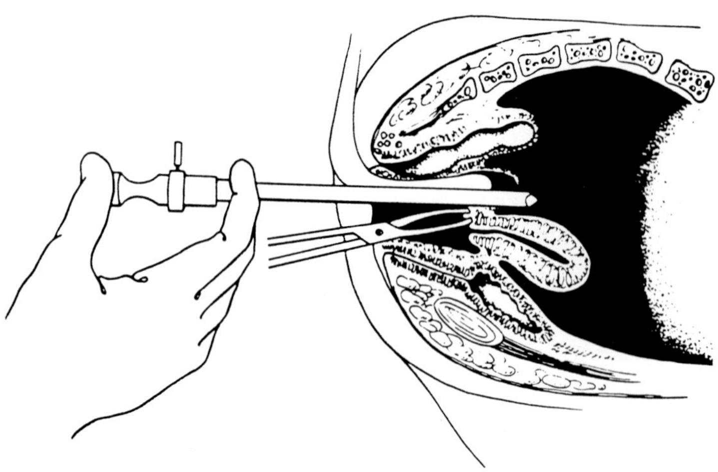

Fig. 31-3

Culdocentesis, first use of optics for vaginal pelvic examination of cul-de-sac (Reprinted with permission from Jones[2]).

Hysterosalpingogram (HSG); normal uterus and tubes.

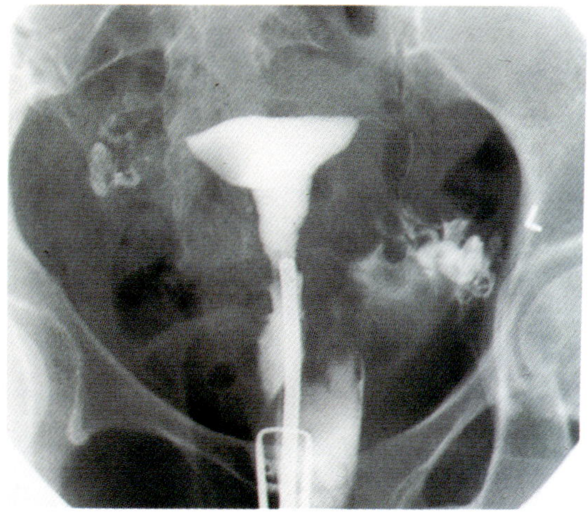

Fig. 31-4

HSG; normal uterus, hydrosalpinx.

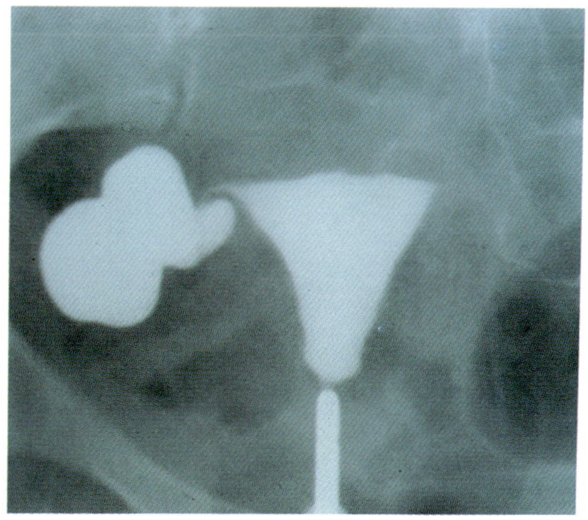

Fig. 31-5

HSG; blocked proximal tube, filling defect, right.

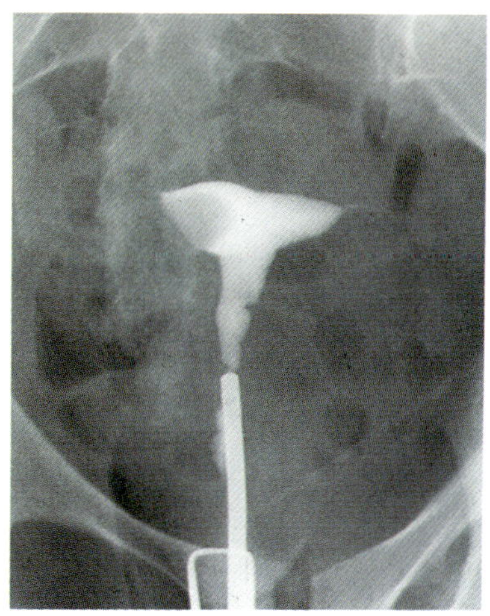

Fig. 31-6

HSG; large uterine cavity with myoma.

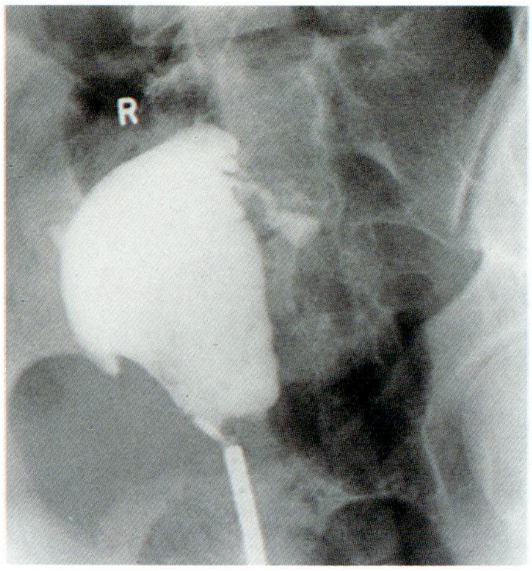

Fig. 31-7

Bicornuate uterus in retroflexion.

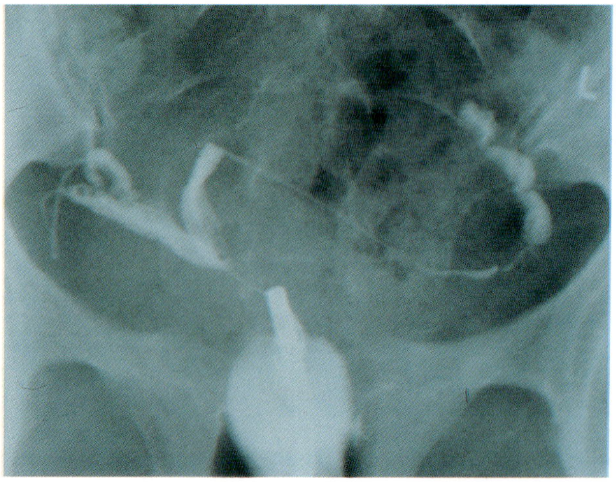

Fig. 31-8

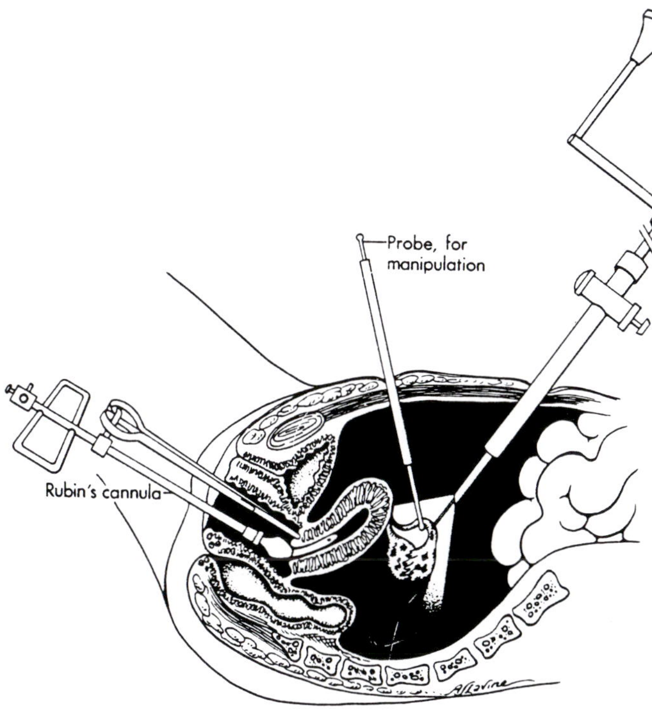

Lateral view, diagnostic laparoscopy (Reprinted with permission from Jones[2]).

Fig. 31-9

Endometrioma of ovary.

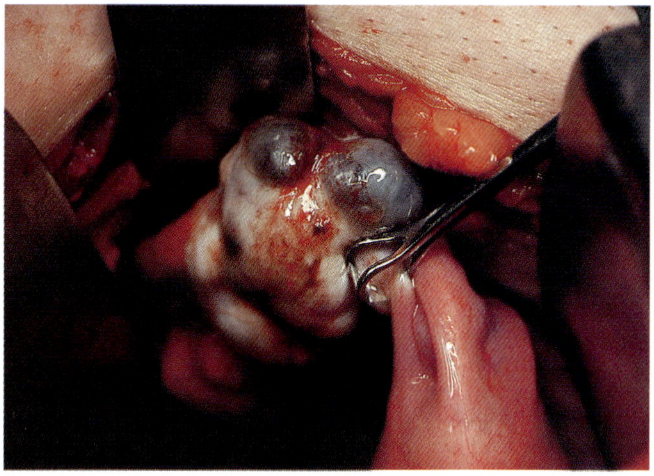

Fig. 31-10

Varicosity of the lateral ovarian ligament.

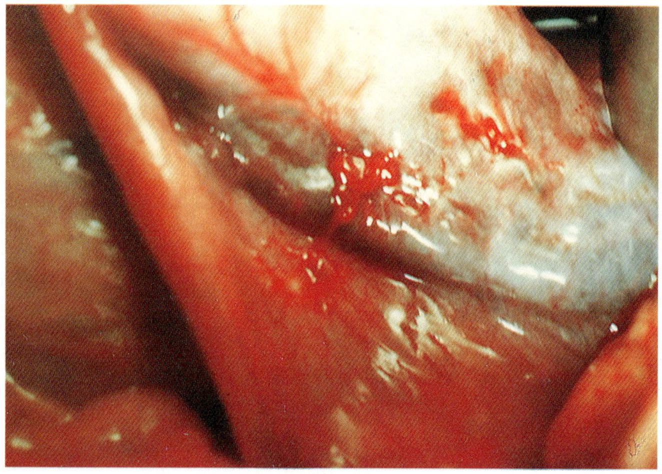

Fig. 31-11

Fimbrial destruction.

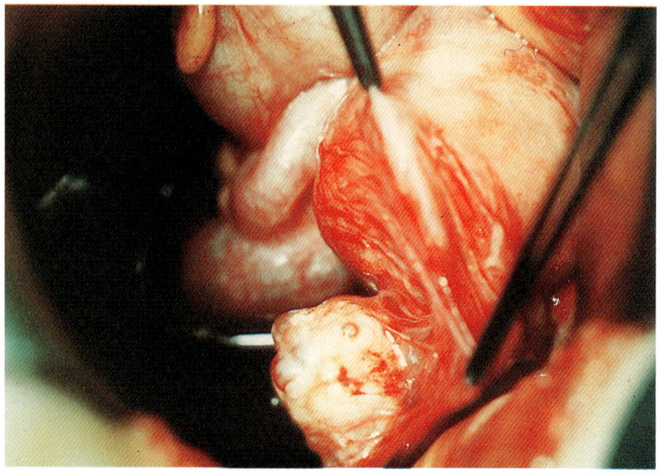

Fig. 31-12

Spontaneous regeneration of fimbria, after fimbriectomy (Figs. 31-13 through 31-16 reprinted with permission from Phillips[3]).

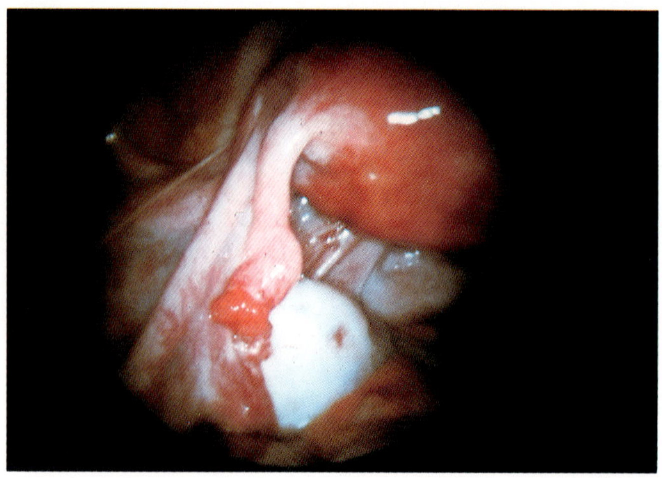

Fig. 31-13

Recanalization of tubal ligation.

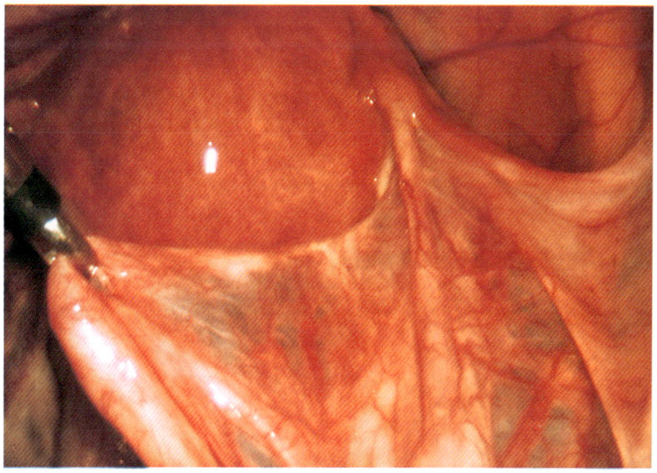

Fig. 31-14

Postoperative salpingostomy, open tube and adhesions.

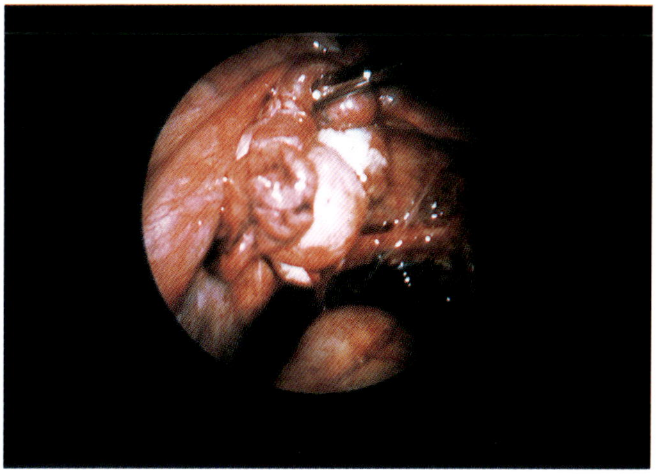

Fig. 31-15

Adnexal adhesions, postsurgical.

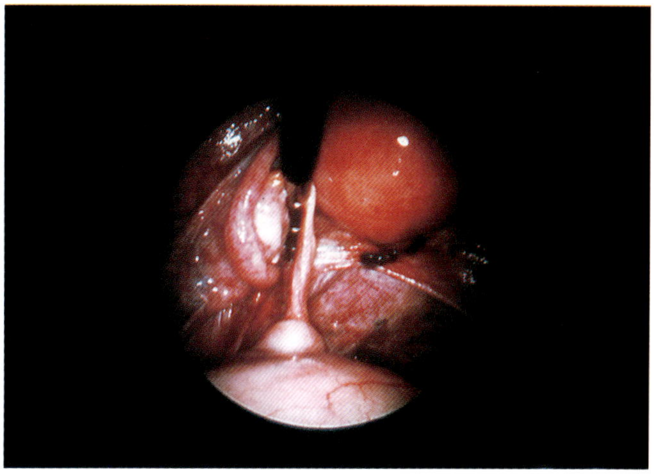

Fig. 31-16

Salpingitis isthmica nodosa.

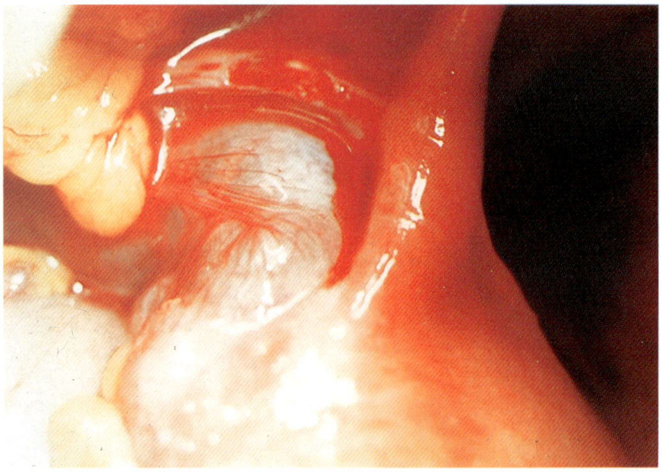

Fig. 31-17

Tubointestinal adhesions.

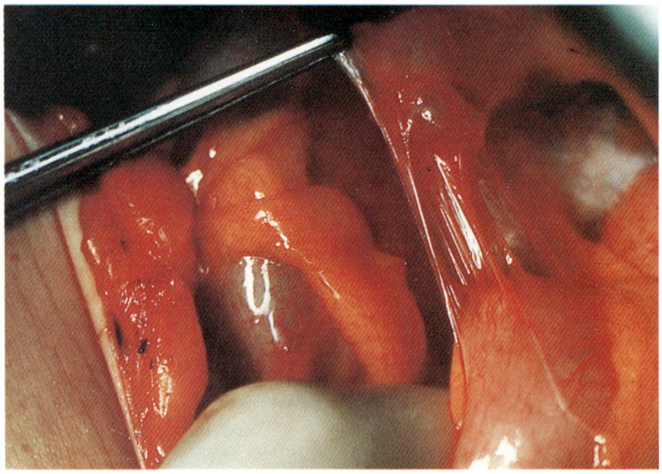

Fig. 31-18

Laparoscopy; paraovarian cysts (Figs. 31-19 through 31-22 reprinted with permission from Phillips[3]).

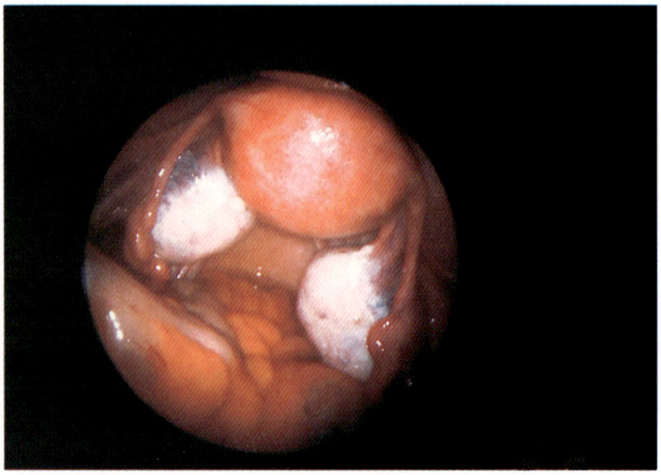

Fig. 31-19

Double uterus with peritoneal fold.

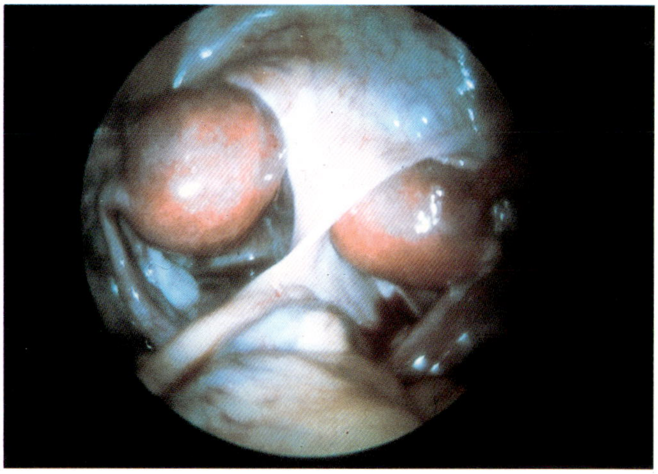

Fig. 31-20

Uterine horn.

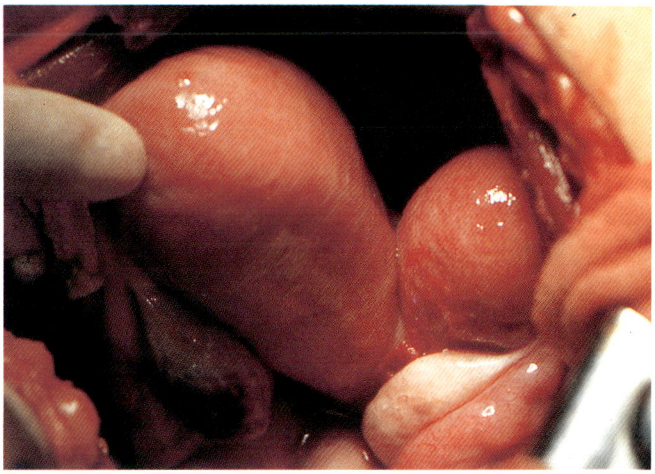

Fig. 31-21

Fimbrial, intestinal adhesions.

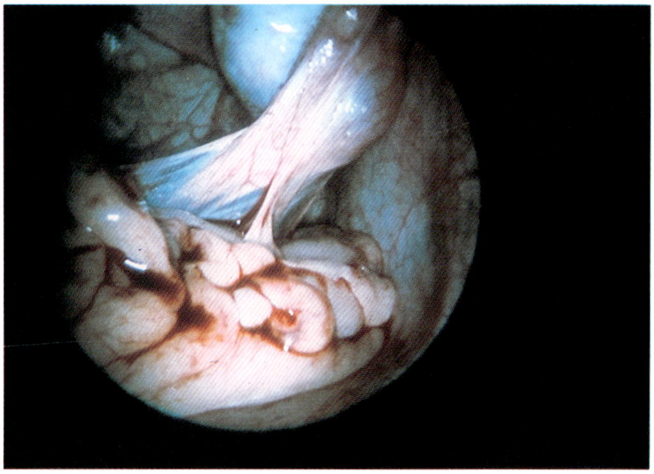

Fig. 31-22

Instrument setup for hysteroscopy.

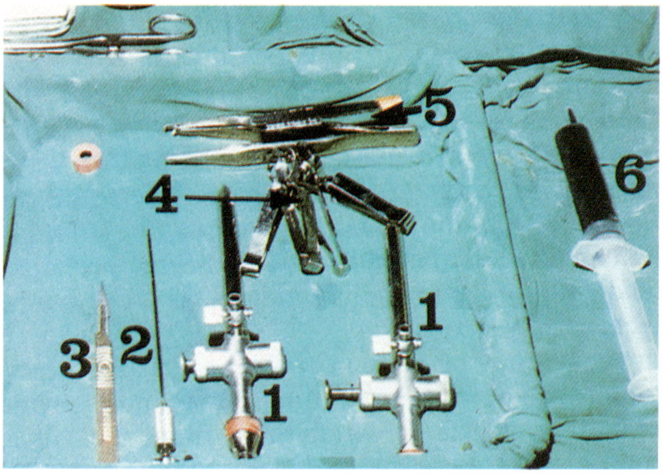

Fig. 31-23

Hasson cannula for open laparoscopy.

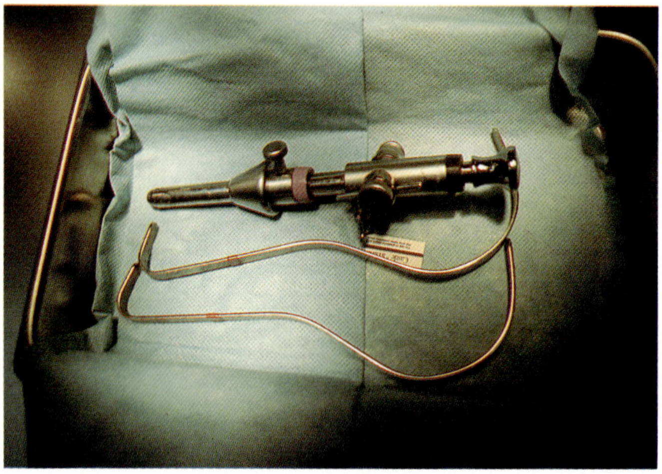

Fig. 31-24

Hamou hysteroscope and flexible instruments (Hunt).

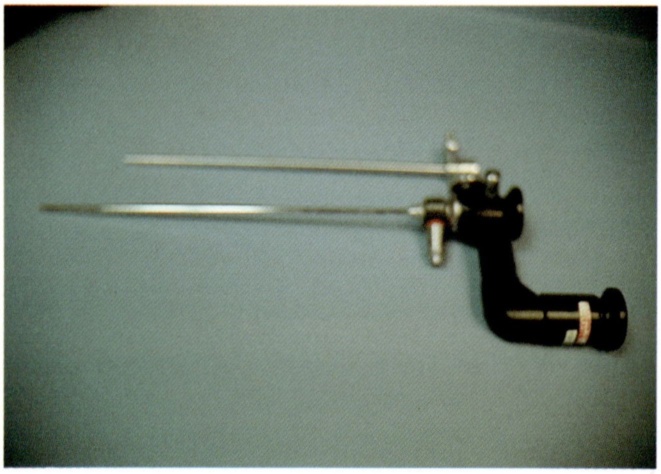

Fig. 31-25

Hysteroscope.

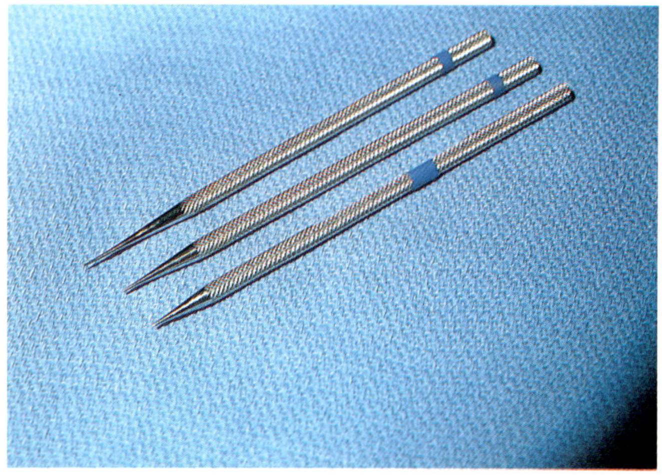

Fig. 31-26

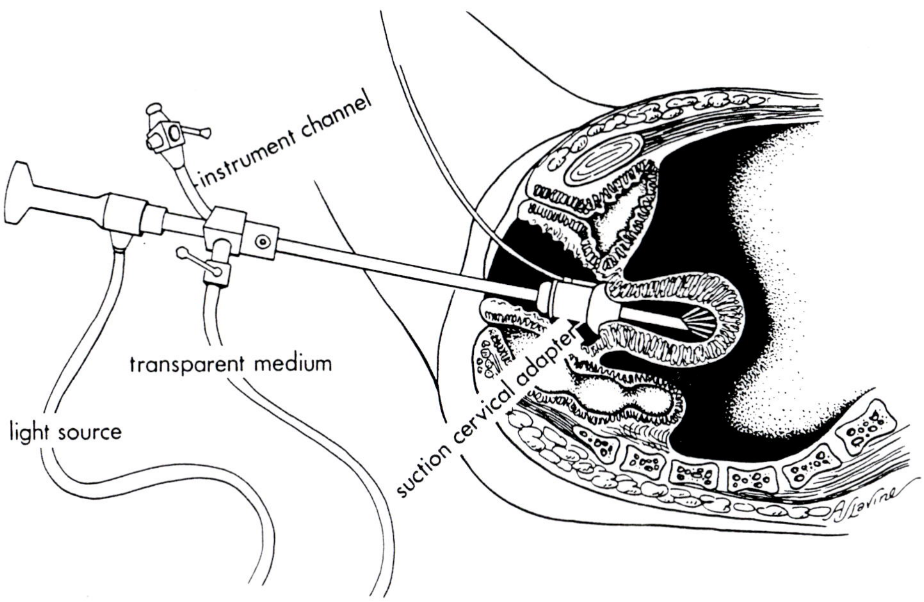

Fig. 31-27

Hysteroscopy using dextran, may use carbon dioxide also (Reprinted with permission from Jones[2]).

Cervical canal (Figs. 31-28 through 31-30 reprinted with permission from Semm[4]).

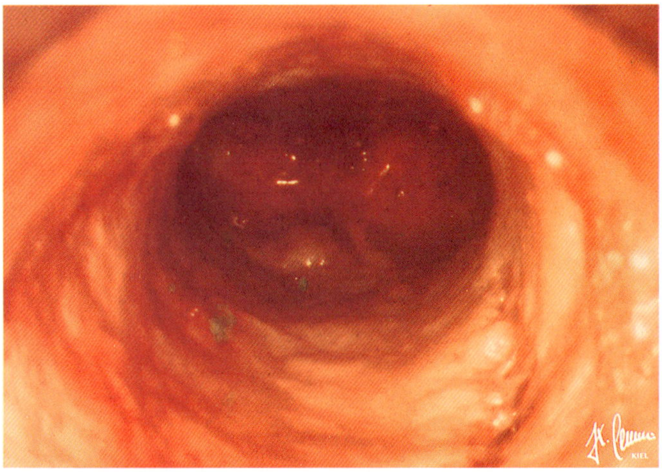

Fig. 31-28

Arcuate uterine cavity.

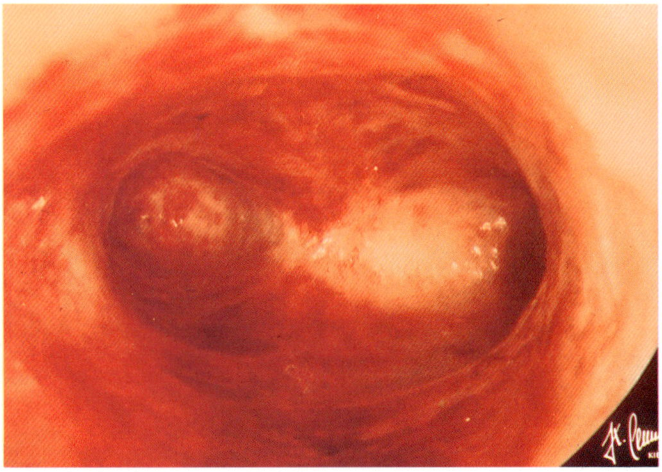

Fig. 31-29

Internal tubal os.

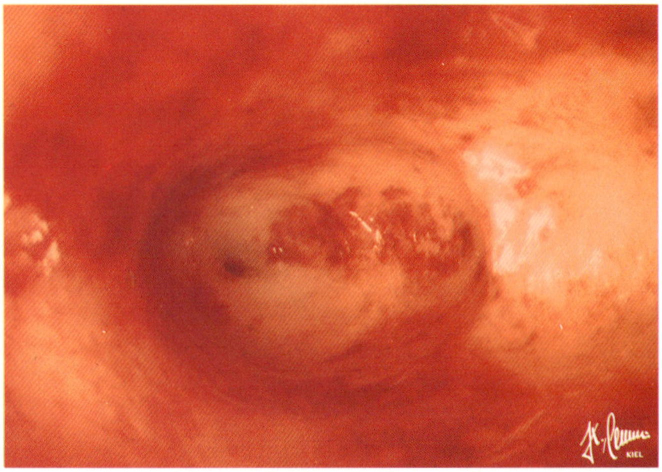

Fig. 31-30

Intracavitary myoma (Figs. 31-31 through 31-36 reprinted with permission from Phillips[3]).

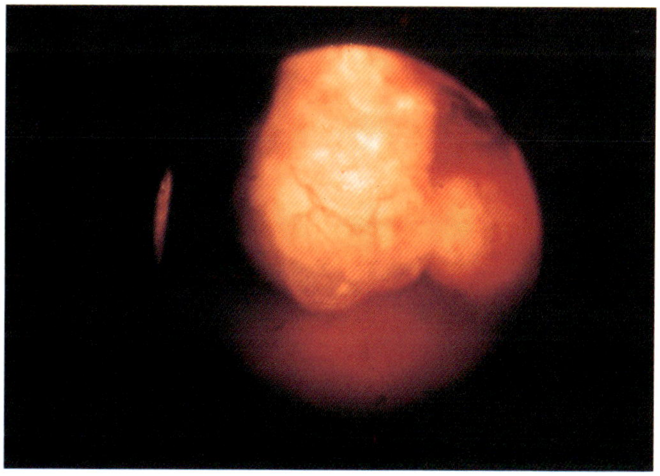

Fig. 31-31

Endometrial polyps.

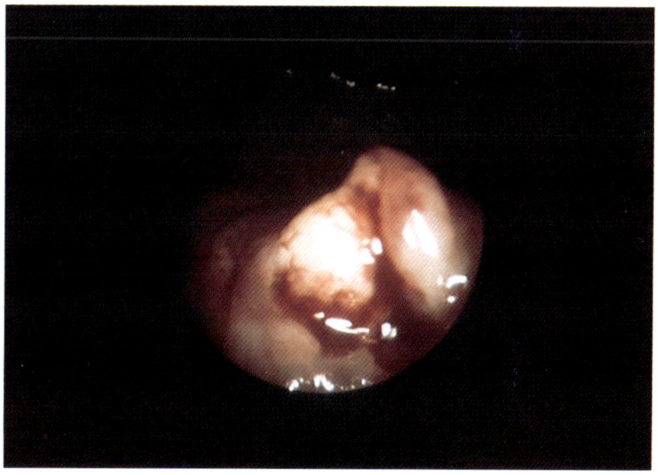

Fig. 31-32

Uterine intracavitary adhesions.

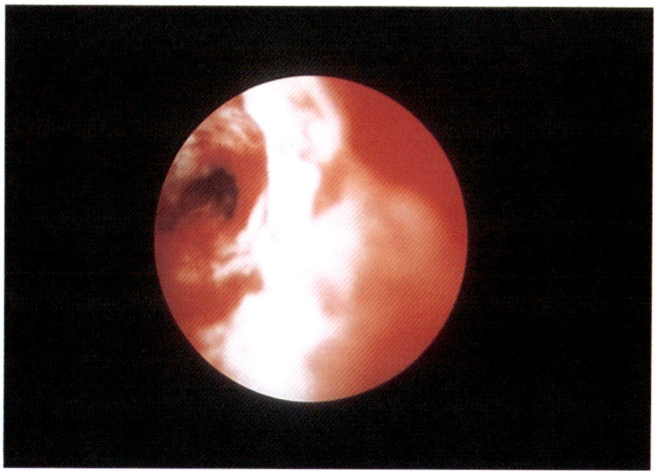

Fig. 31-33

Early pregnancy implantation.

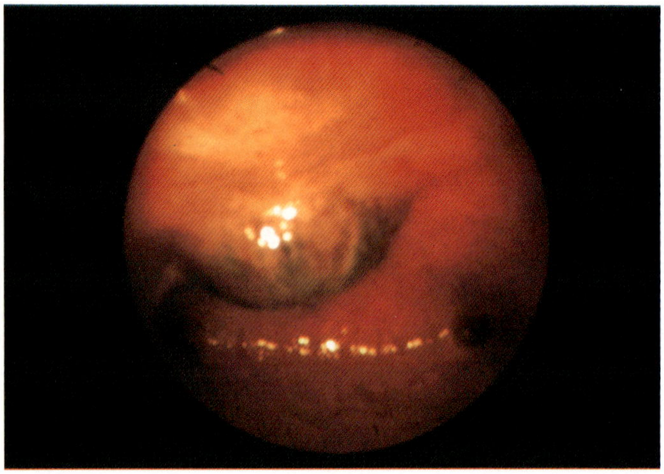

Fig. 31-34

Septate uterus.

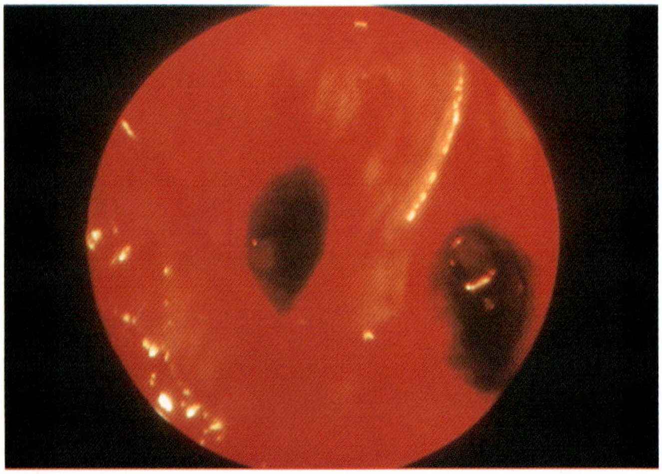

Fig. 31-35

Decidual reaction.

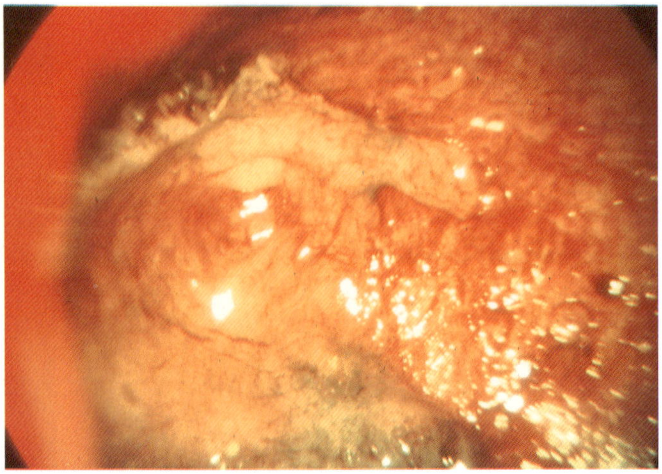

Fig. 31-36

Uterine tubal lavage using Buxton clamp and intracath and blue dye (Reprinted with permission from Patton[5]).

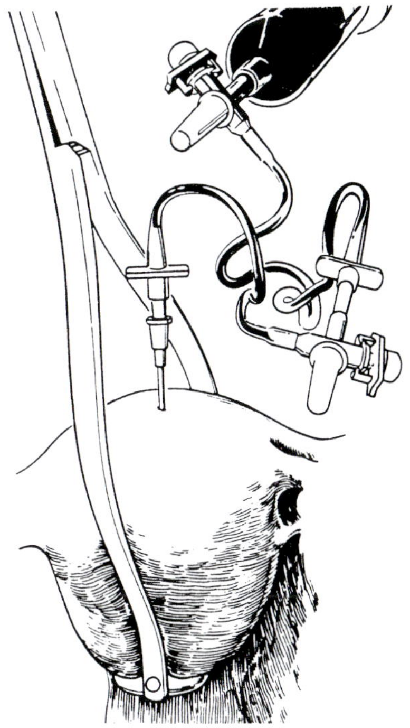

Fig. 31-37

Actual appearance.

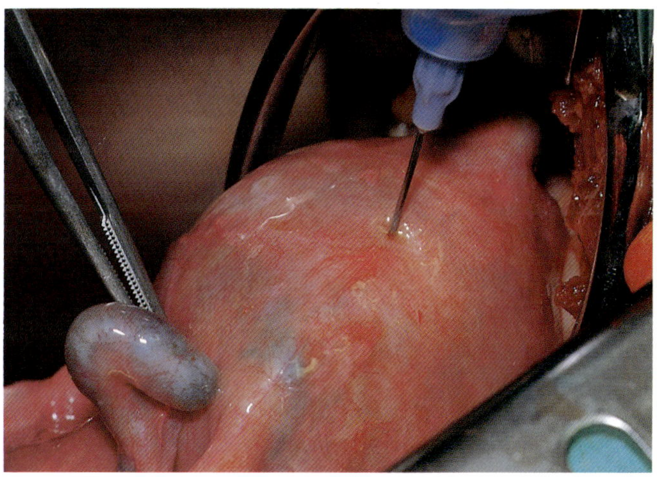

Fig. 31-38

Uterotubal lavage using Harris uterine injector (Figs. 31-39 and 31-40 reprinted with permission from Patton[5]).

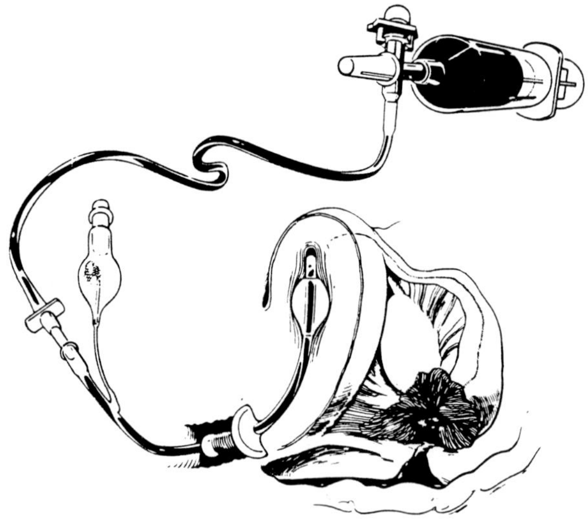

Fig. 31-39

Retrograde tubal injection instead of Stengel tubes.

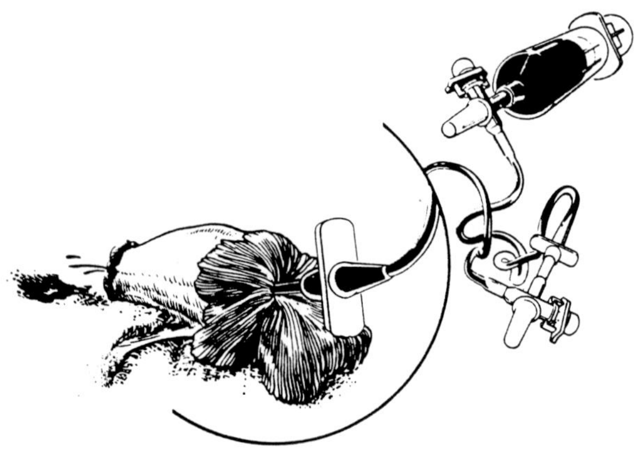

Fig. 31-40

All black and white line art is from Patton and Kistner. The use of either methylene blue or indigo carmine dyes is extremely useful for many situations either by laparoscopy, during microtubal procedures, or immediately following anastomoses to determine tubal patency. The staining of the tubal mucosa by these dyes is very helpful in finding the lumen either in the cornua or in the isthmic portion of the tube. See Figs. 31-45 and 31-46.

Setup using Buxton clamp, fundal needle, intratubal stent, rubber pad (Reprinted with permission from DeCherney[6]).

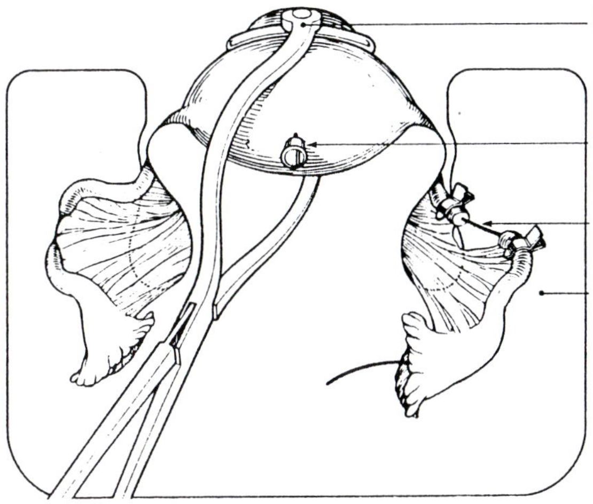

Fig. 31-41

Distal adhesions at laparoscopy (Reprinted with permission from Phillips[3]).

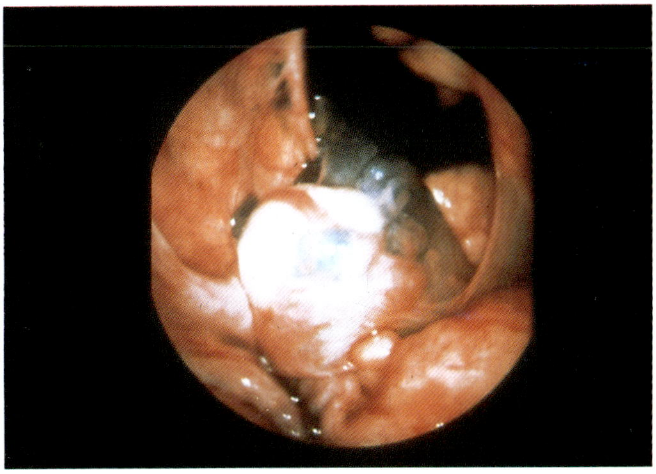

Fig. 31-42

Distal adhesions and hydrosalpinx at laparotomy.

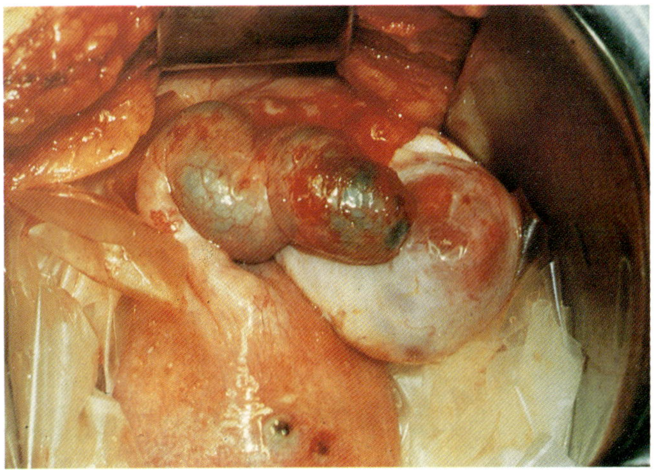

Fig. 31-43

Proximal tubal patency to end of stump.

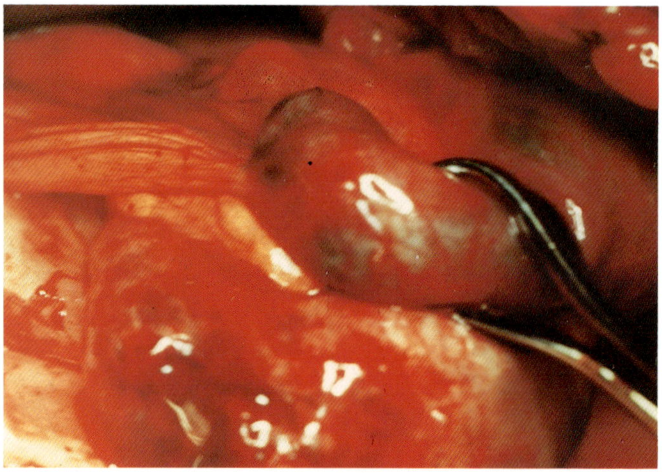

Fig. 31-44

Proximal tubal patency for anastomosis.

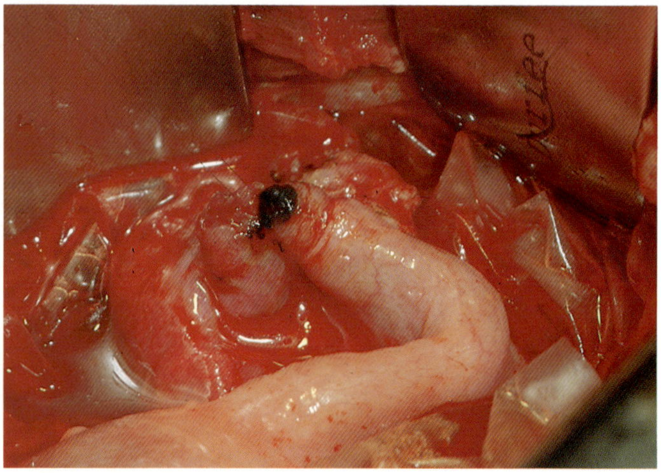

Fig. 31-45

Identifying tubal mucosa in difficult situation.

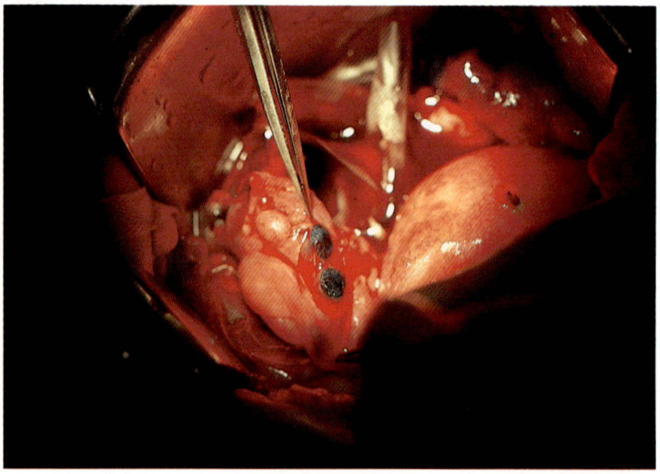

Fig. 31-46

Extensive inflammatory distal adhesions.

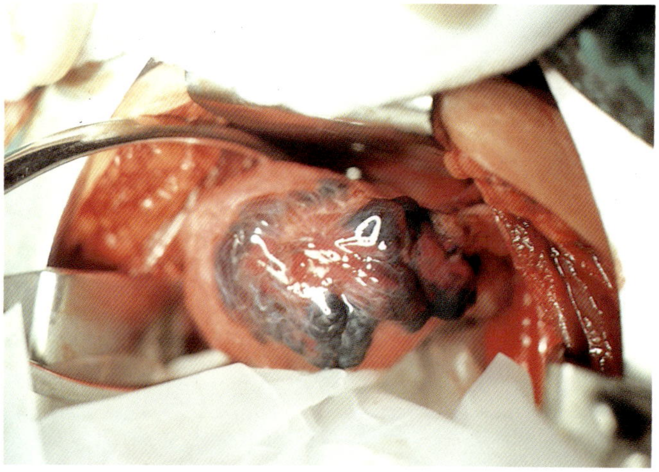

Fig. 31-47

Identification of interstitial lumen.

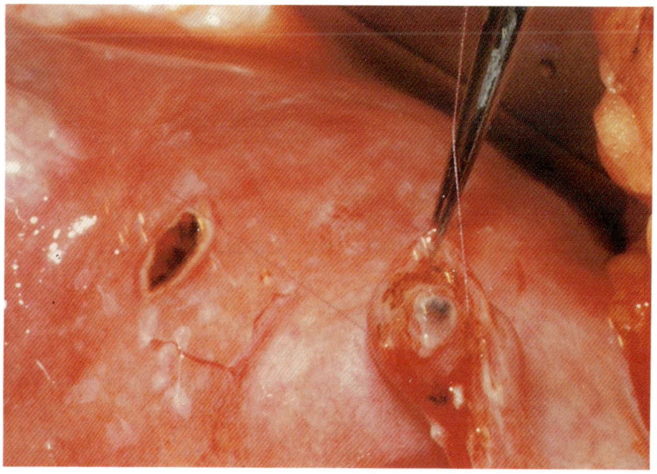

Fig. 31-48

Facilitates cornual isthmic anastomosis, blue mucosa.

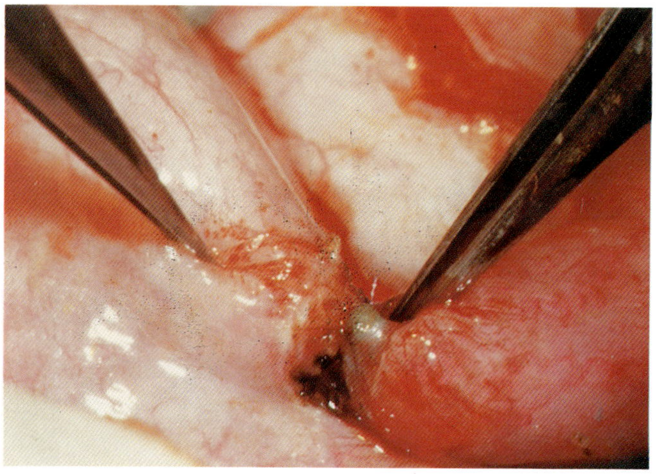

Fig. 31-49

Tubal patency after neosalpingostomy.

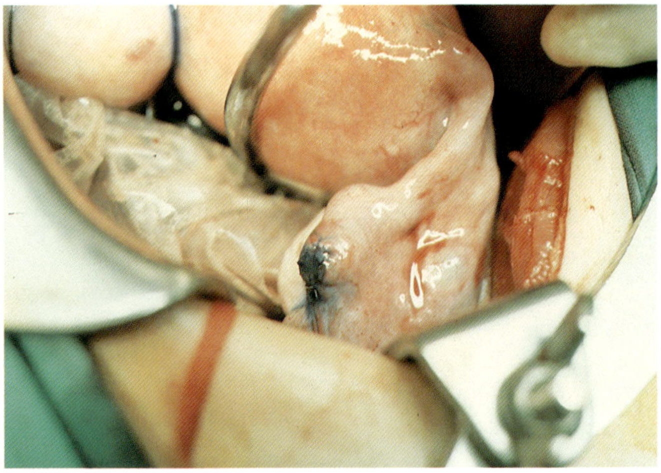

Fig. 31-50

Indicates patent tube, note repaired ovary in background.

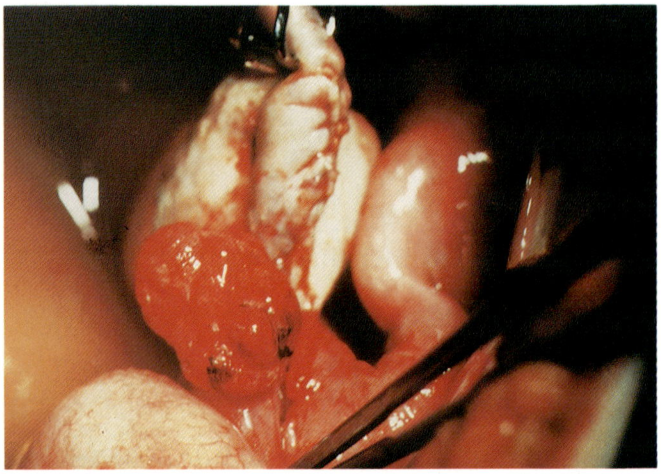

Fig. 31-51

Dye extruding from opened fimbria.

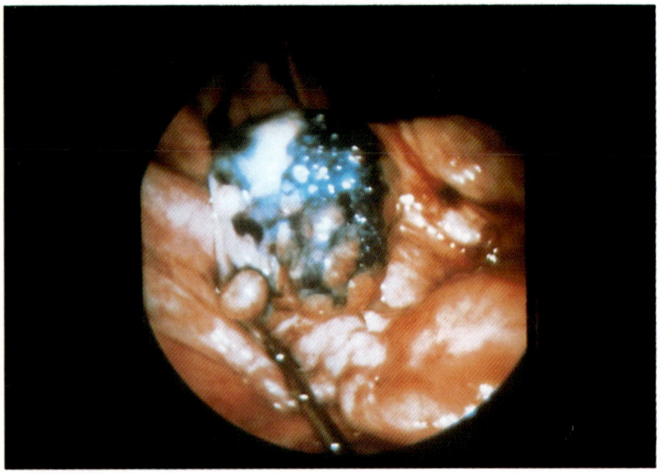

Fig. 31-52

Undiagnosed external tubal adhesions also involving the ovary.

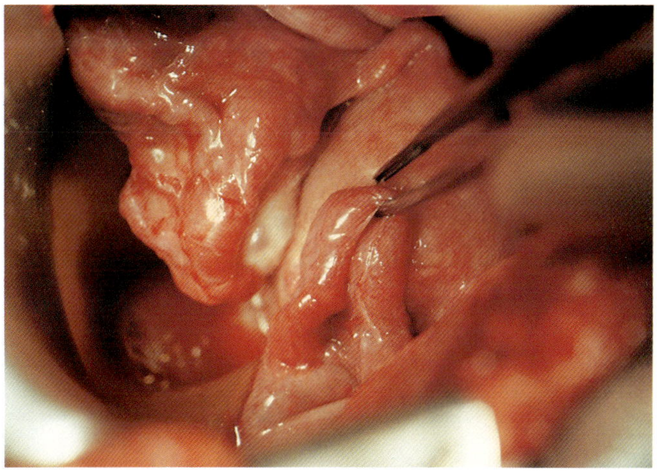

Fig. 31-53

Tubal ovarian adhesions.

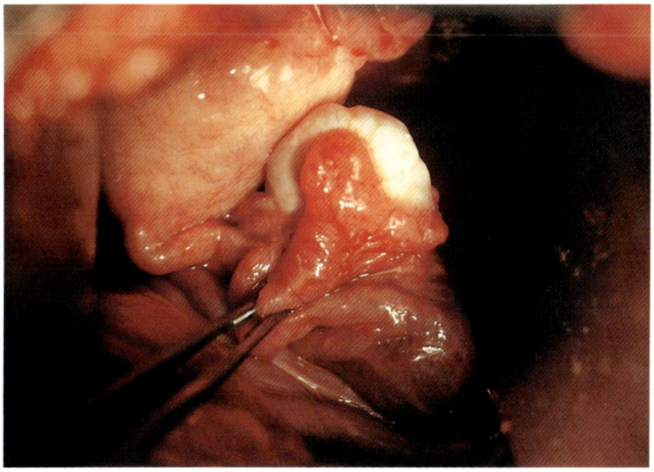

Fig. 31-54

Postfimbriectomy tube with mild hydrosalpinx.

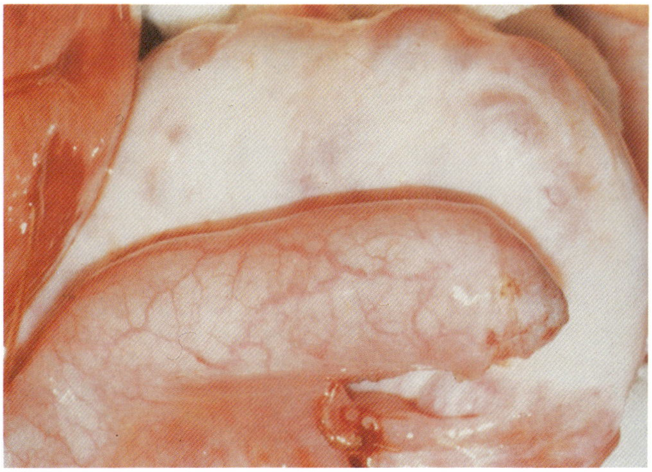

Fig. 31-55

Peritubal and ovarian inflammatory cysts.

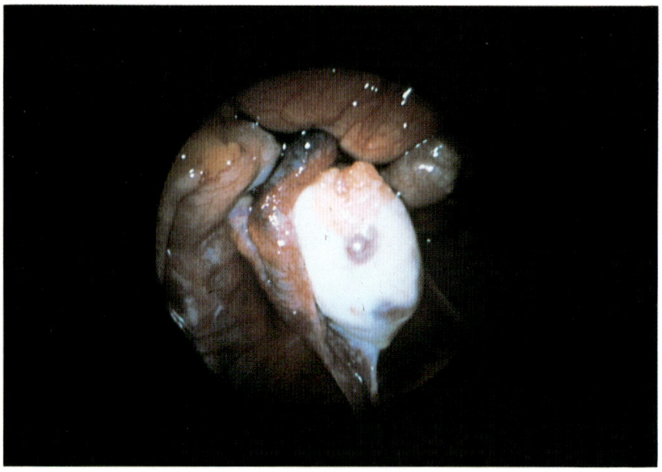

Fig. 31-56

Blood-filled Fallopian tube.

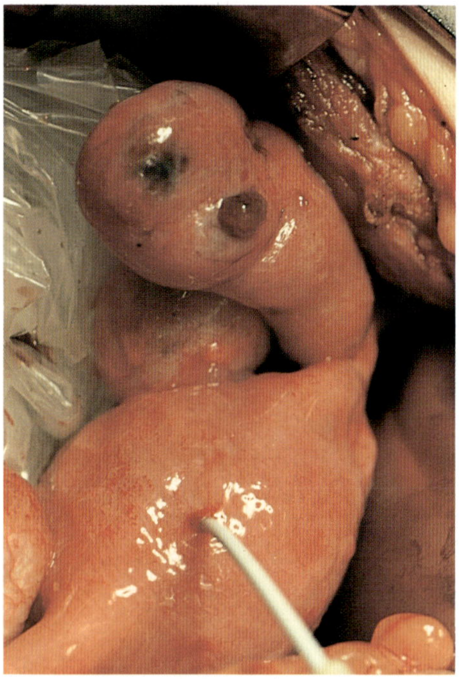

Fig. 31-57

Ultrasound machine with vaginal applicator added.

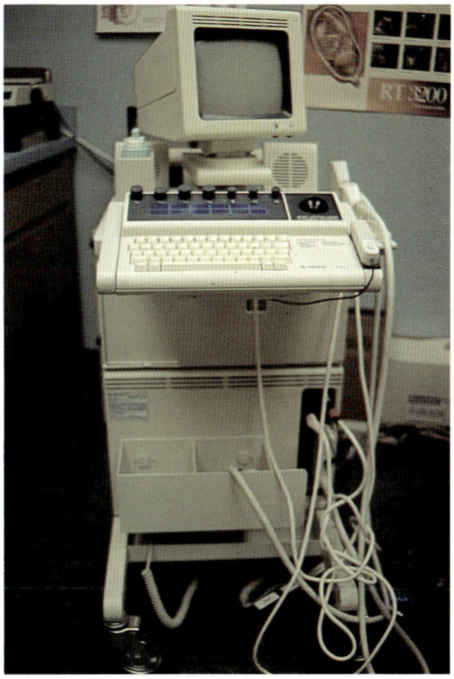

Fig. 31-58

Ultrasound picture of tubo-ovarian abscess.

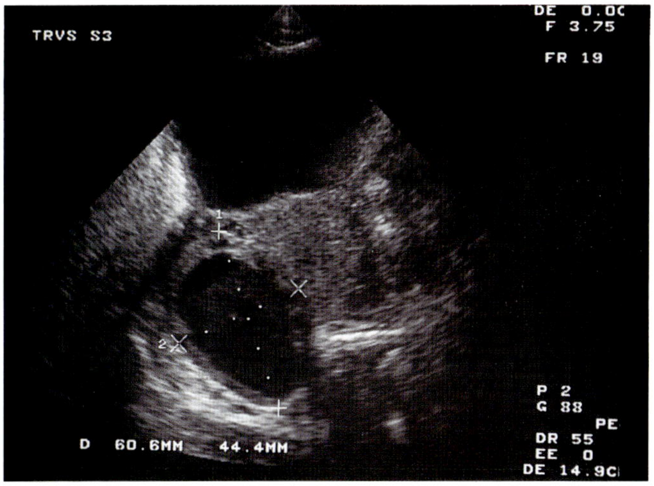

Fig. 31-59

Ultrasound picture of follicle cyst of the ovary.

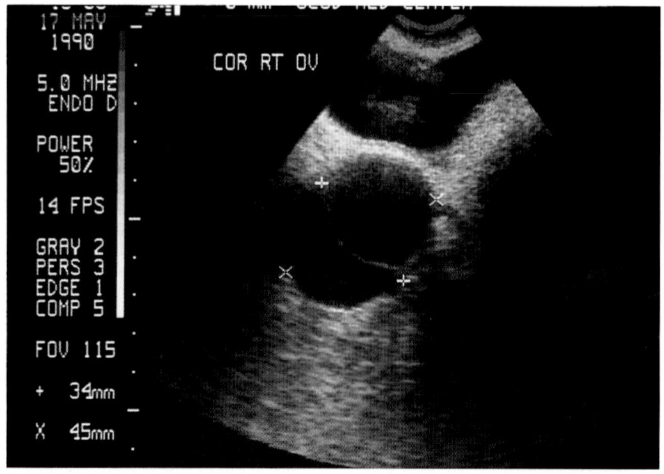

Fig. 31-60

Ultrasound picture of a myoma.

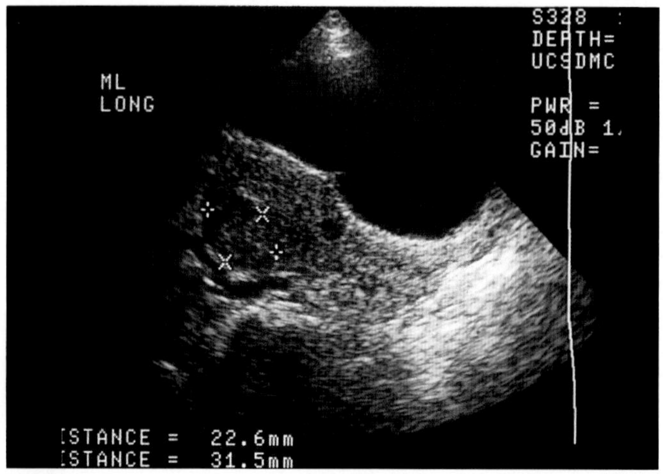

Fig. 31-61

Ultrasound picture of pelvic abscess.

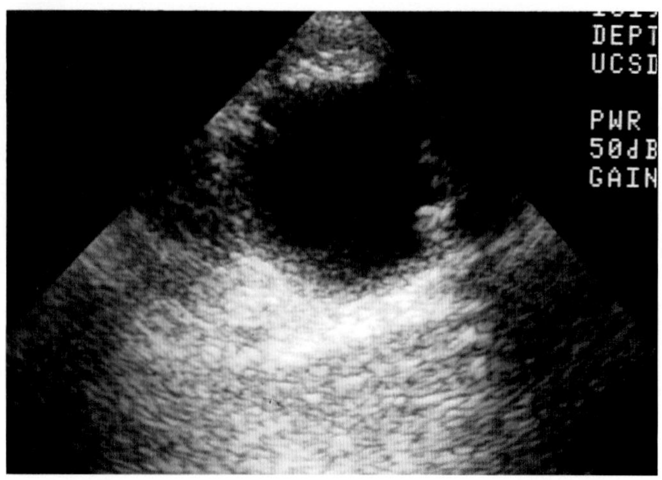

Fig. 31-62

Ultrasound picture of hemorrhagic corpus luteum.

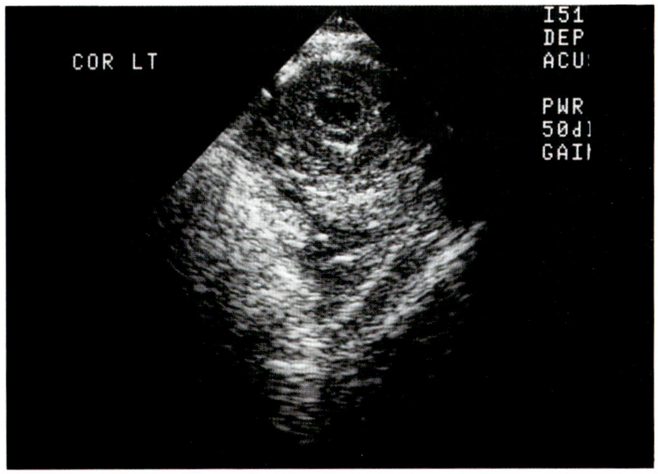

Fig. 31-63

If either laparoscopy, HSG, or ultrasound had been used in most of these cases, these surprises would not have existed.

Stein-Leventhal ovary.

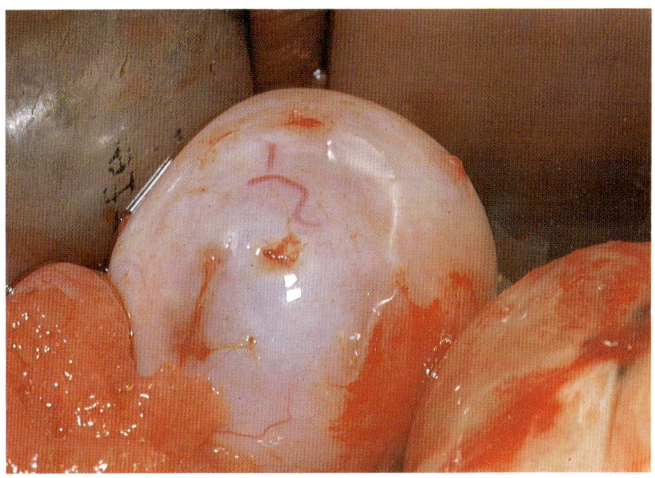

Fig. 31-64

Hemorrhaging corpus luteum.

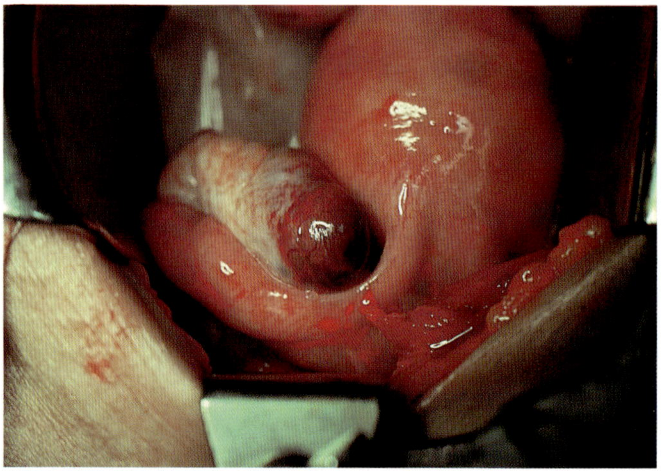

Fig. 31-65

Hemorrhagic corpus luteum.

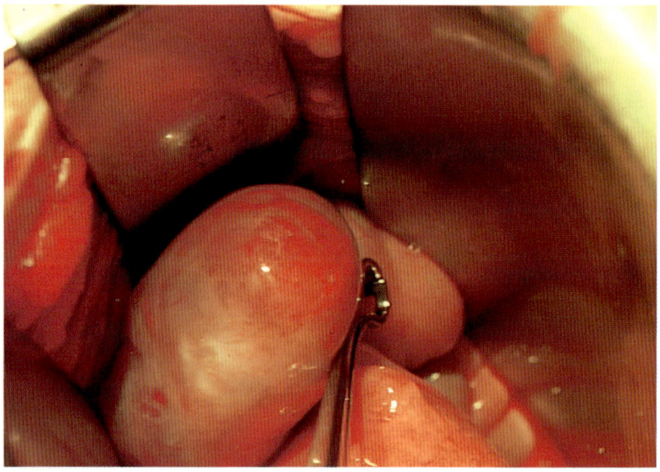

Fig. 31-66

Extra long, but patent tubes.

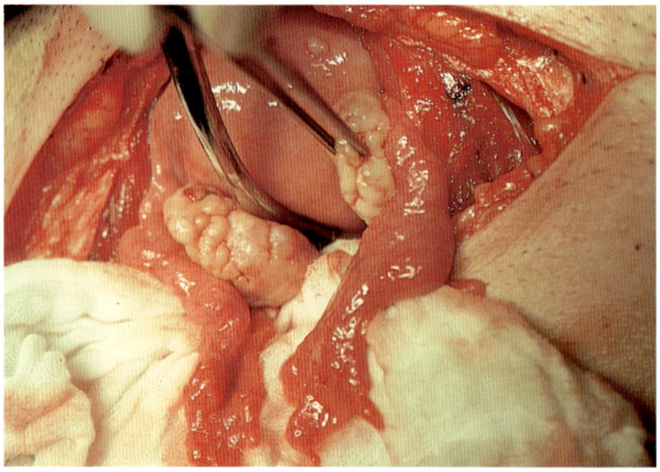

Fig. 31-67

Accessory fimbria.

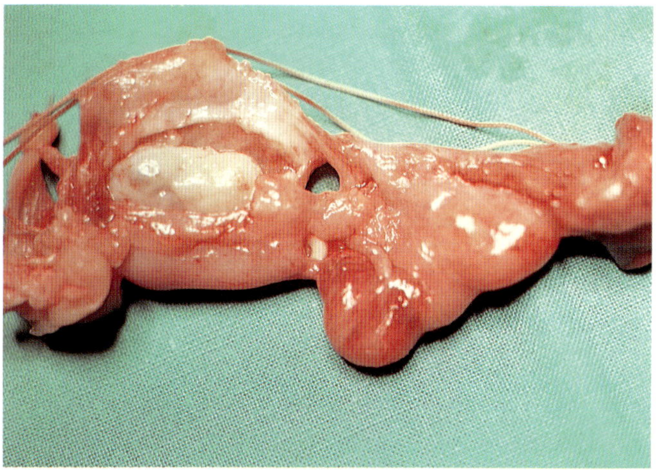

Fig. 31-68

Separate uterine fundi.

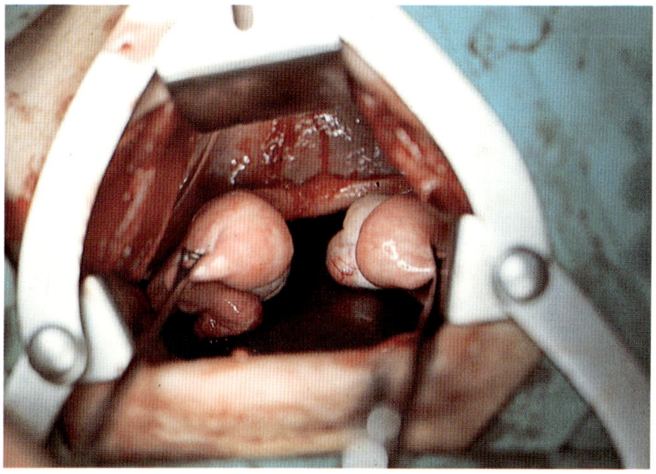

Fig. 31-69

References

1. Kelly H. *Operative Gynecology*. Vol I. New York, NY: D. Appleton; 1898.
2. Jones H, Rock J. *Reparative and Constructive Surgery of the Female Generative Tract*. Baltimore, Md: Williams and Wilkins; 1983.
3. Phillips J. Instructional slides from: *Endoscopy in Gynecology*. Published by A.A.G.L., Downey, Calif; 1985.
4. Semm K. *Atlas of Gynecology and Hysteroscopy, Slide-Atlas*. Philadelphia, Penn: WB Saunders Company; 1980.
5. Patton G, Kistner R. *Atlas of Infertility Surgery*. 2nd ed. Boston, Mass: Little, Brown and Company; 1984.
6. DeCherney A. *Reproductive Failure*. New York, NY: Churchill Livingstone; 1986.

Chapter 32

Lysis of Adhesions, Fimbrial Release and Repair

Raphael B. Durfee, MD

LYSIS OF ADHESIONS

A high percentage of cases that are subjects for various uses of microsurgery are found to have adhesions to some degree. The real problem with lysis of adhesions is that unless the fibrinous base of the adhesion is completely removed from the underlying tissue, the adhesion will re-form. This may be even more severe than the original formation. Until the advent of the laser, the total removal of an adhesive process was almost impossible without removing the surface layer of tissue. Now, however, using the unfocused low to moderate intensity of the CO_2 laser, only the surface layer of cells is removed, together with the adhesion base. The addition of hypertonic solutions has been somewhat successful, but the combination is very effective.

FIMBRIAL RELEASE

Coagulated, even phimotic, fimbria are a challenge for the microsurgeon. If the feathery tissues are comparatively normal when released, their function of ovum collection may be renewed. If the tissues are too severely damaged, however, reconstruction may be abandoned in favor of creating a neosalpingostomy using the ampullary portion for this purpose. If the ampulla is also badly damaged, a successful neosalpingostomy is very doubtful. These adhesions may be lysed with needle tip electrodissection or the laser. Fimbriaplasty involves very exacting fine suturing with 9 or 10-0 polyglycolic material. If prolene is used, it should be very sparingly applied, and inversion of the knot is essential.

Hydrosalpinx, Post Inflammatory or Endometriosis Related

Almost all post pelvic inflammatory disease hydrosalpinx cases are not readily repaired. Regeneration of mucosa is not frequently sufficient to heal the damaged mucosal surface, and since these fragile ciliated cells are apparently necessary for tubal ovum transport, no amount of skillful microplasty will restore normal function. In our opinion, moderately or severely damaged tubes should be removed and the ovaries placed so that ovum harvesting for in vitro fertilization at a later date provides a potentially better opportunity for intrauterine pregnancy. Diseased tubes provide an ideal region for the development of tubal pregnancy.

Manual control, coagulation and cutting with modified Bovie, can use micro-tips.

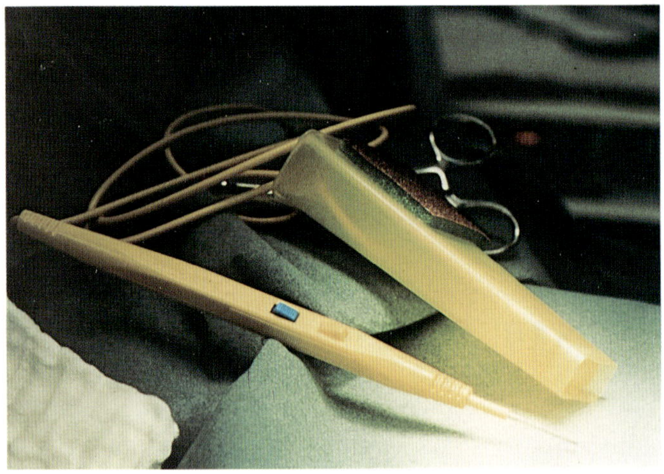

Fig. 32-1

Elmed micro-tips; insulated, cutting (Reprinted with permission from Elmed[1]).

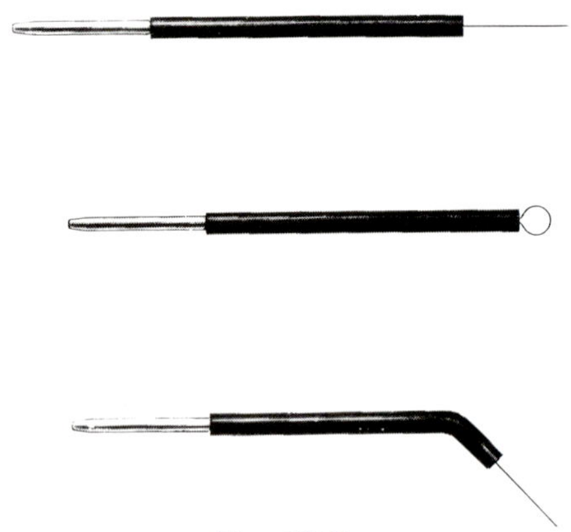

Fig. 32-2

Elmed micro-tips; non-insulated, cutting, fine.

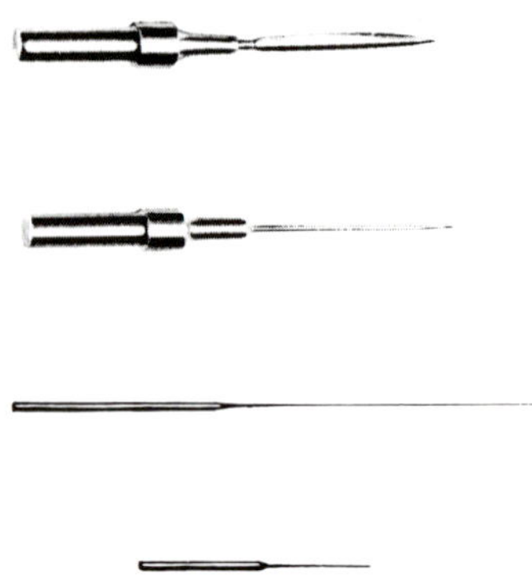

Fig. 32-3

Local hemostasis using coagulation tip, pulsatile irrigation (Reprinted with permission from Hunt[2]).

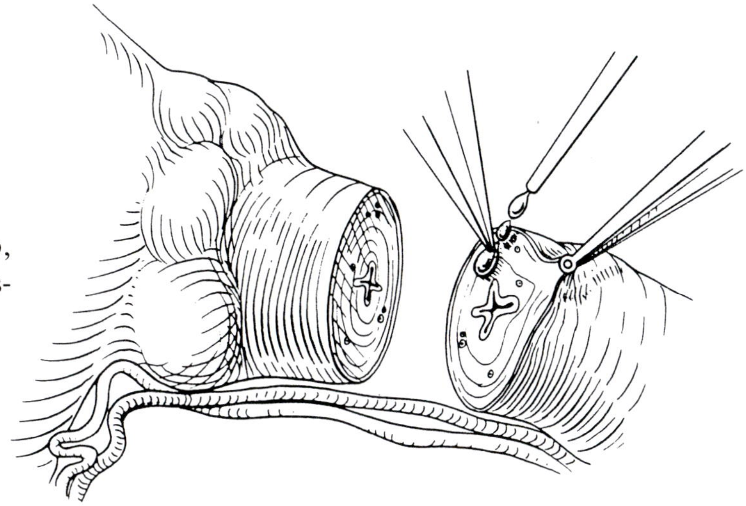

Fig. 32-4

Tip in action with irrigator.

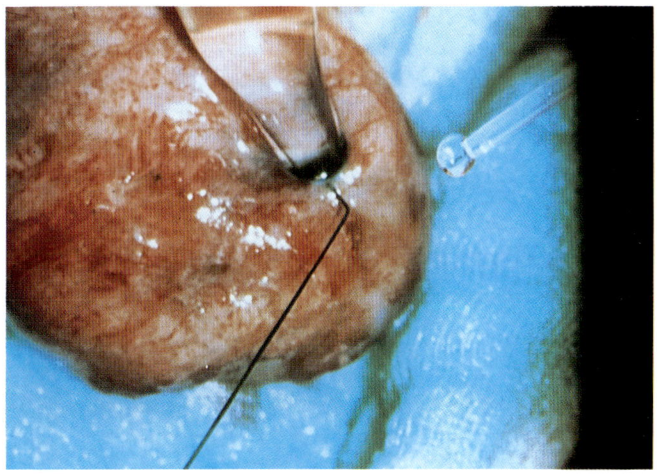

Fig. 32-5

Elmed coagulation micro-tips, insulated, and not (Reprinted with permission from Elmed[1]).

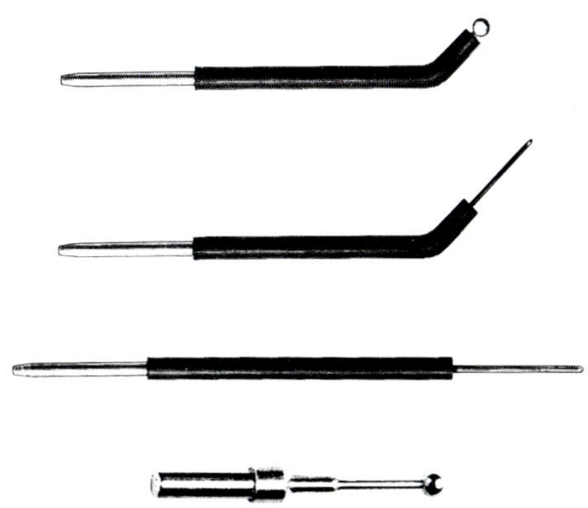

Fig. 32-6

Fine electrocoagulation, adhesion lysis, adnexal structures (Reprinted with permission from Patton[3]).

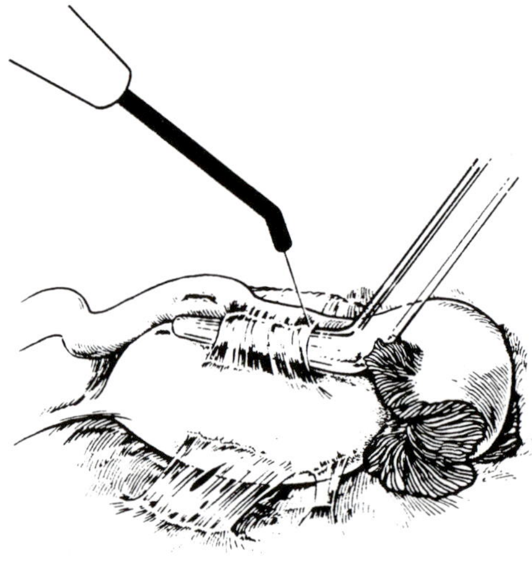

Fig. 32-7

Adnexal adhesions to anterior abdominal wall (Reprinted with permission from Phillips[4]).

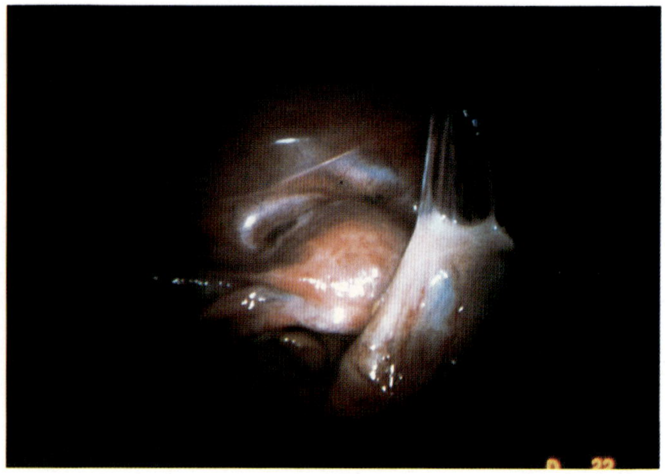

Fig. 32-8

Scissors dissection, adnexal adhesions, using fine sharp scissors (Figs. 32-9 and 32-10 reprinted with permission from Patton[3]).

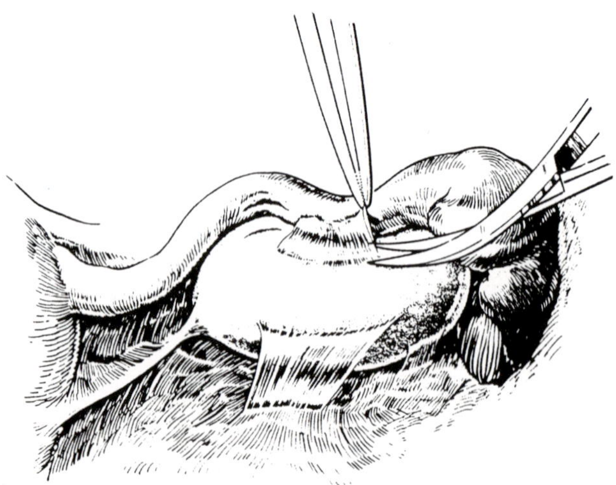

Fig. 32-9

Same, fimbrial adhesions with glass rod.

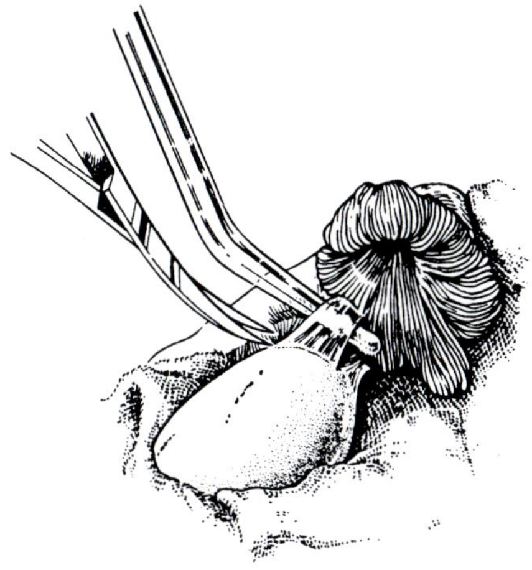

Fig. 32-10

Post-surgical tubal adhesions (Reprinted with permission from Phillips[4]).

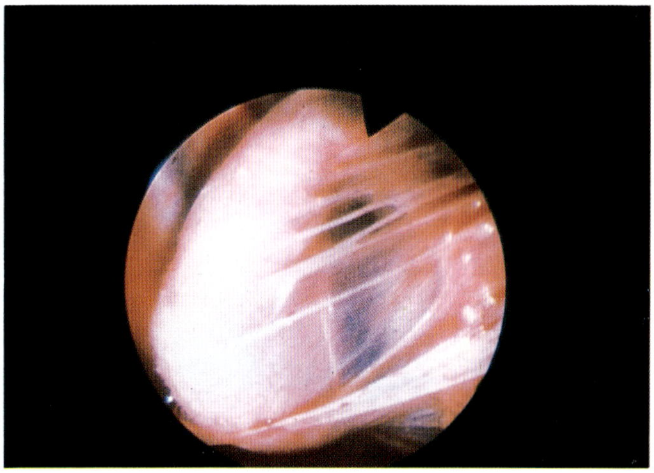

Fig. 32-11

Suture of mucosal defect using 8-0 or 9-0 (Reprinted with permission from Patton[3]).

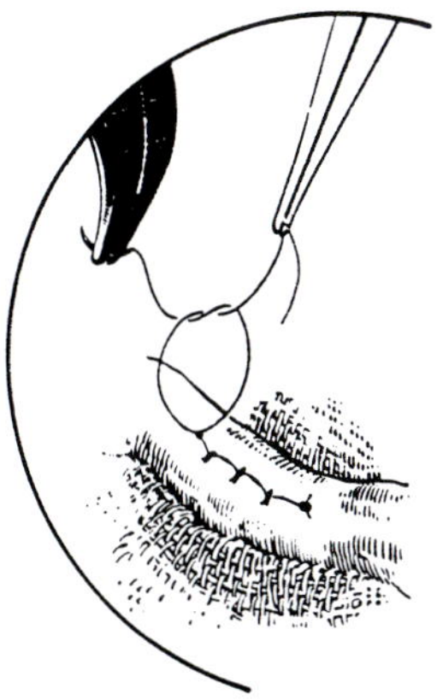

Fig. 32-12

The degree of involvement of the fimbria and distal tube with adhesions in hydrosalpinx, intrafimbrial adhesions, and damage to the endosalpinx determines the extent to which fimbriaplasty and fimbrial release can be successfully accomplished. Past a certain point, post inflammatory changes are irreversible from a functional viewpoint. The high risk of intratubal pregnancy (ectopic) following repair of a tube damaged by bacterial infection does not justify the effort to really repair these tubes. A better choice is to arrange the ovaries for easy follicle aspiration for in vitro fertilization attempts.

Postgonorrheal PID with distal hydrosalpinx partial phimosis of the fimbria and partial obstruction of the other one.

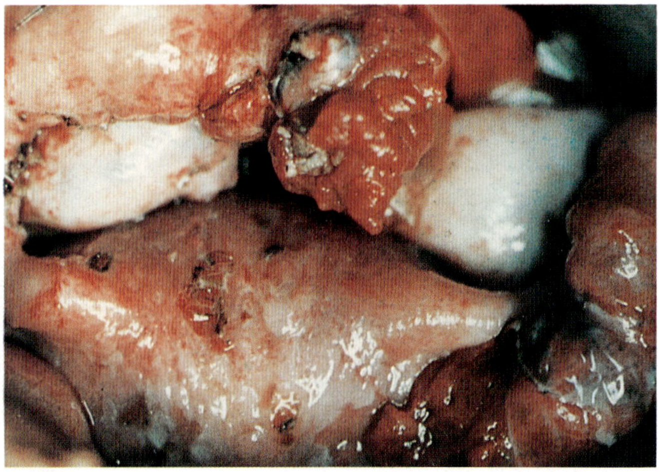

Fig. 32-13

Fimbrialovarian adhesion.

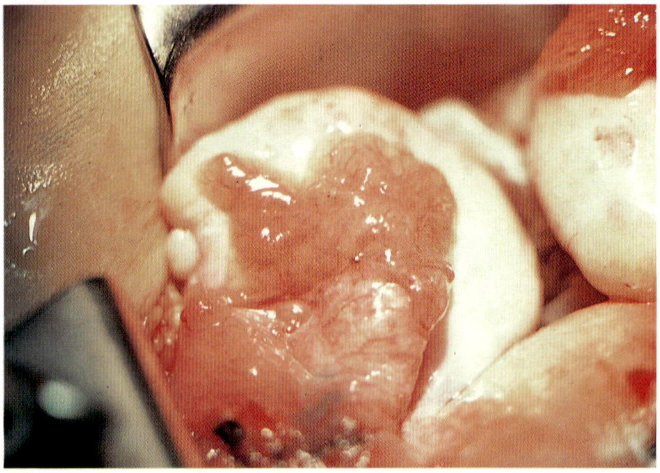

Fig. 32-14

Ovarian adhesions (Reprinted with permission from Phillips[4]).

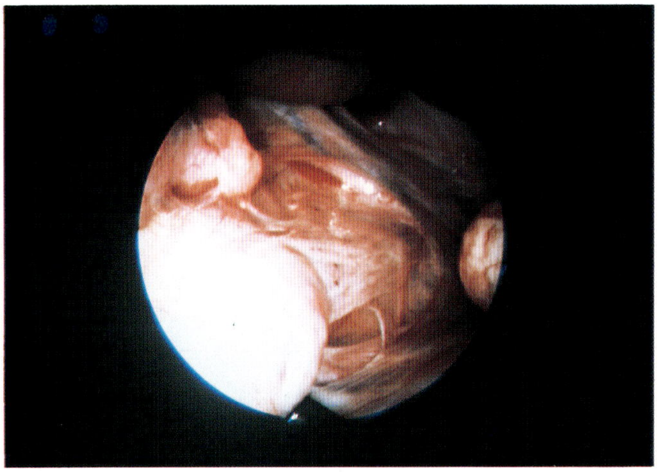

Fig. 32-15

Electro-dissection of ovarian adhesions (Reprinted with permission from Patton[3]).

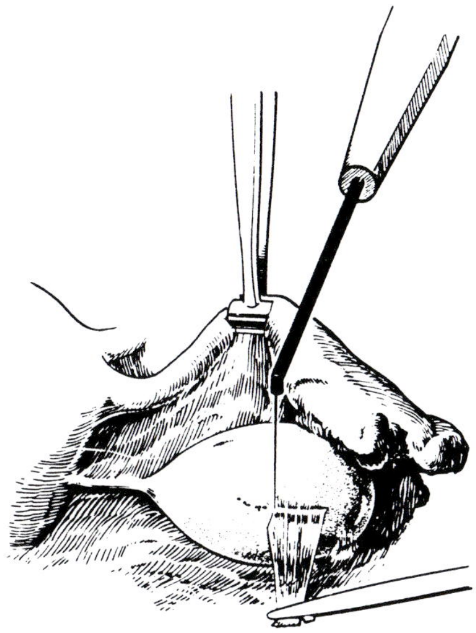

Fig. 32-16

PID, hydrosalpinx, closed fimbria, first incision (Figs. 32-17 through 32-19 reprinted with permission from Rock[5]).

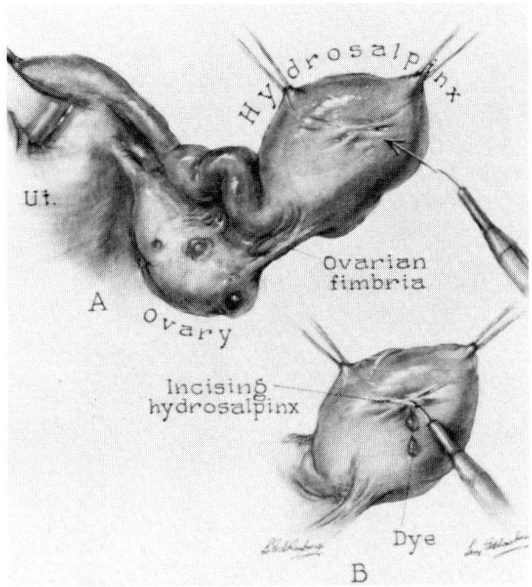

Fig. 32-17

Next four steps in treatment.

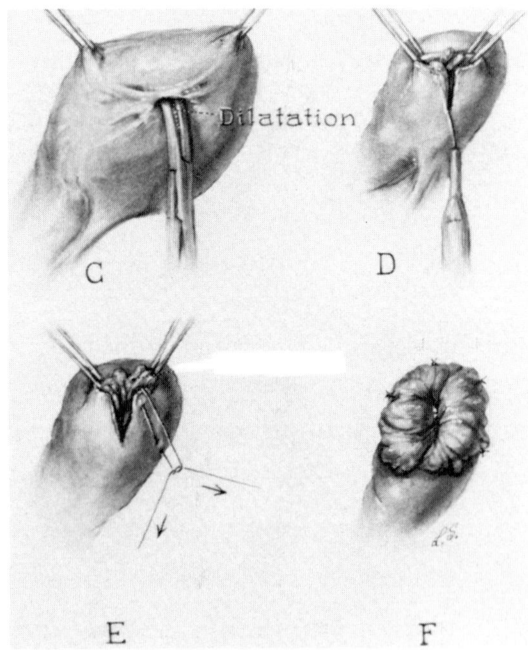

Fig. 32-18

Lateral view of same process.

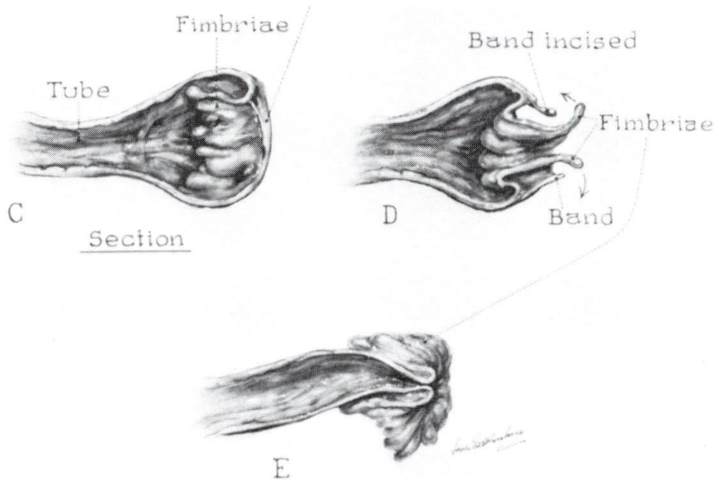

Fig. 32-19

Dye-filled, obstructed fimbria with hydrosalpinx.

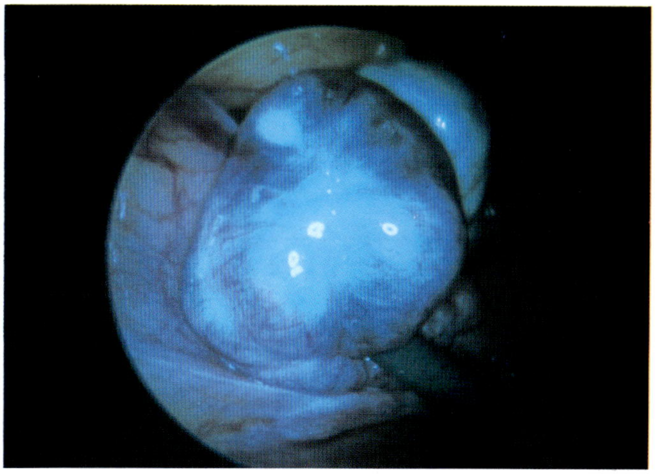

Fig. 32-20

Lysis of peri-tubal adhesions (Figs. 32-21 through 32-25 reprinted with permission from Patton[3]).

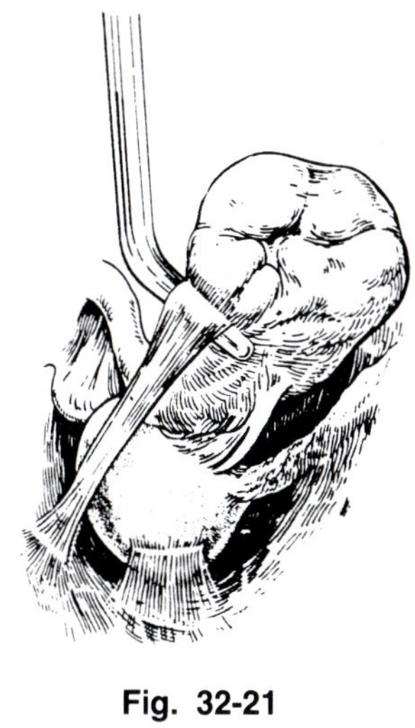

Fig. 32-21

Lysis of adhesions, both tubal and ovarian.

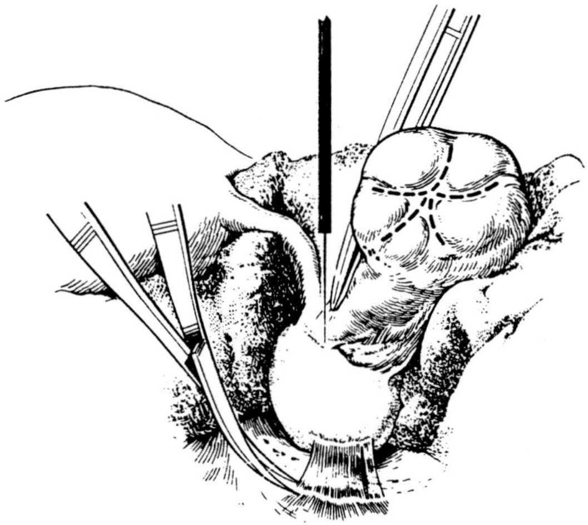

Fig. 32-22

Incisions made by fine electrodissection at areas delineated in Fig. 32-22.

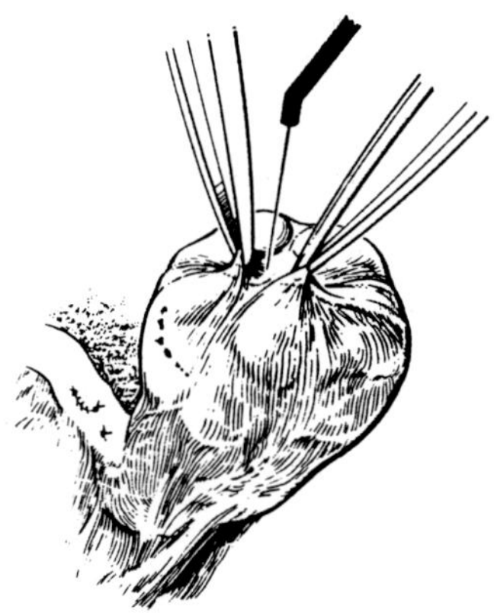

Fig. 32-23

Final release of fimbria by sharp dissection.

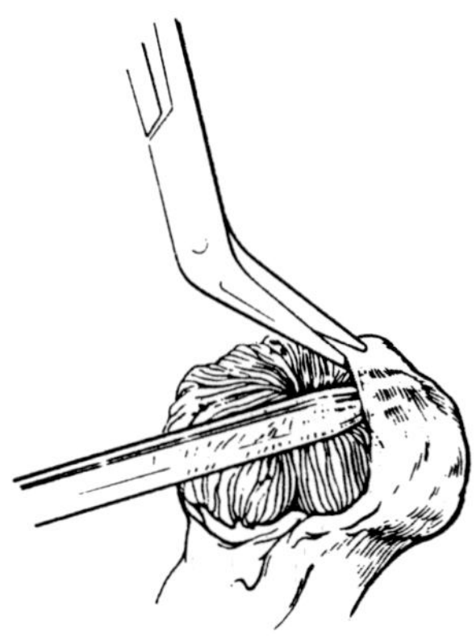

Fig. 32-24

Everting sutures, and serosal closure.

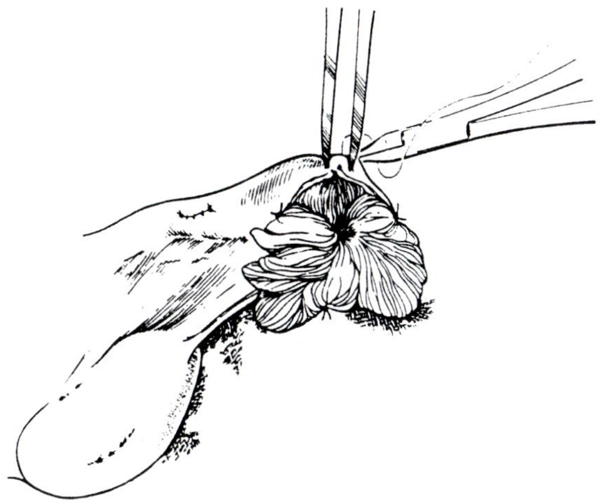

Fig. 32-25

Electrodissection, lysis of adhesions, fimbrial release, fimbriaplasty.

Peritubular adhesions, phimotic fimbria.

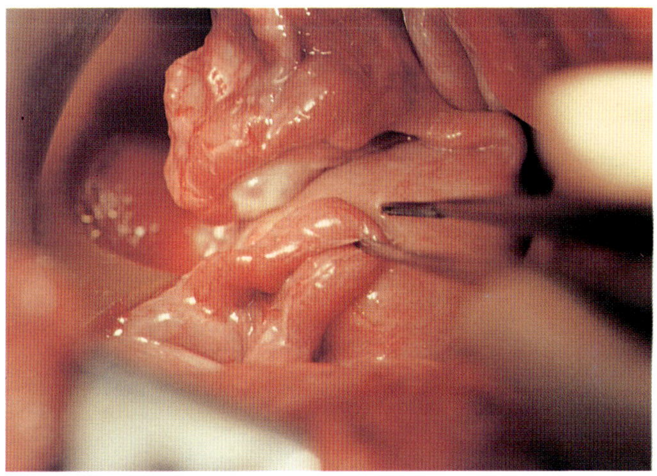

Fig. 32-26

Peritubular cysts, occluded fimbria.

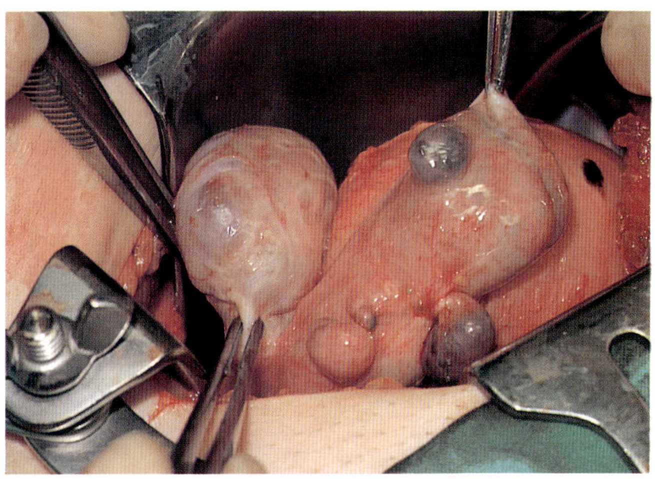

Fig. 32-27

Mild hydrosalpinx, obscured fimbria, tube open (blue dye).

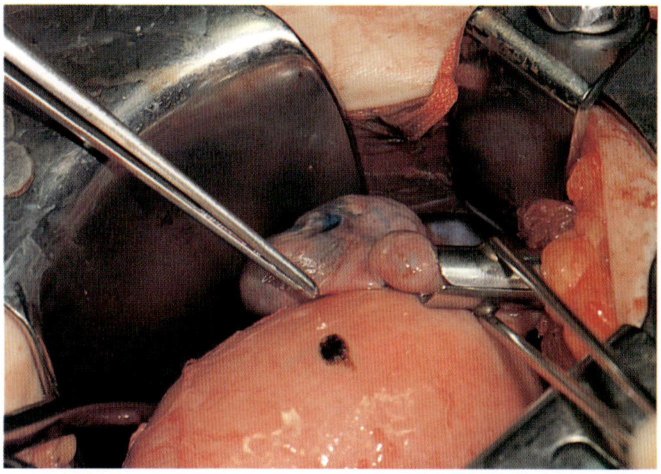

Fig. 32-28

Tubo-ovarian adhesions.

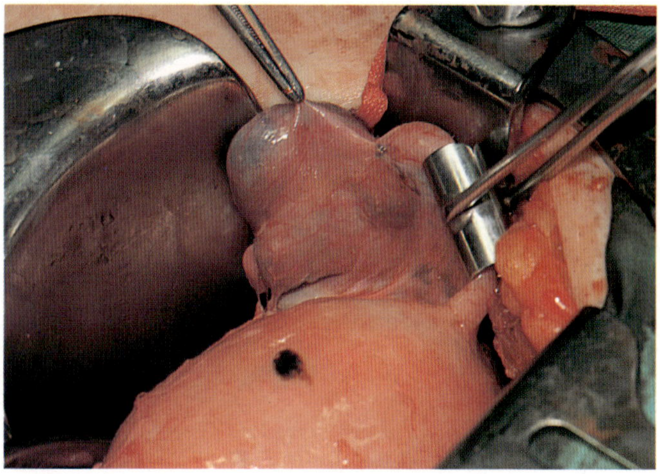

Fig. 32-29

Fimbrial and tubo-ovarian adhesions.

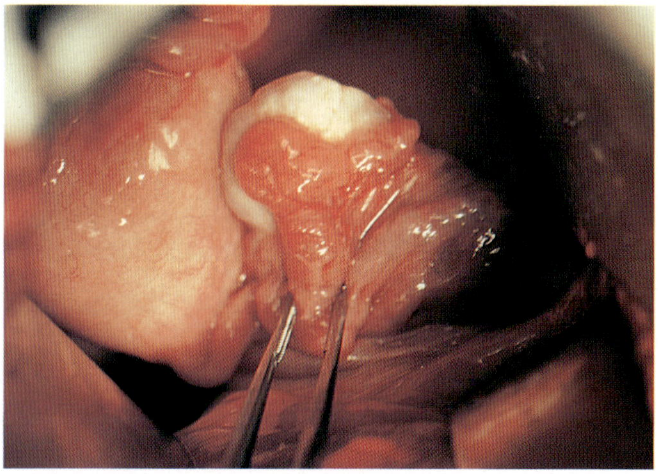

Fig. 32-30

Fimbrial phimosis, tubo-ovarian adhesions.

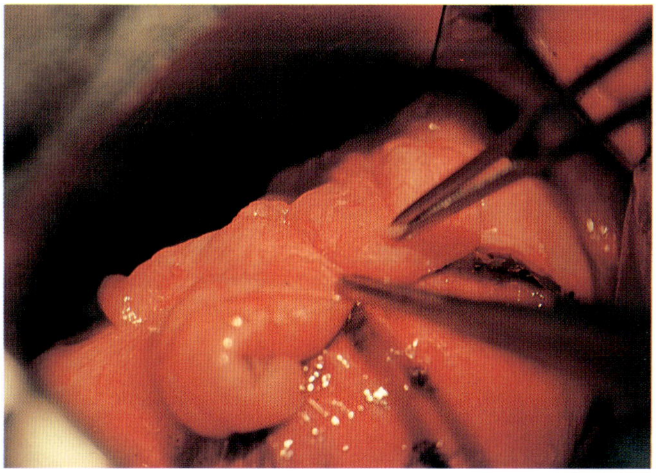

Fig. 32-31

Tiny phimosis, closed fimbria, ampullar buried Fallope ring.

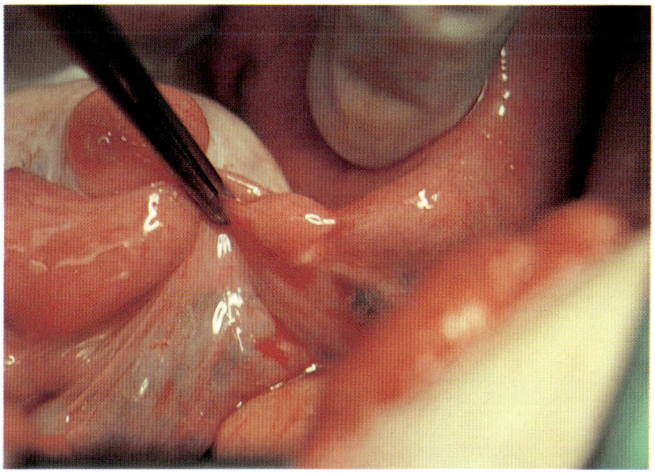

Fig. 32-32

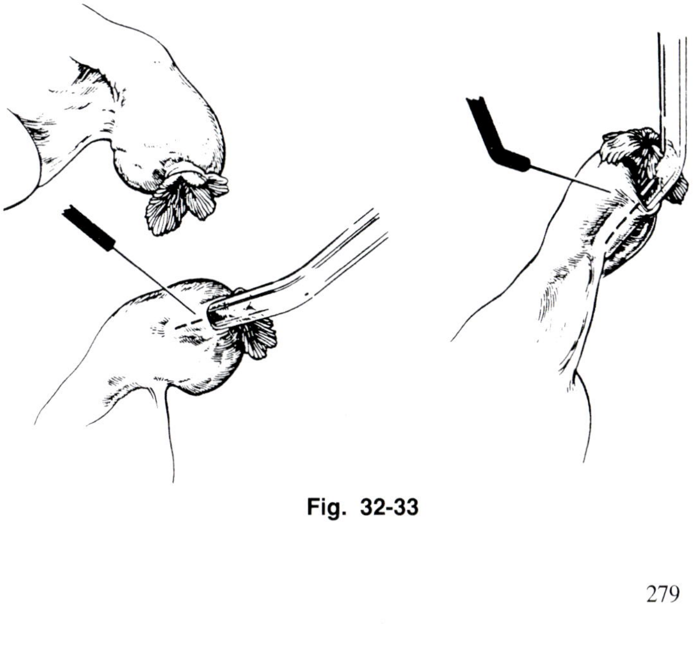

Fig. 32-33

Opening of phimosis (Figs. 32-33 through 32-37 reprinted with permission from Patton[3]).

Fimbrial deagglutination.

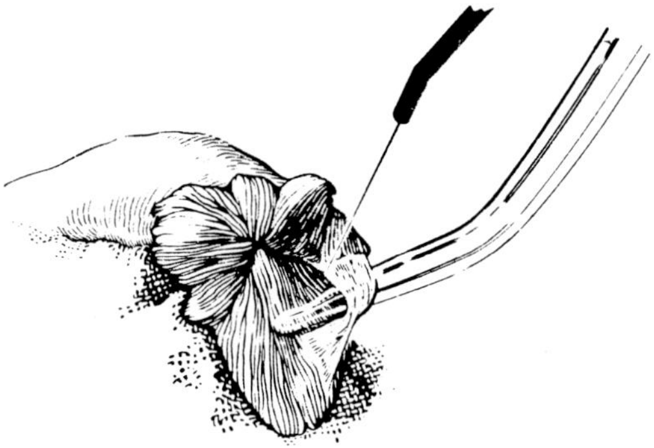

Fig. 32-34

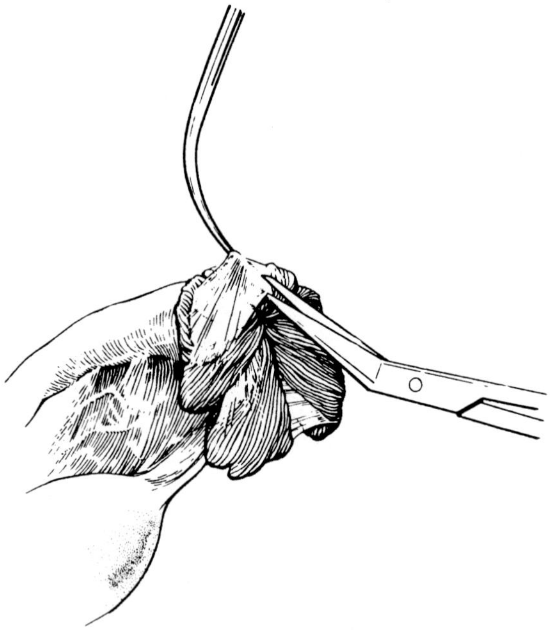

Fig. 32-35

Final release of fimbria.

Everting sutures, size 7-0.

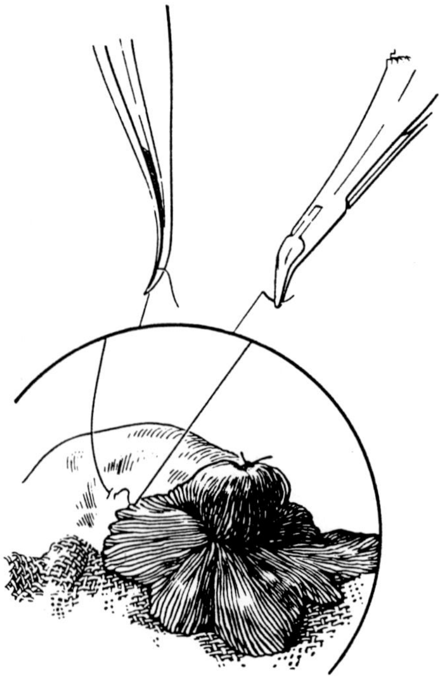

Fig. 32-36

Can be done by laser or at two-stick laparoscopy.

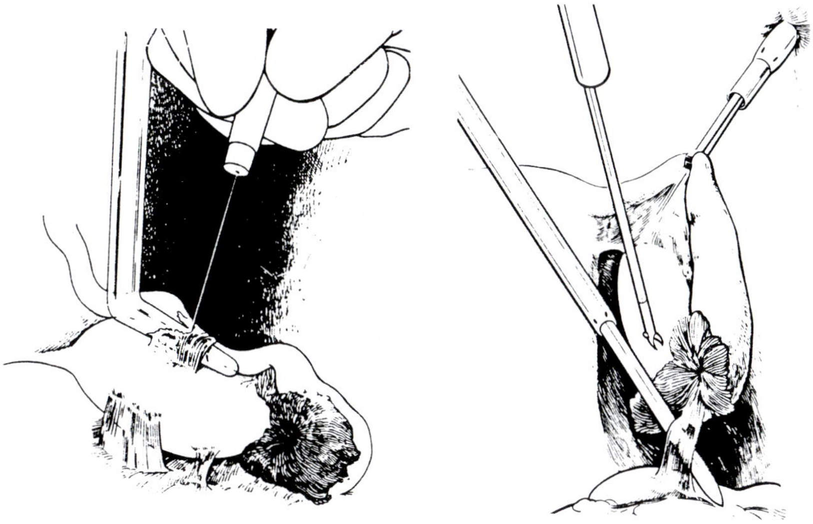

Fig. 32-37

Remnant of adhesion, must be cleared by laser, one cell deep.

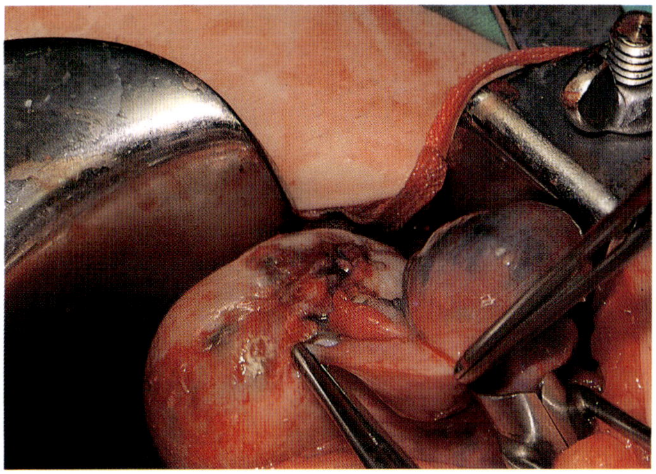

Fig. 32-38

May repair serosal damage with 8-0 or 9-0 suture (Reprinted with permission from Patton[3]).

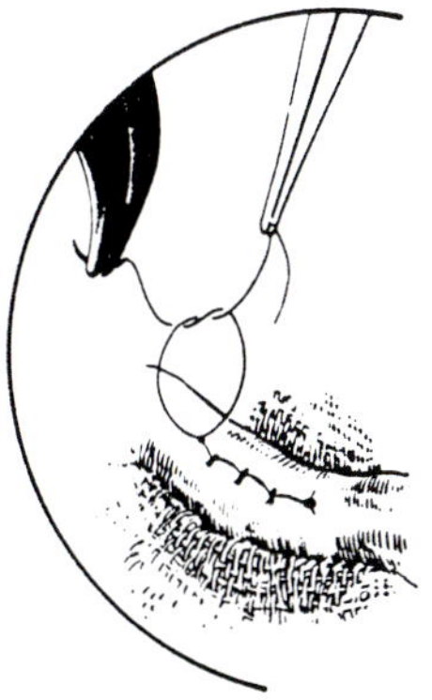

Fig. 32-39

Probable cause of some adhesions exposed, heated, dried serosal surface (left), inflammatory cell infiltration.

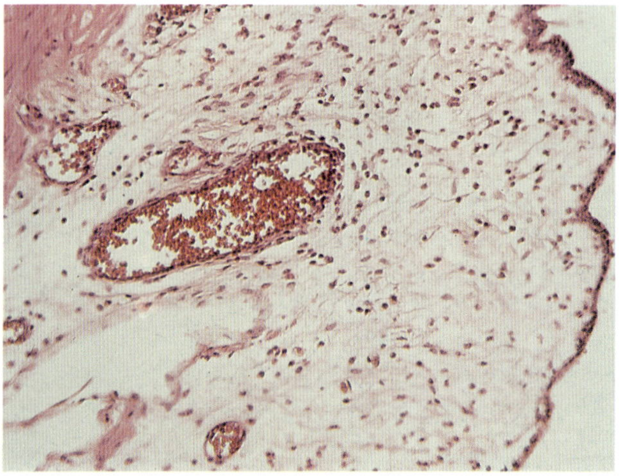

Fig. 32-40

Serosal fibrin formation adhesion source, cleared best with laser only.

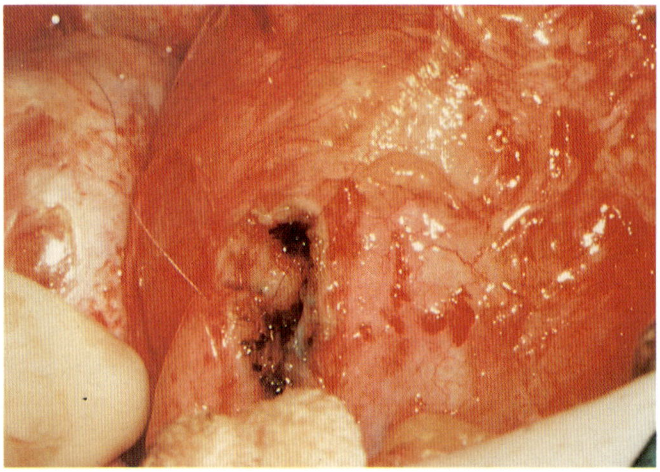

Fig. 32-41

Heavy adhesions, clear with electrodissection first, then unfocused laser, surface of all organs.

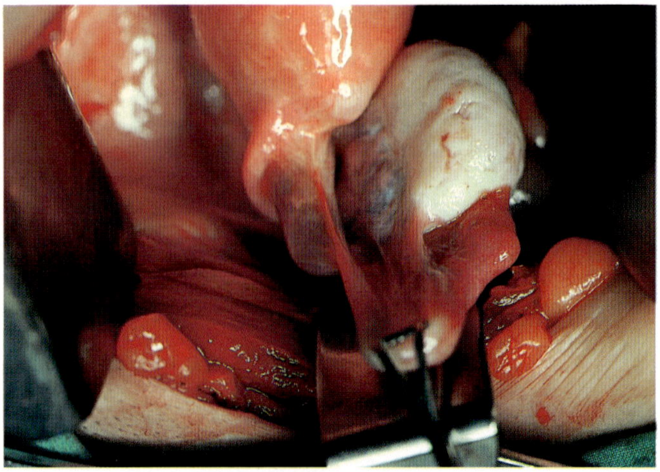

Fig. 32-42

Sharp dissection, ovarian adhesion.

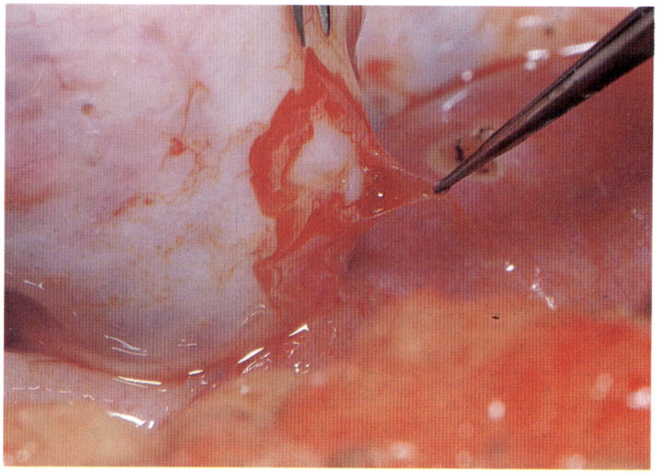

Fig. 32-43

Sharp dissection near the cornua, prior to anastomosis (Figs. 32-44 through 32-46 reprinted with permission from Phillips[4]).

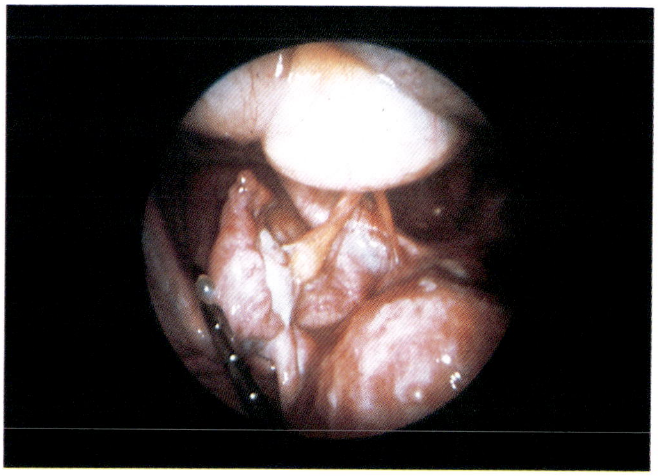

Fig. 32-44

Dissection with fine tip and dropper wash.

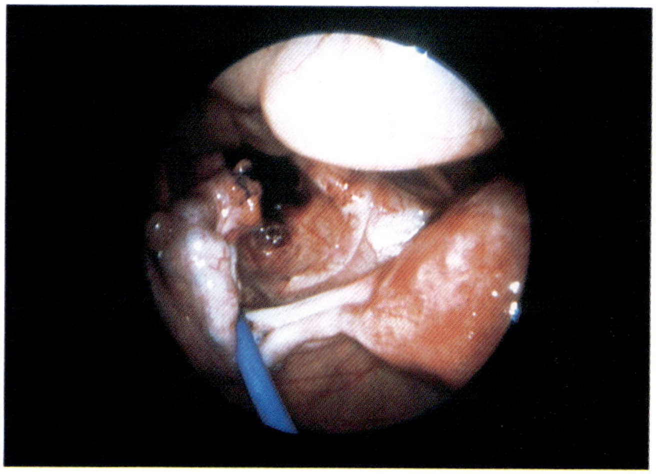

Fig. 32-45

Use of fine tip near the fimbria.

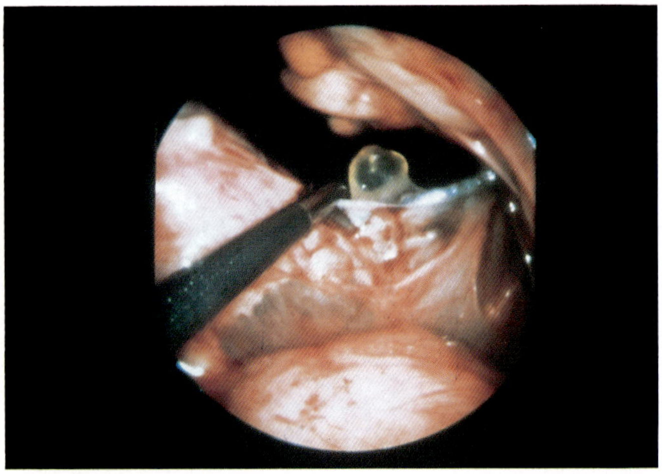

Fig. 32-46

Several charred areas, after hemostasis coagulation they disappear rapidly.

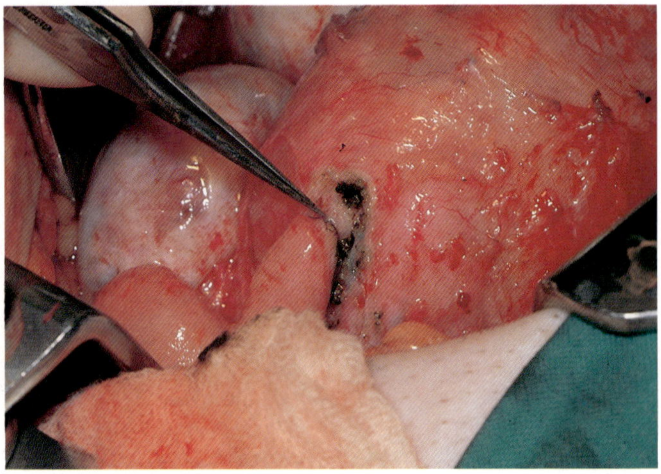

Fig. 32-47

Charred areas disappearing.

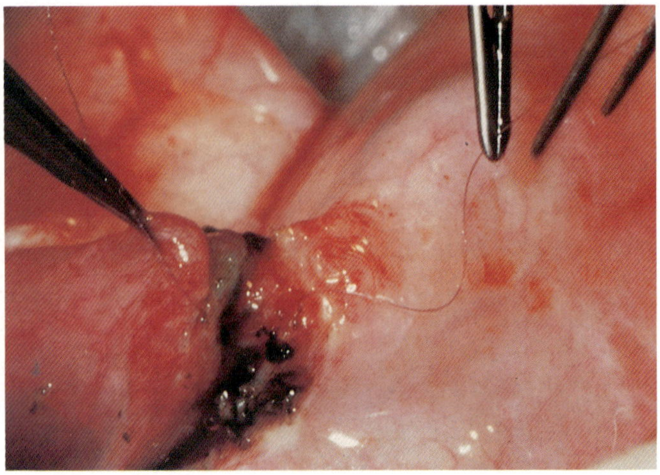

Fig. 32-48

Sharp dissection of adhesions (Figs. 32-49 through 32-50 reprinted with permission from Phillips[4]).

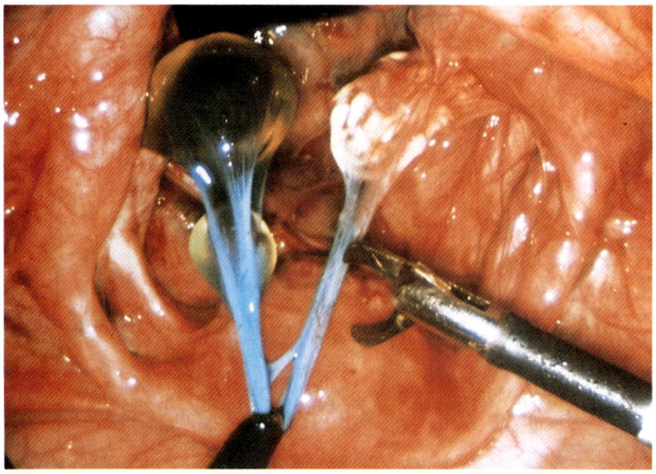

Fig. 32-49

Adhesion release yields blue-dyed fluid.

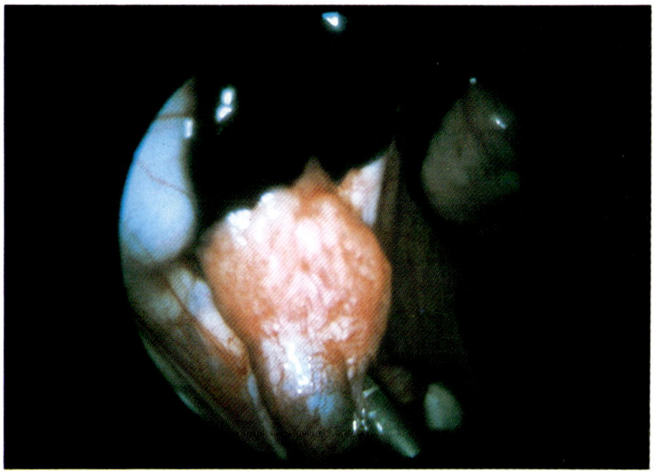

Fig. 32-50

Unfocused laser clears ovarian surface.

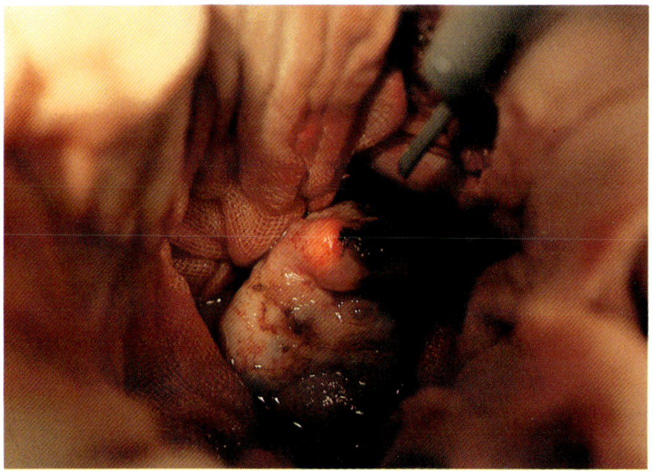

Fig. 32-51 A

Unfocused laser, next step.

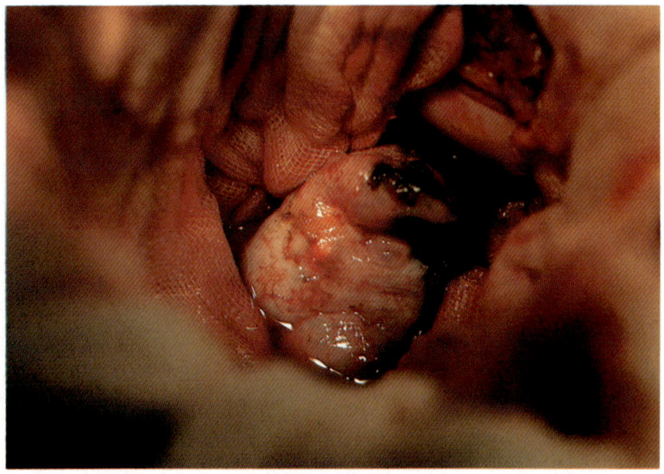

Fig. 32-51 B

Surface almost clear, repeat if necessary.

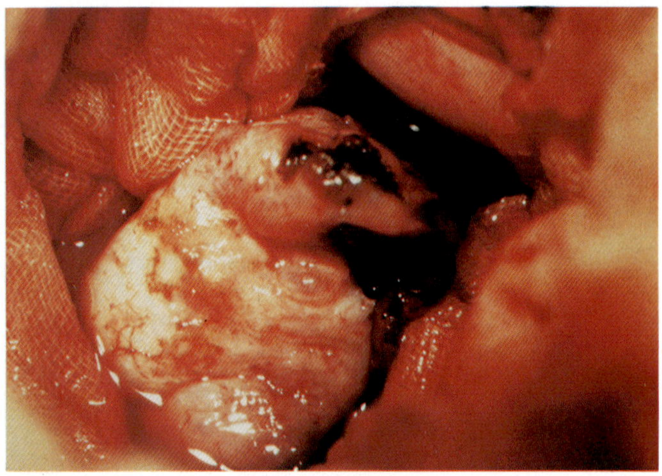

Fig. 32-52 A

Ovary clear, patent tube, no adhesions.

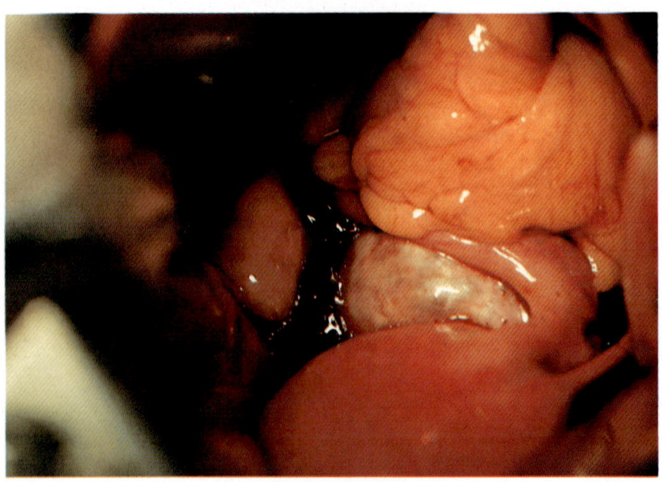

Fig. 32-52 B

Final appearance, ovary clear.

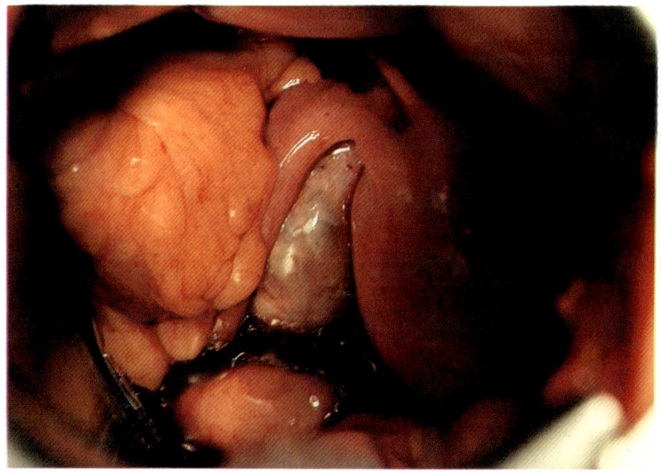

Fig. 32-53

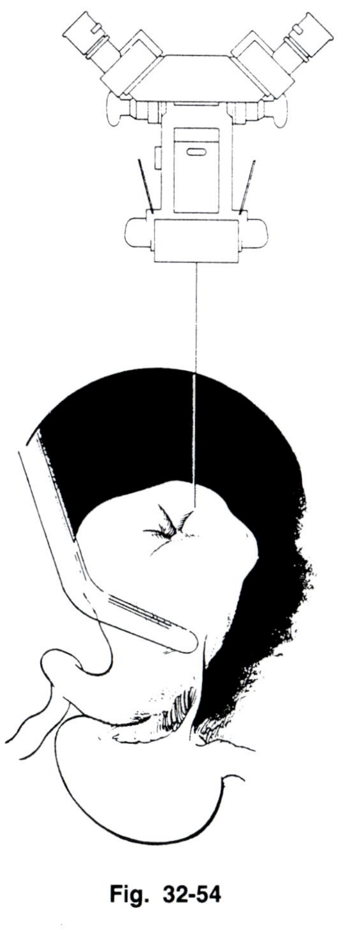

Fig. 32-54

Laser use in fimbrial adhesion release (Figs. 32-54 through 32-57 reprinted with permission from Patton[3]).

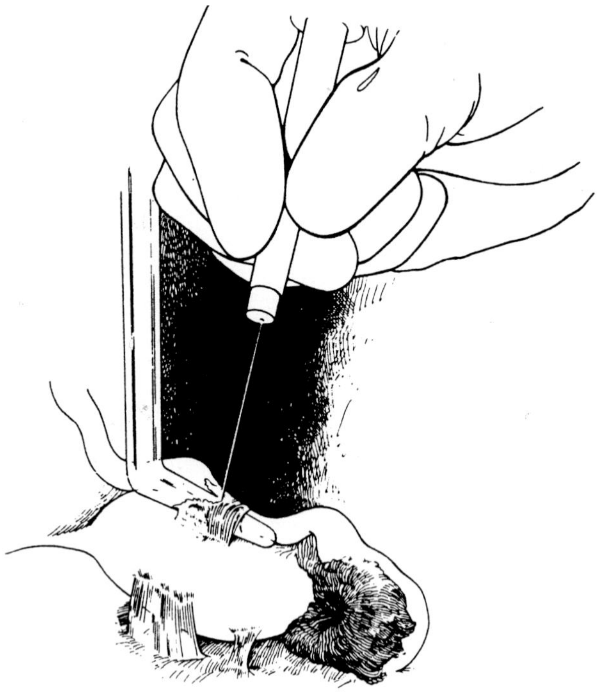

Fig. 32-55

Laser in adhesion lysis.

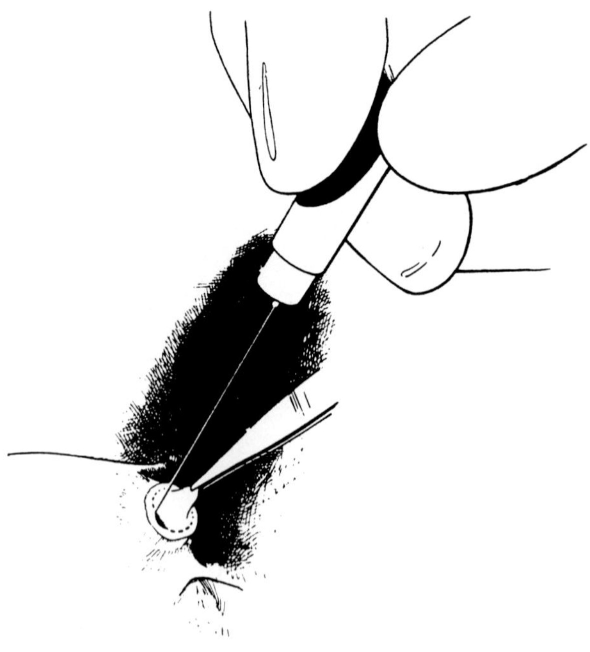

Fig. 32-56

Laser for cornual dissection, either anastomosis or implants.

Laser use with mirror in obscure areas.

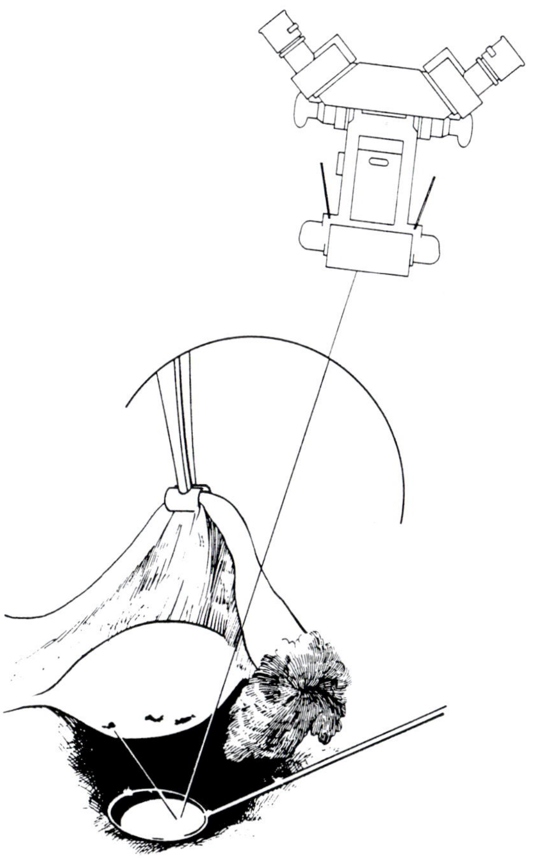

Fig. 32-57

Fimbrial release in progress, note patent tube.

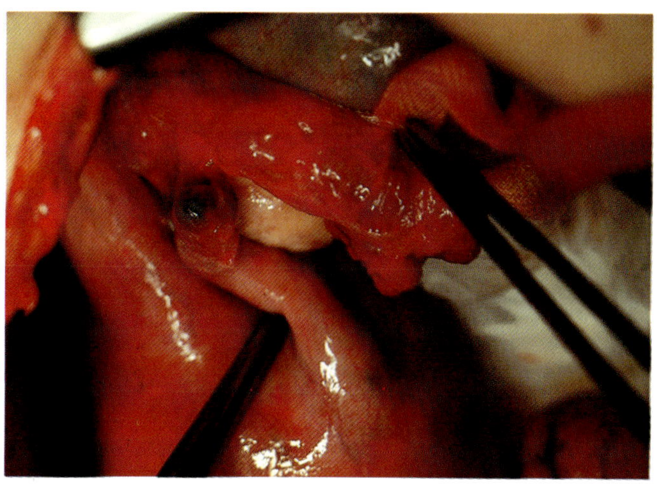

Fig. 32-58 A

Fimbrial release other side, tube to be opened.

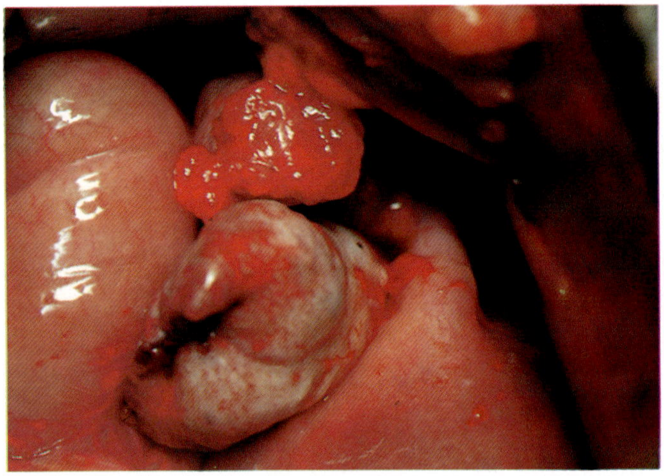

Fig. 32-58 B

The two figures above indicate combined anastomosis of isthmus-to-isthmus bilaterally, fimbrial release, ampulla-isthmus anastomoses, all bilateral, in the same case.

Completed fimbrial release prior to lavage.

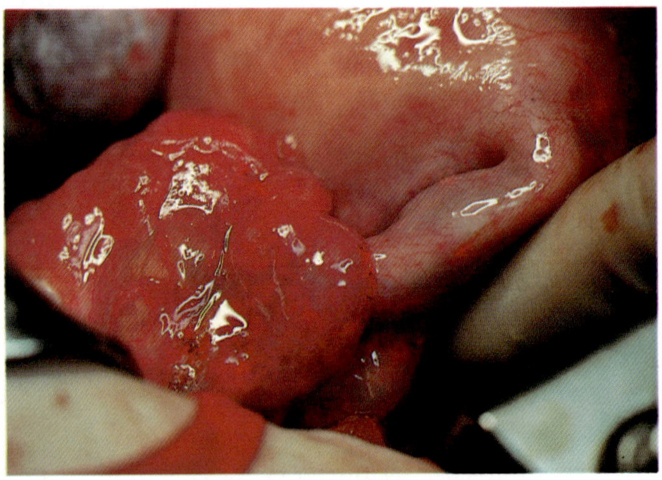

Fig. 32-59

Final appearance, fimbrial release.

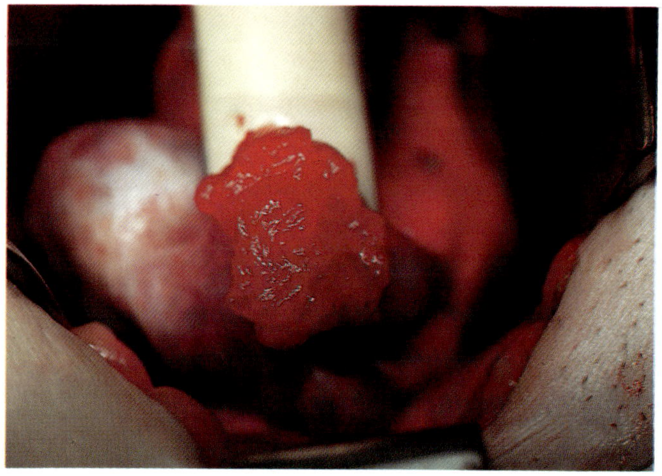

Fig. 32-60

Fimbrial release and cornua-isthmus anastomosis.

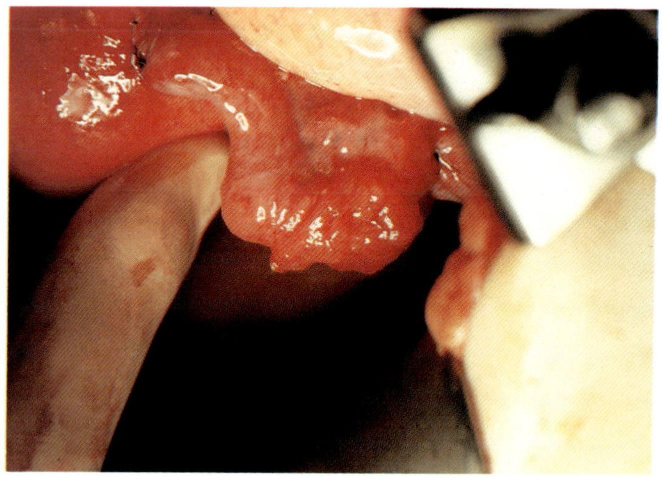

Fig. 32-61

References

1. Elmed Catalogue. Elmed Incorporated, 60 West Fay Avenue, Addison, Illinois
2. Hunt R. *Atlas of Female Infertility Surgery*. Chicago, Ill: Year Book Publishers; 1986.
3. Patton G, Kistner R. *Atlas of Infertility Surgery*. 2nd ed. Boston, Mass: Little, Brown and Company; 1984.
4. Phillips J. Instructional slides from: *Endoscopy in Gynecology*. Published by A.A.G.L., Downey, Calif; 1985.
5. Jones H, Rock J. *Reparative and Constructive Surgery of the Female Generative Tract*. Baltimore, Md: Williams and Wilkins; 1983.

Chapter 33

Microsurgical Tubouterine Implantation

Raphael B. Durfee, MD

Tubouterine implantation is not universally performed because of the poor intrauterine pregnancy yield. Implantation is somewhat complicated and there is frequently considerable tissue manipulation and trauma. Some of this is noticeable in the following photographs. Complications are: postoperative hematoma, failure of tubouterine union, elevated incidence of abortion, interstitial and isthmic uterine rupture, and postdelivery placental adherence. Indication for the operation is the presence of totally obstructed interstitial canals bilaterally. Some surgeons use the ampulla instead of the isthmus for this procedure. Occasionally there is a "blowout" at the implantation site.

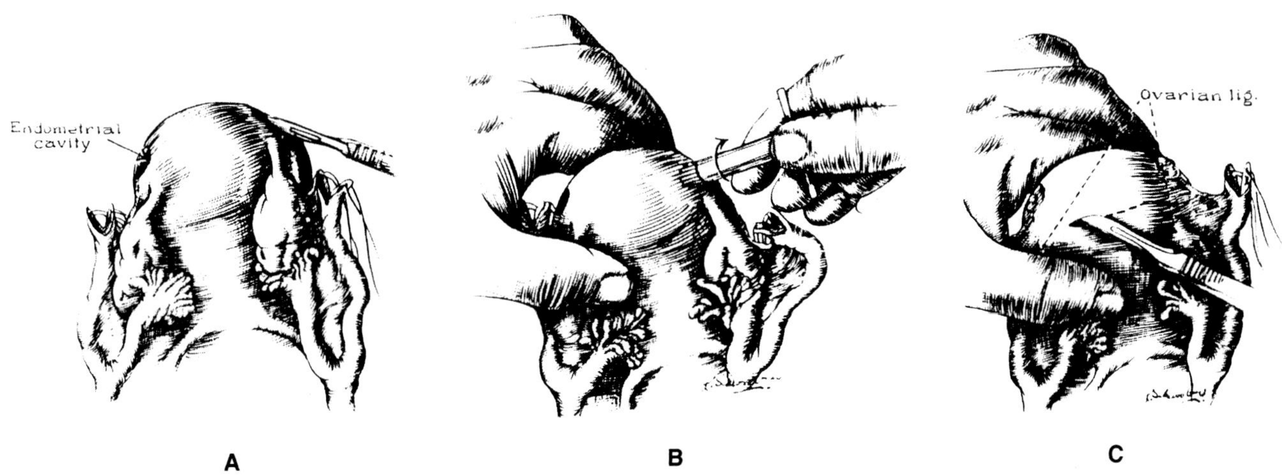

Fig. 33-1 A, B, and C indicates the three most commonly used approaches to the uterine cavity. Hunt bores two holes in the posterior upper uterine wall, as will be shown later. **A**, a sharp incision in the cornua into the uterine cavity. **B**, the use of a borer to remove the interstitial tissue entirely. **C**, a posterior fundal transverse incision (Reprinted with permission from Jones[1]).

Total cornual obstruction, some hydrosalpinx.

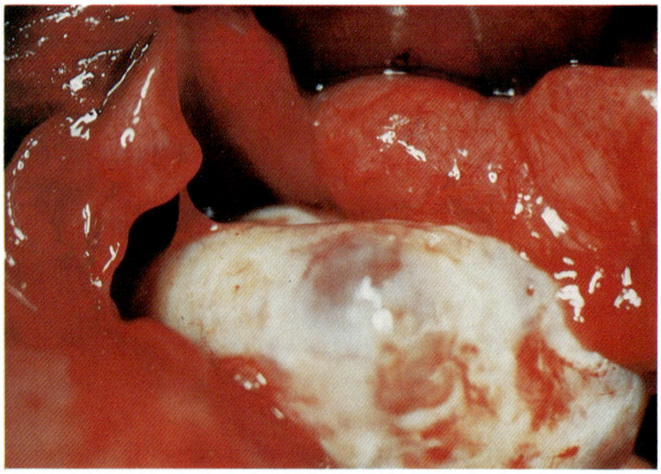

Fig. 33-2

Final result, ampullary cornual implant, uterine tubal anchoring sutures not visible.

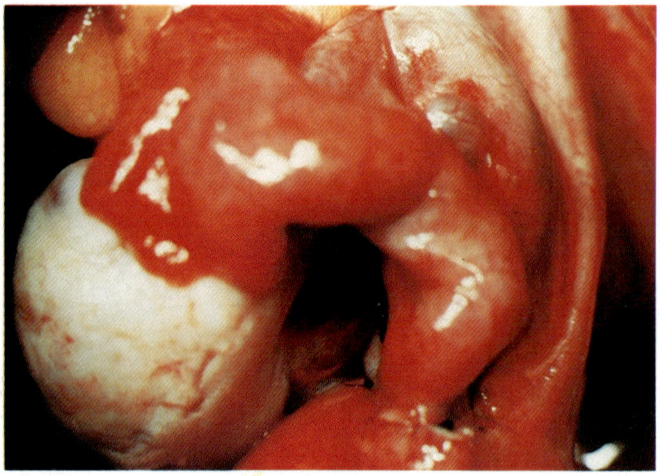

Fig. 33-3

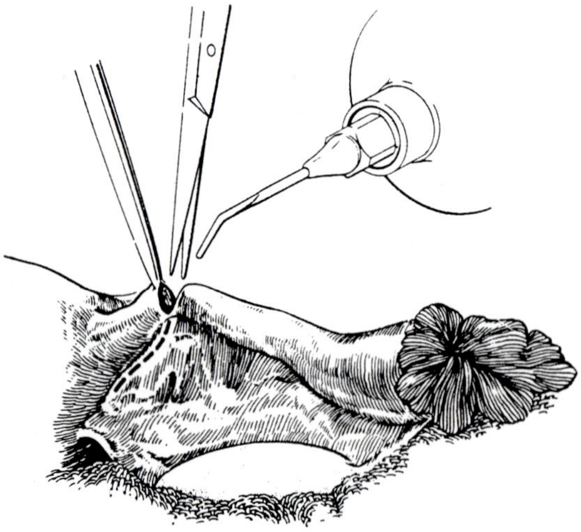

Fig. 33-4

Tube is amputated, usually at the isthmic-ampullary junction (Figs. 33-4 through 33-8 reprinted with permission from Patton[2]).

Cornual tissue shaved back, area injected with dilute Pitressin (circle).

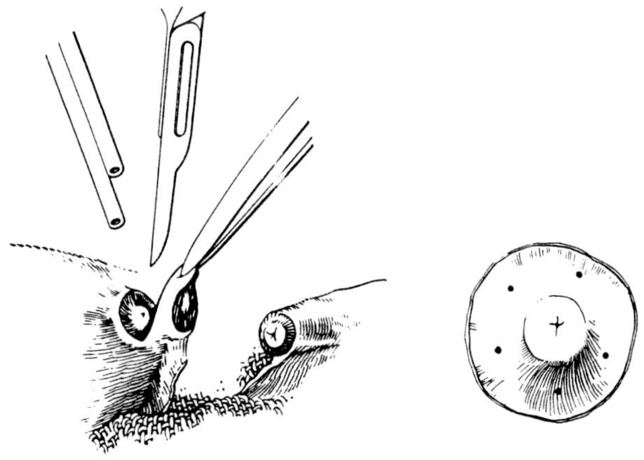

Fig. 33-5

Interstitial area cut out to endometrial cavity; this may also be done with the laser.

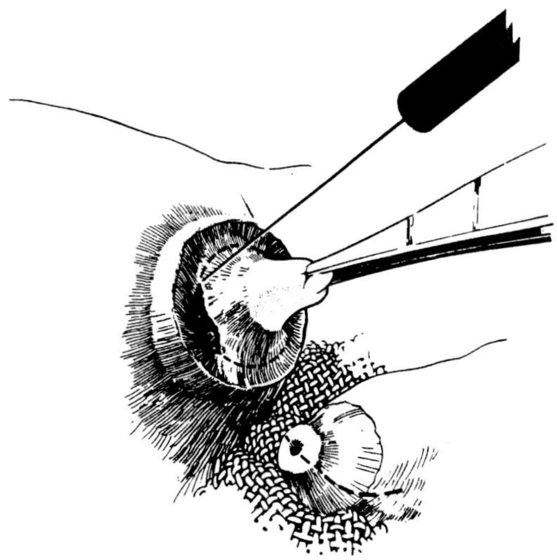

Fig. 33-6

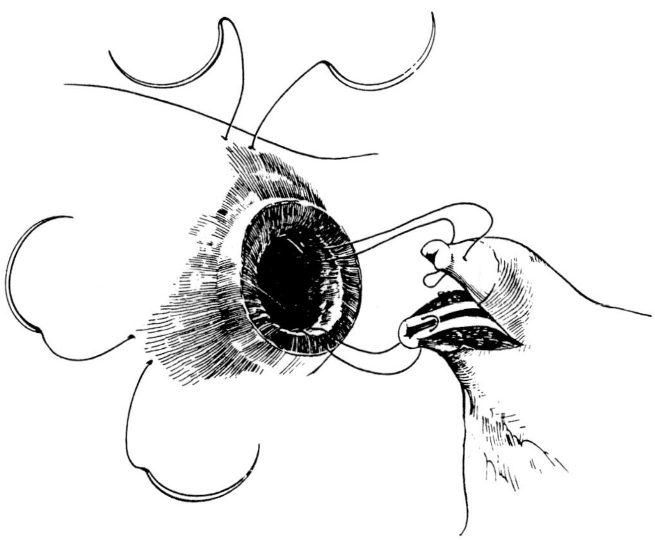

Fig. 33-7

Previously prepared tube is sutured into the uterine cavity as illustrated.

Sutures are tied and the area is closed, including the mesosalpinx. A 2-0 absorbable synthetic suture should be placed at least 1.5 cm deep horizontally, below the round ligament in the uterine wall, to obstruct the anterior branches of the uterine artery to partially control bleeding. The mesosalpinx should be sutured to the uterine wall early.

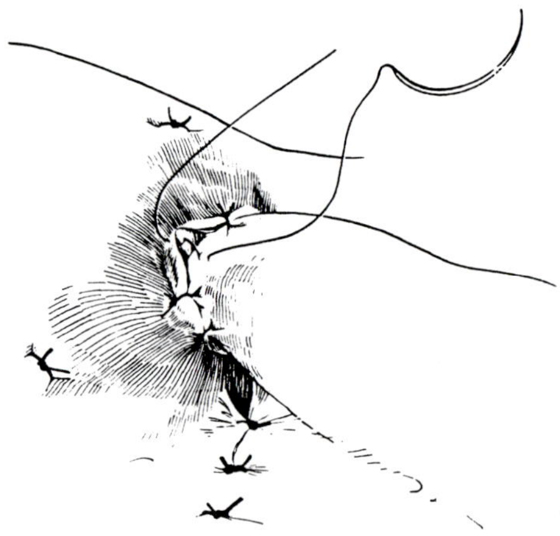

Fig. 33-8

Total interstitial obstruction plus small myoma (not the cause).

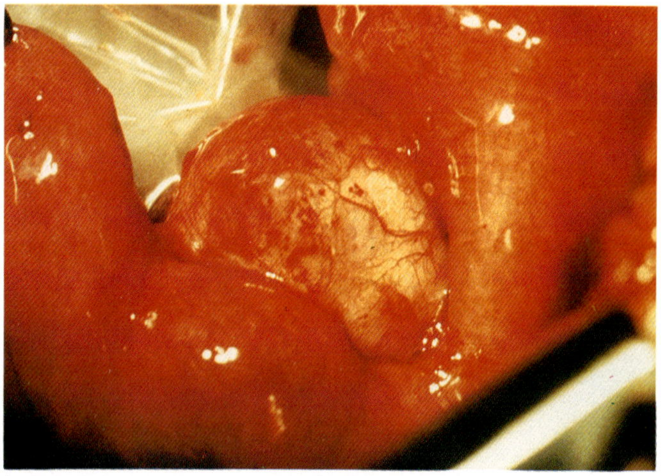

Fig. 33-9

Final appearance.

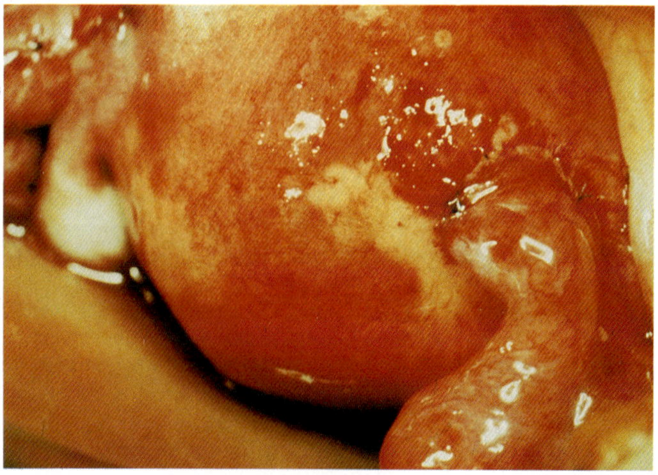

Fig. 33-10

Tube and interstitial area are prepared (Figs. 33-11 through 33-16 reprinted with permission from Jones[1]).

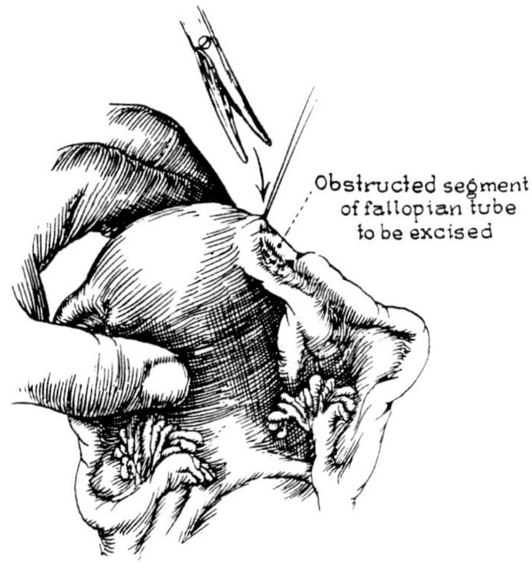

Fig. 33-11

Cornua is bored, tube is split.

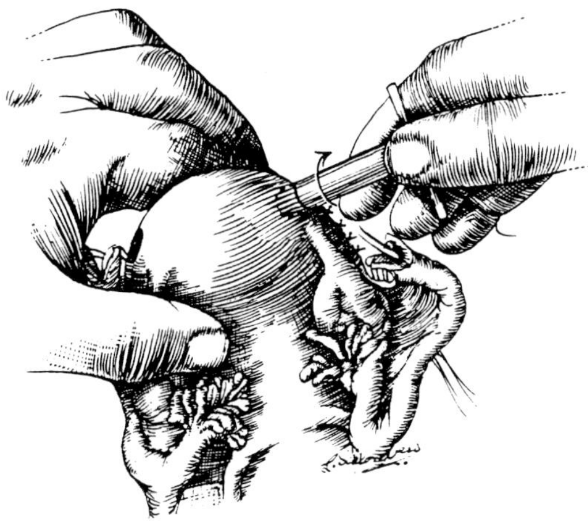

Fig. 33-12

Stent is prepared.

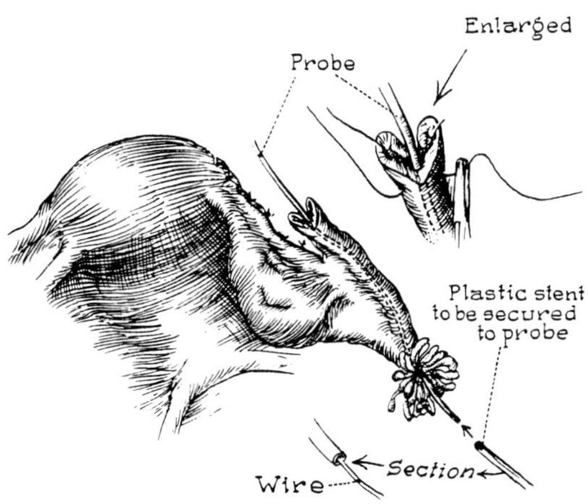

Fig. 33-13

Stent is pulled into uterus.

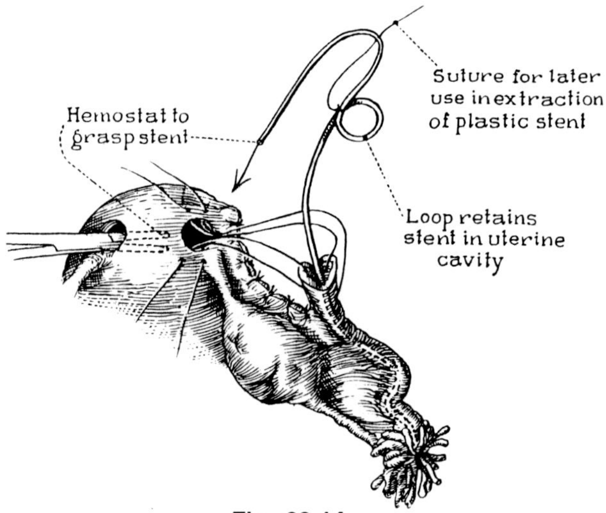

Fig. 33-14

Tube is sutured on one side, stent is pulled into the opposite tube.

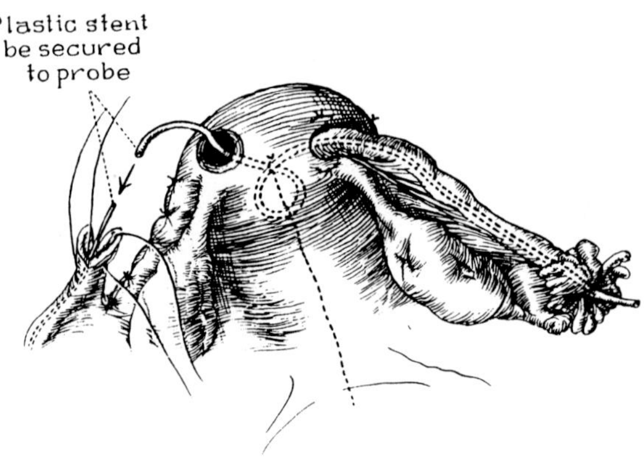

Fig. 33-15

Final appearance, stents are removed later.

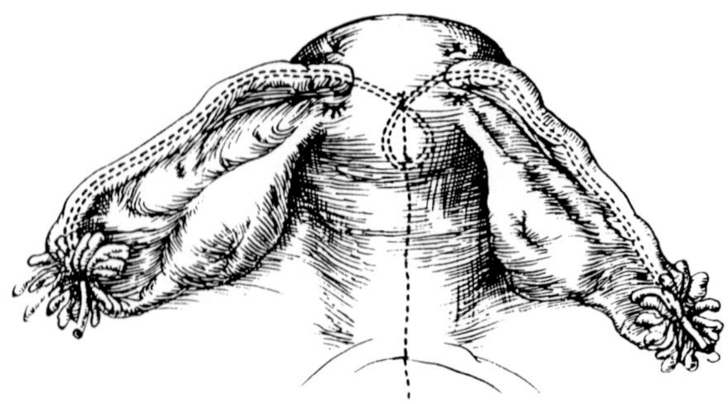

Fig. 33-16

Final appearance in which stents were used.

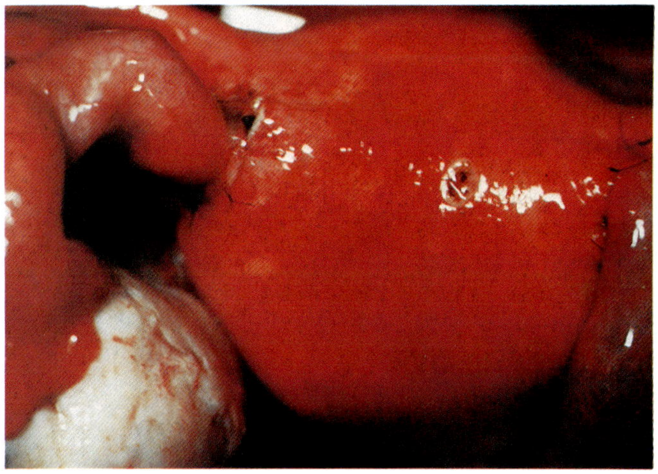

Fig. 33-17

Fundal traction suture, corneal areas closed, tubes prepared, Pitressin injected (Figs. 33-18 through 33-22 reprinted with permission from Jones[1]).

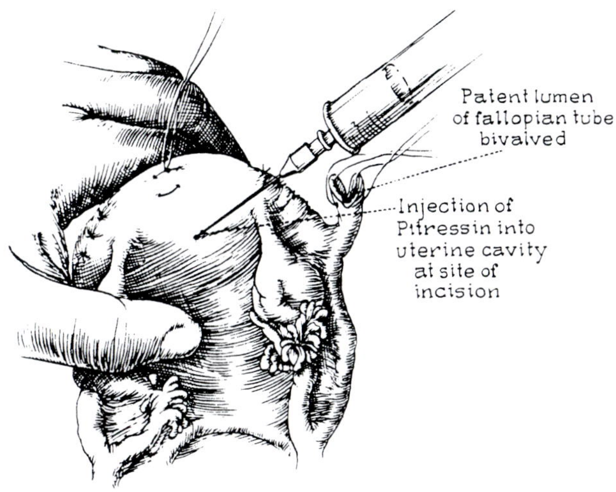

Fig. 33-18

Posterior fundal incision.

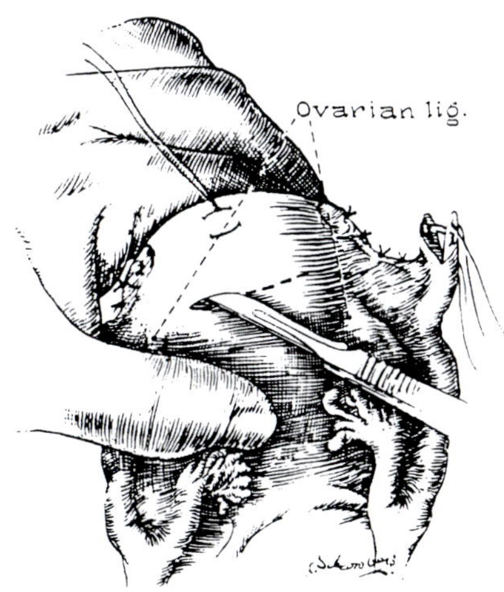

Fig. 33-19

Tubes are implanted through the incision.

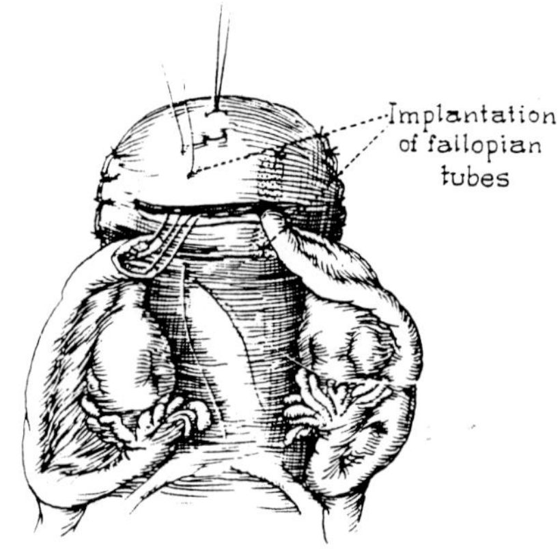

Fig. 33-20

Tubes are tied in place, incision closed.

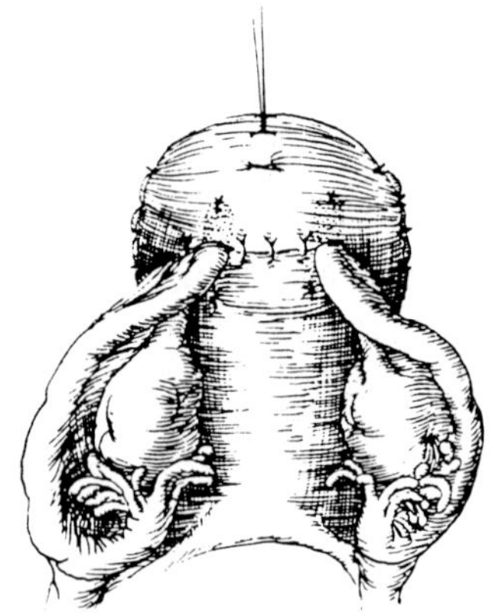

Fig. 33-21

Peritoneum sutured over the uterine fundal incision line (all of this procedure is after Behrman).

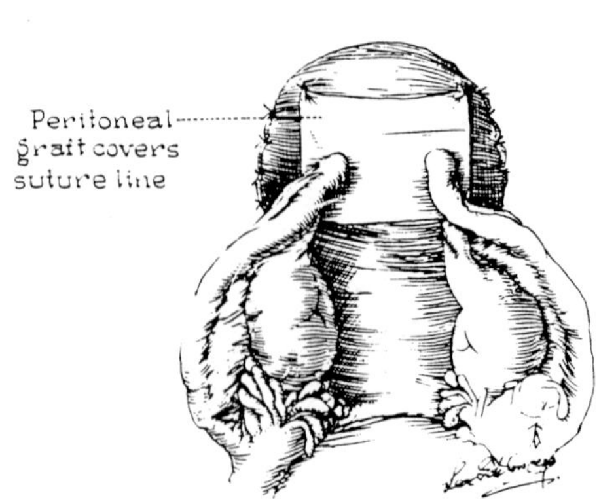

Fig. 33-22

Tubes split, Pitressin injected, cornua closed (Figs. 33-23 through 33-26 reprinted with permission from Hunt[3]).

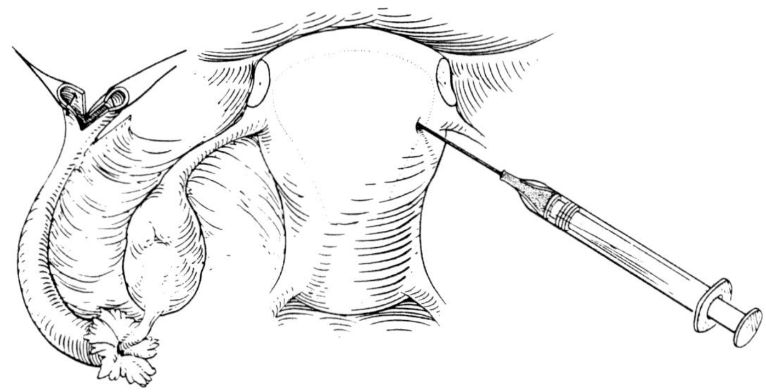

Fig. 33-23

Plug of tissue taken from posterior uterine wall.

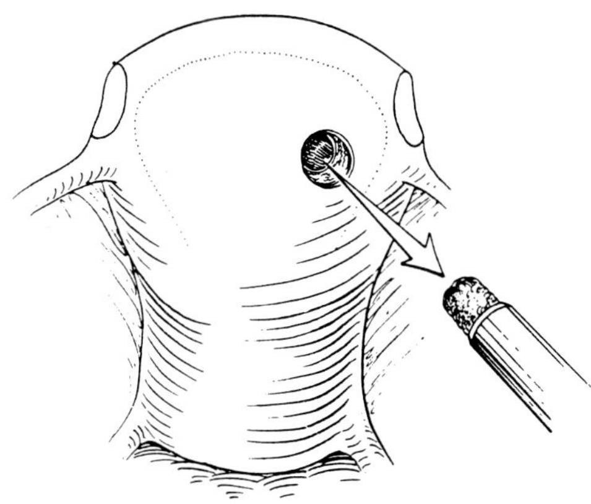

Fig. 33-24

Tubes implanted in uterine cavity.

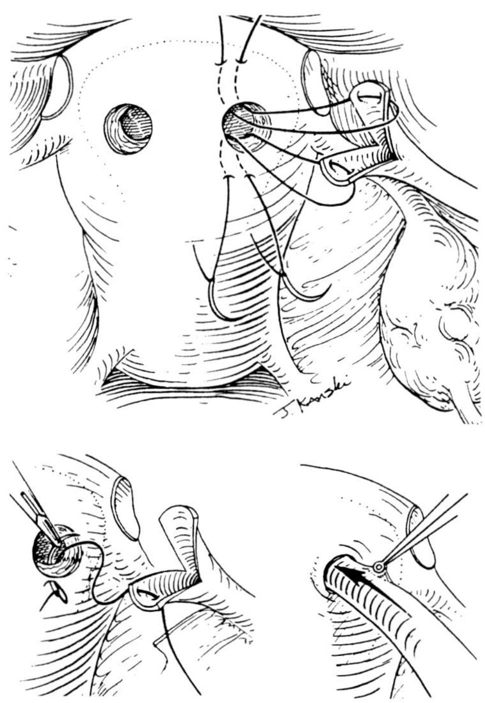

Fig. 33-25

Serosa to serosa, 2. Mucosa to mucosa, 3.

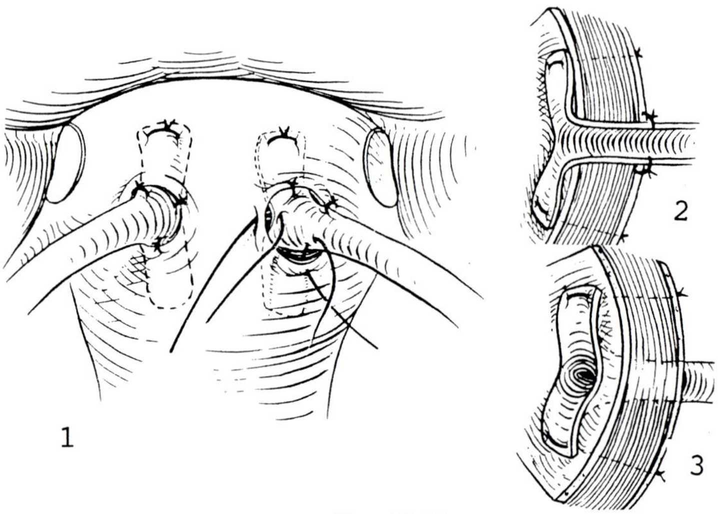

Fig. 33-26

Superior fundal incision, tubal lumen just beyond tip of the probe.

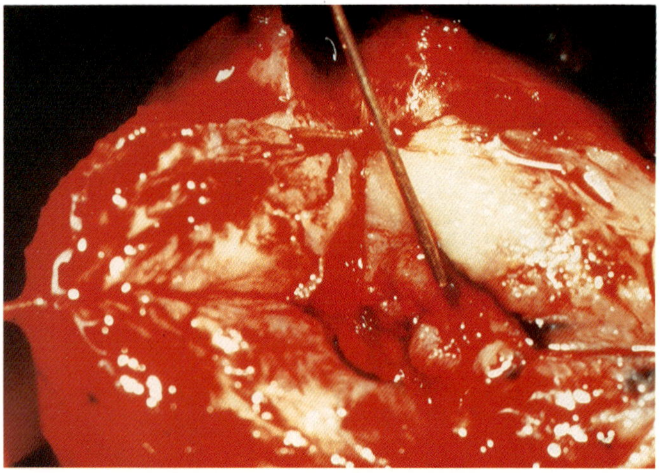

Fig. 33-27

Final appearance.

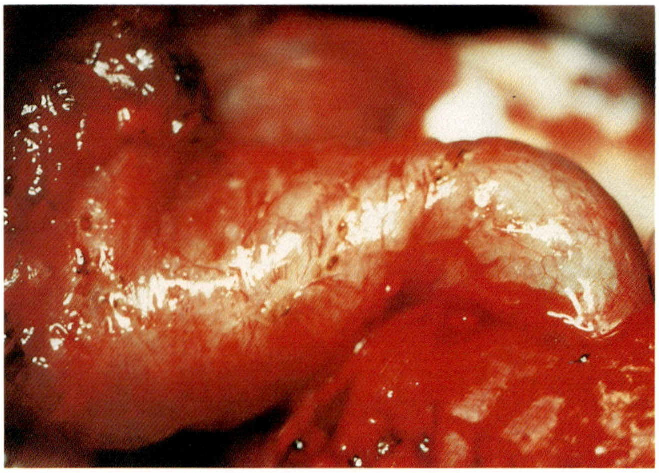

Fig. 33-28

References

1. Jones H, Rock J. *Reparative and Constructive Surgery of the Female Generative Tract*. Baltimore, Md: Williams and Wilkins; 1983.

2. Patton G, Kistner R. *Atlas of Infertility Surgery*. 2nd ed. Boston, Mass: Little, Brown and Company; 1984.

3. Hunt R. *Atlas of Female Infertility Surgery*. Chicago, Ill: Year Book Publishers; 1986.

Chapter 34

Ampullary Neosalpingostomy

Raphael B. Durfee, MD

Reversal of fimbriectomy is partially based upon the ability of tubal mucosal cells to proliferate spontaneously. This growth, combined with the necrosis produced by a permanent silk ligature (which allows the formation of a small foramen through the serosa into the tubal lumen), accounts for the failure rate of both the Kroener fimbriectomy and the Madlener tubal ligations.

When reversal of the fimbriectomy is desired, the creation of a reasonably large opening at the distal end of the proximal segment of tube should provide a functional os. If the mucosal cells proliferate in this area, as they should, intrauterine pregnancy should be feasible. The work of Dr. Miles Novy of Portland, Oregon in this regard is presented with his personal permission and cooperation.[1,2] See also Case #2 in Chapter 38.

HSG shows distal tubal obstruction with mild hydrosalpinx (Figs. 34-1 through 34-9 courtesy Dr. Miles Novy).

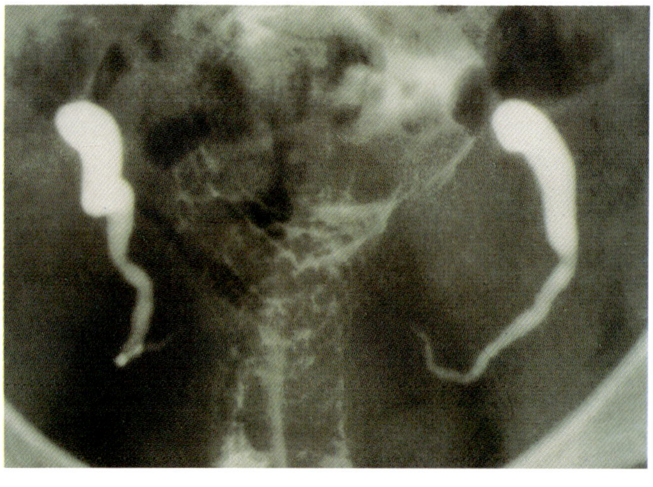

Fig. 34-1

Ultrasound shows tubal obstruction.

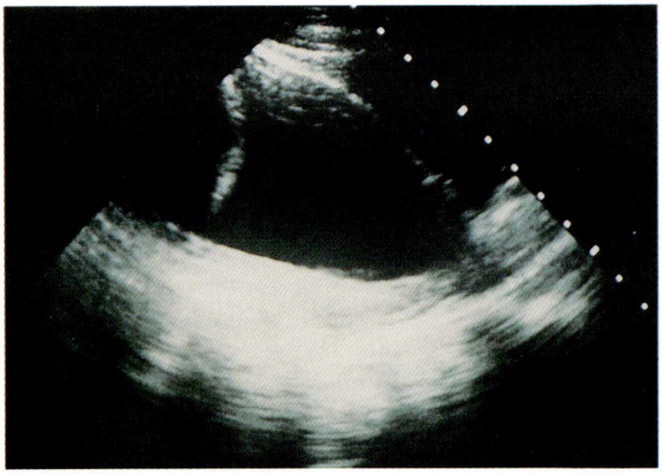

Fig. 34-2

Tube at surgery, patent to the end, with adhesion.

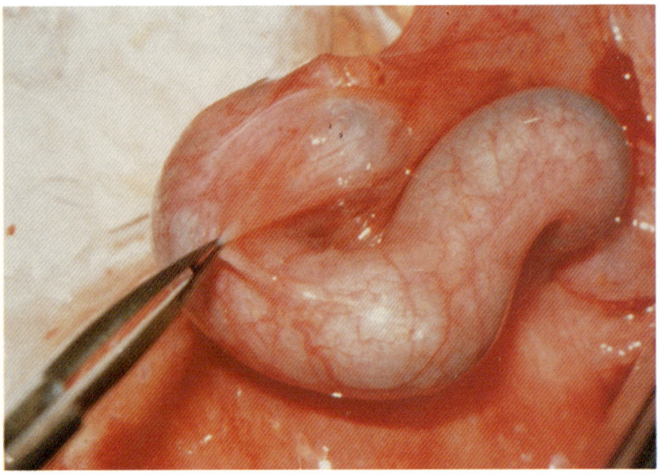

Fig. 34-3

Mucosa after tubal incision, can be mobilized.

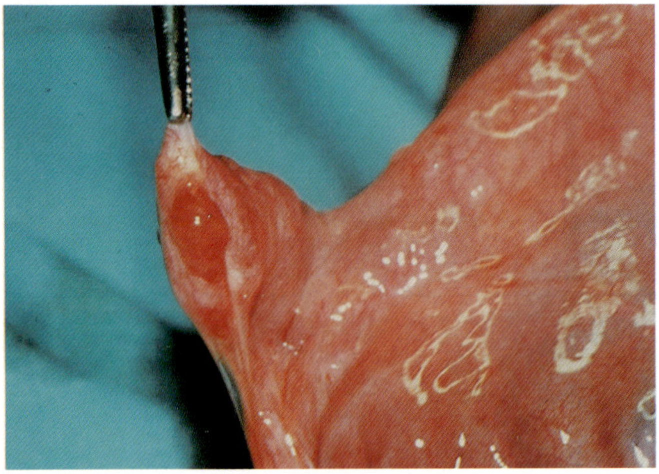

Fig. 34-4

Excision of adhesions with eversion of mucosa.

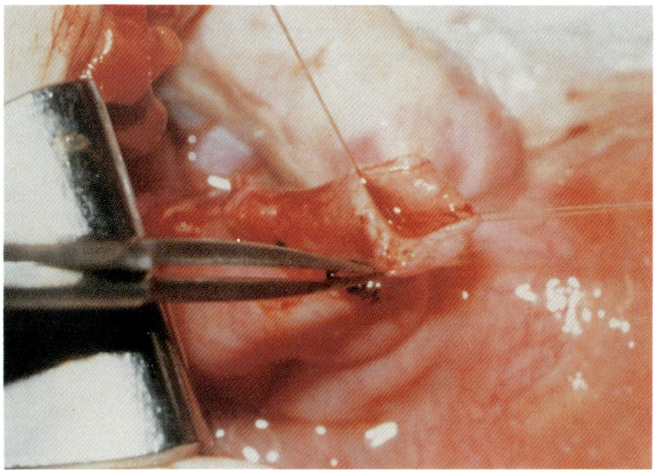

Fig. 34-5

Good available tissue.

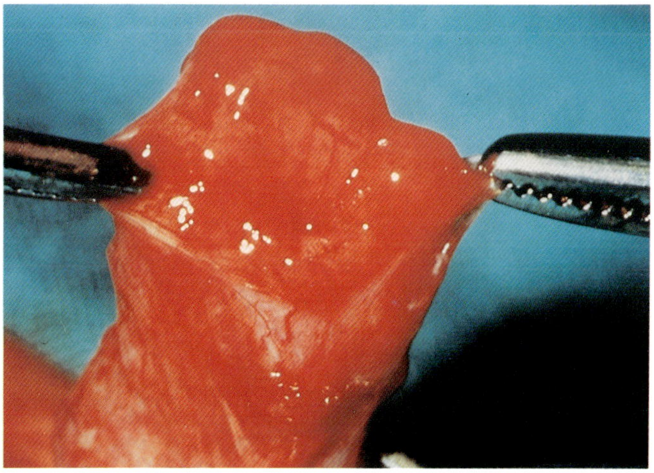

Fig. 34-6

Fine suture eversion of tubal mucosa.

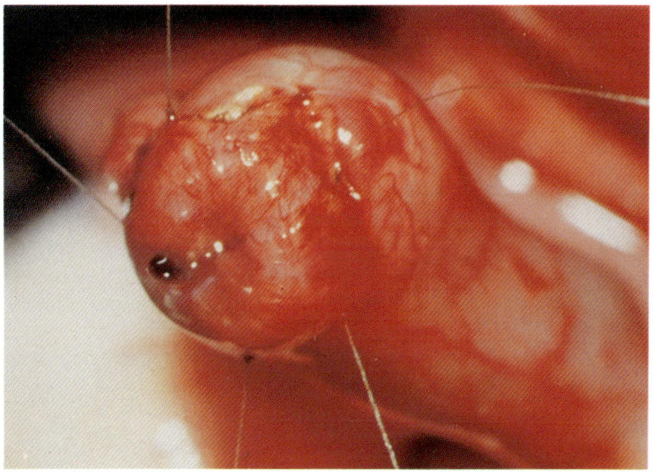

Fig. 34-7

Final appearance, with excellent open os.

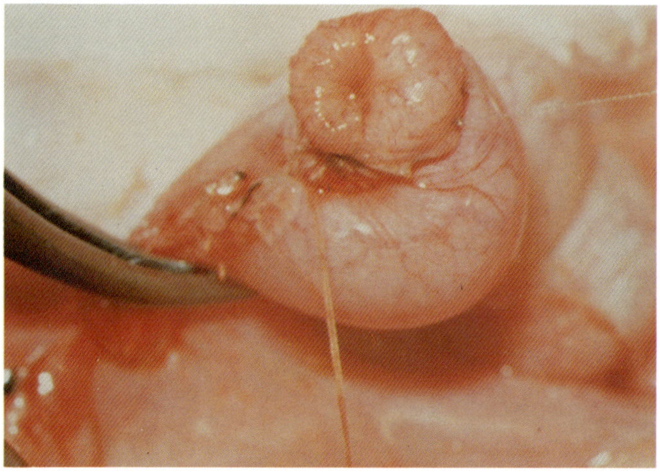

Fig. 34-8

Patent tube, good relationship to ovary. (See Ch 31, Fig. 31-13 for spontaneous fimbrial regeneration.)

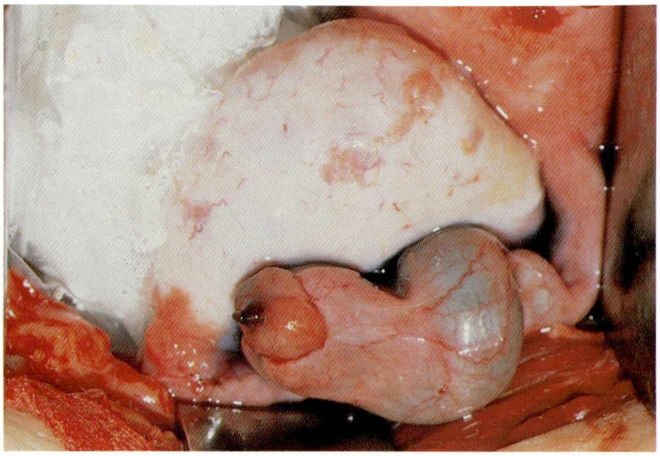

Fig. 34-9

References

1. Novy M. Neosalpingostomy after Fimbriectomy. Personal communication.
2. Novy M. Reversal of Kroener fimbriectomy sterilization. *Am J Obstet Gynecol.* 1980;137:198-206.

Chapter 35

Microsurgical and Laser Treatment of Endometriosis

Raphael B. Durfee, MD

The application of microsurgical methods to the management of endometriosis, enhanced by microlaser techniques, has greatly improved the beneficial results. The startling three-dimensional sight through the operating binocular microscope allows for determination of the depth and extent of pelvic endometriotic lesions. It also allows for improved use of retroperitoneal dissection in difficult cases. The preservation of the serosal and peritoneal surfaces, which includes the absence of suturing for closure of peritoneal pelvic and cul-de-sac wounds, has reduced the number and extent of postoperative adhesions. Ovarian reconstruction following adhesion lysis and tumor removal is markedly improved using both the laser and fine nonreactive sutures with efficiently closed superficial surfaces.

The microscope permits finer and more accurate dissection, placement of finer sutures, better hemostasis without ligatures, and amazing use of the laser in most cases.

CO_2 laser.

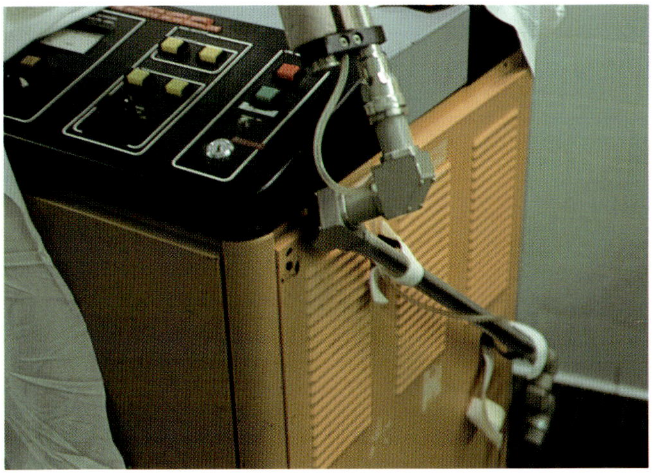

Fig. 35-1

Laser adaptor for the microscope.

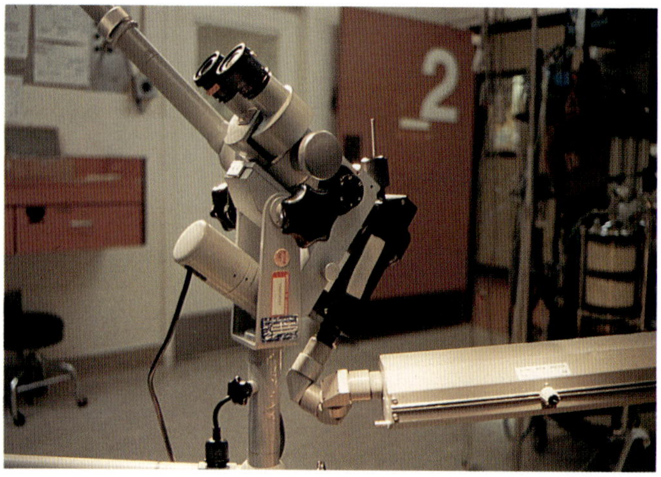

Fig. 35-2

Endometriosis of the cul-de-sac (Figs. 35-3 and 35-4 reprinted with permission from Phillips[1]).

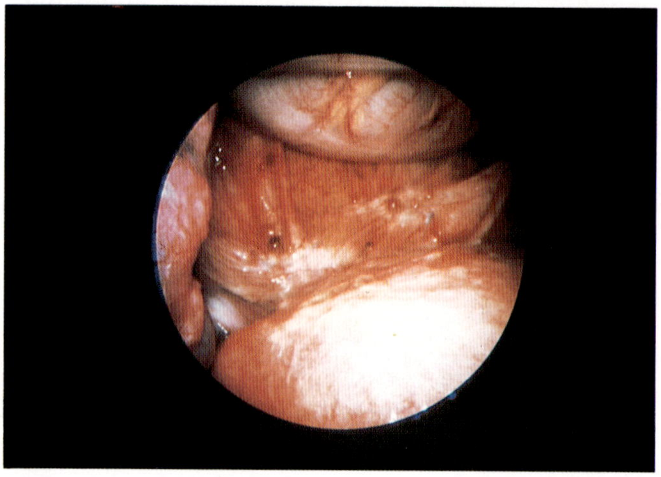

Fig. 35-3

Cul-de-sac endometrioma.

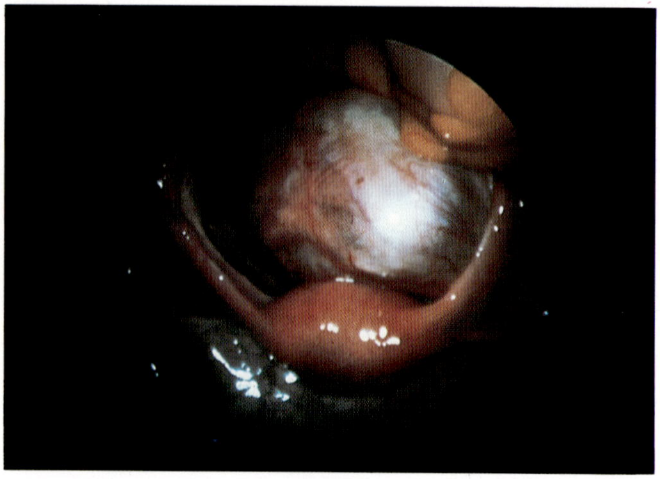

Fig. 35-4

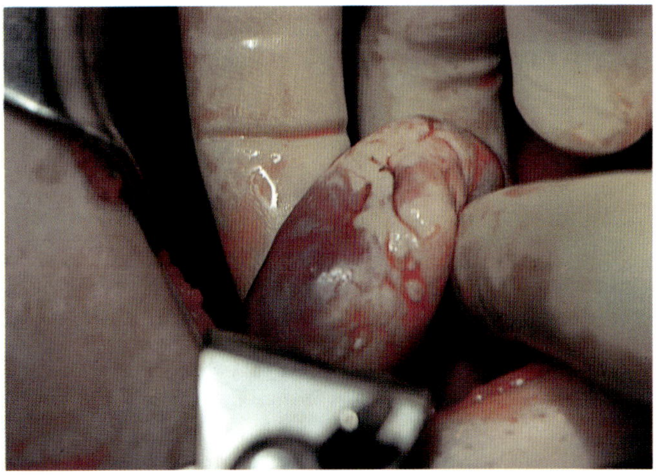

Fig. 35-5

Ovarian endometrioma.

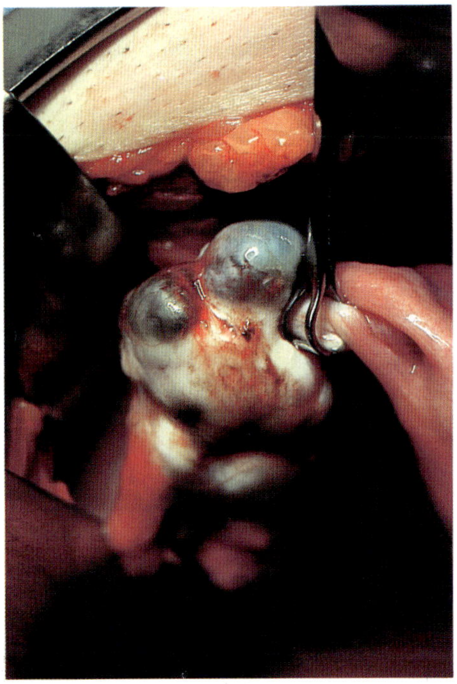

Fig. 35-6

Ovarian endometrioma.

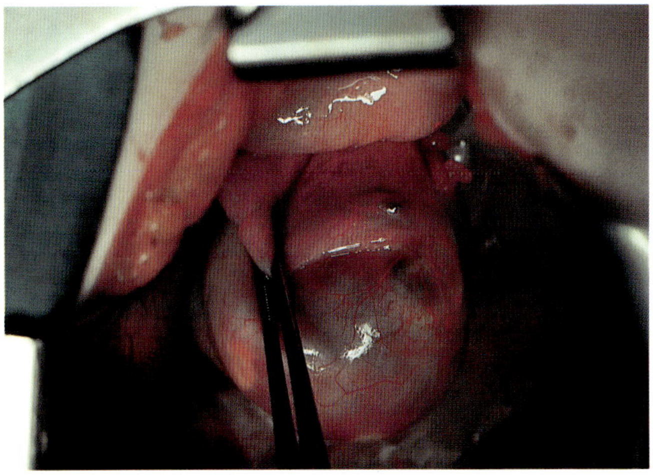

Fig. 35-7

Extensive ovarian involvement.

Bilateral endometriomas, so-called "Kissing Ovaries" (Figs. 35-8 and 35-9 reprinted with permission from Phillips[1]).

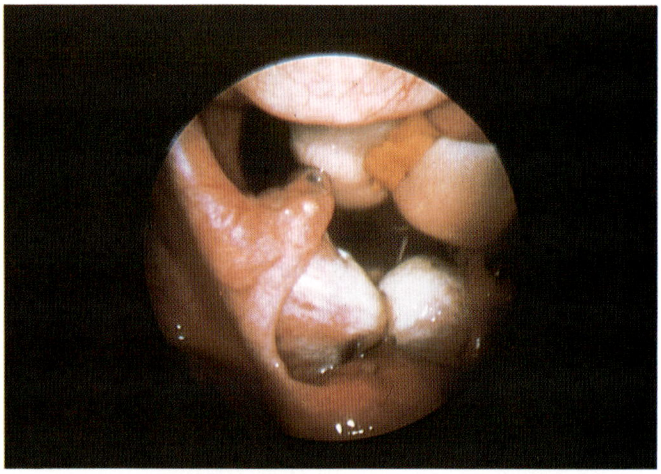

Fig. 35-8

Leaking brown fluid.

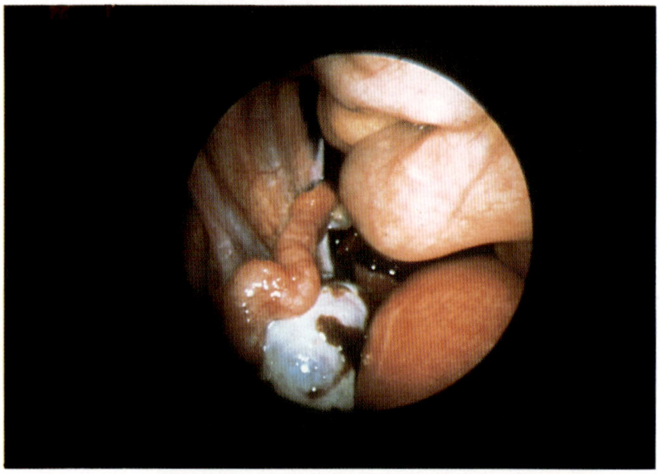

Fig. 35-9

Large ovarian endometrioma.

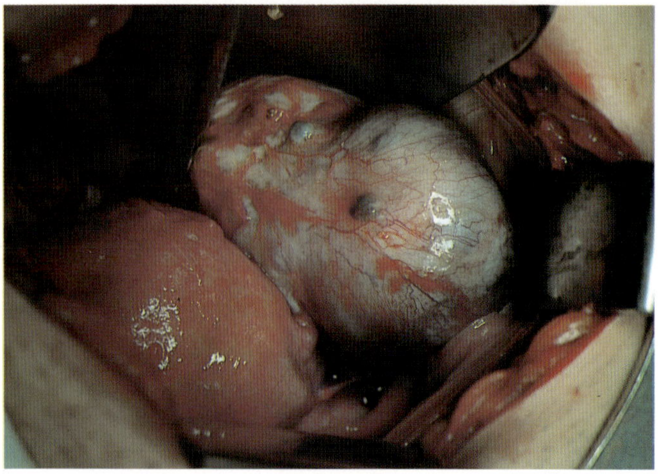

Fig. 35-10

Same, leaking brown fluid.

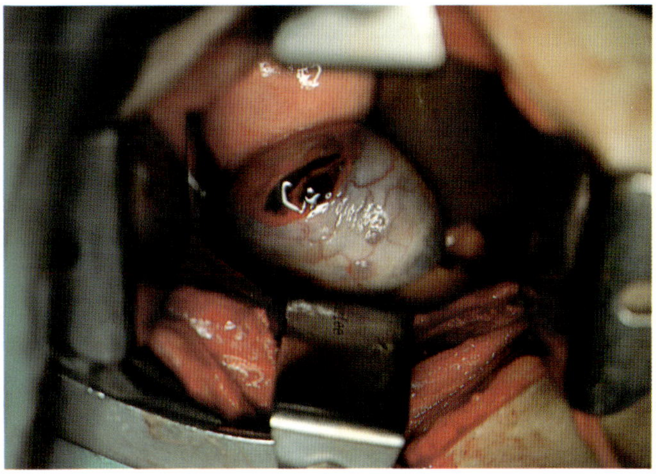

Fig. 35-11

Fallopian tube closed with endometriosis.

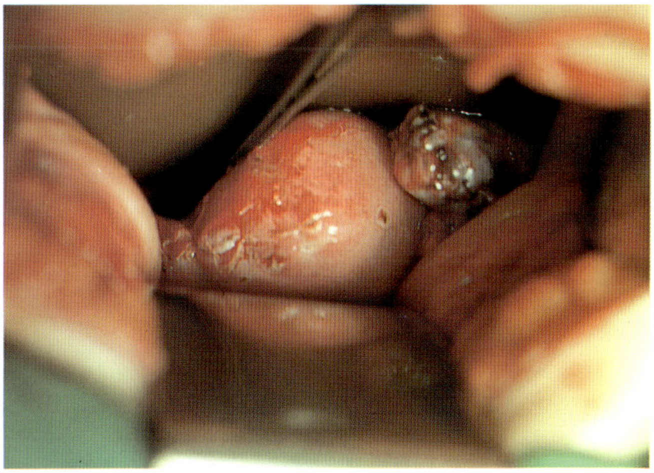

Fig. 35-12

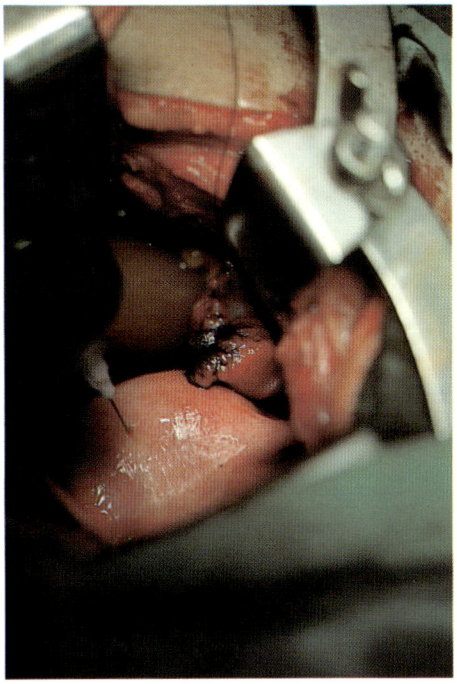

Fig. 35-13

Same, shows patent tube after surgery.

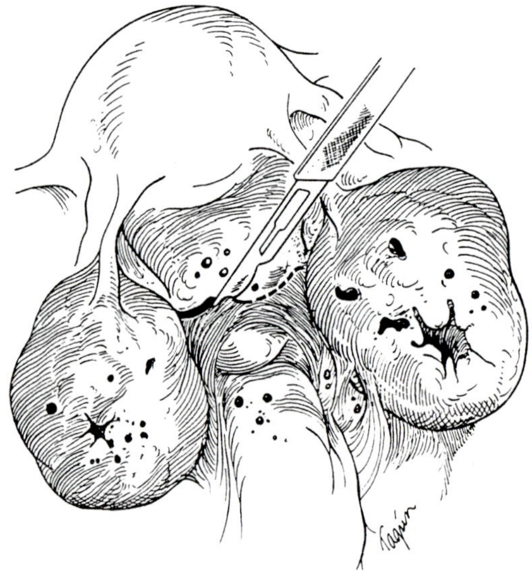

Fig. 35-14

Cul-de-sac incision to release peritoneum and permit dissection (Reprinted with permission from Patton[2]).

Ovarian cystectomy for endometrioma.

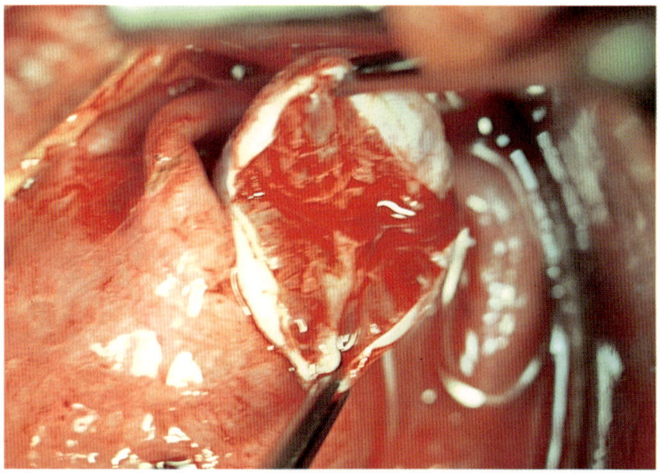

Fig. 35-15

Ovary repaired.

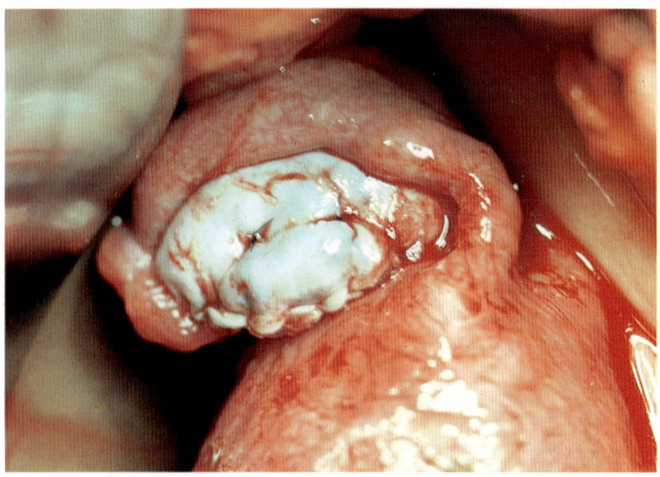

Fig. 35-16

Fimbrial release, final appearance.

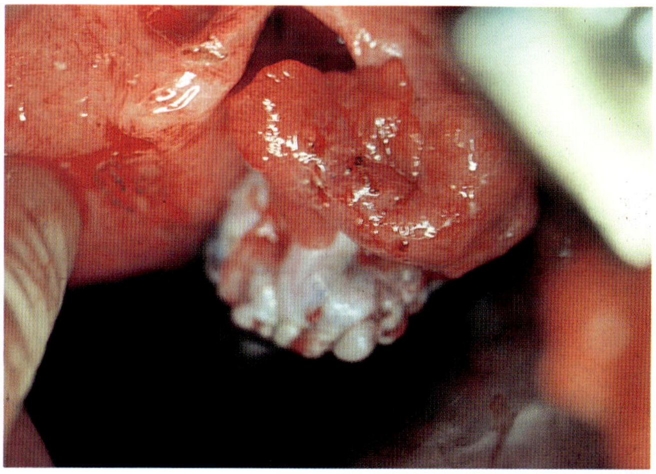

Fig. 35-17

Left, scalpel incision of ovary; right, laser incision of ovary (Figs. 35-18 through 35-21 adapted with permission from McLaughlin[3]).

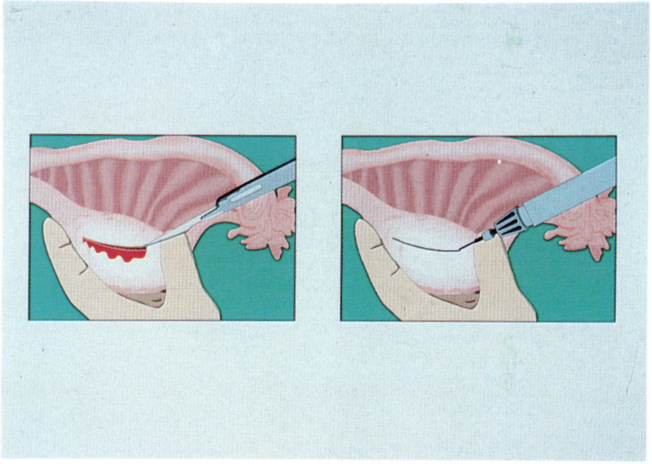

Fig. 35-18

Left, excision of ovarian cyst; right, ovarian bed, instrument removal.

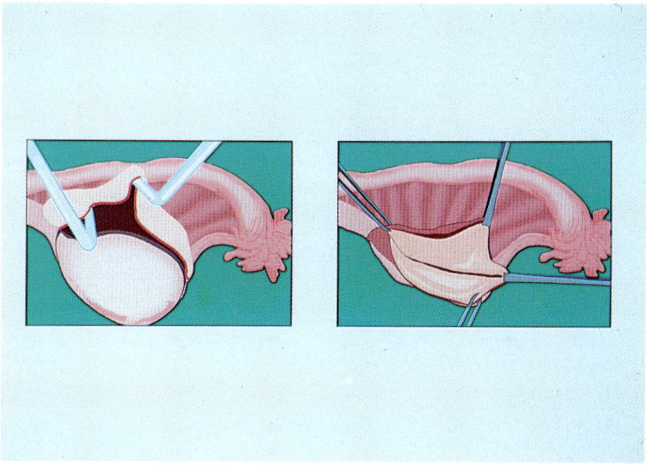

Fig. 35-19

Left, standard closure—macrosuture; right, microclosure—microsuture.

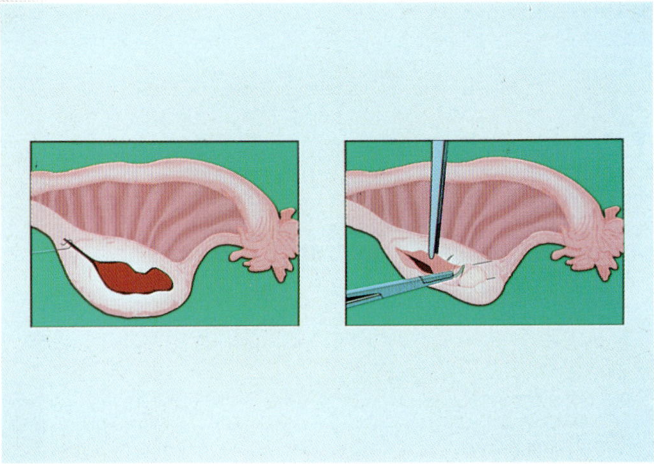

Fig. 35-20

Left, completed microclosure; right, standard macroclosure.

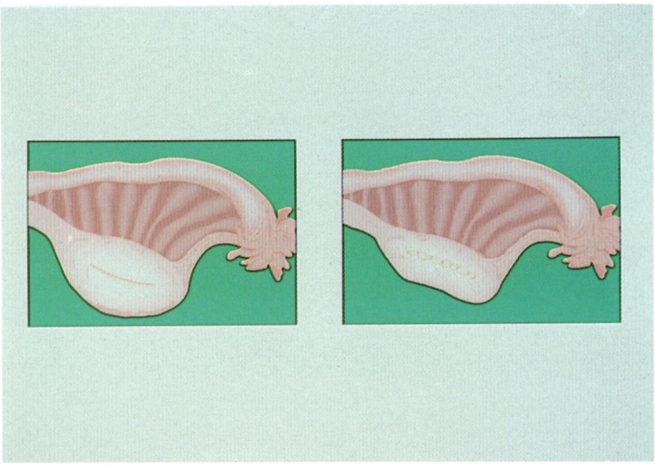

Fig. 35-21

Laparoscopic ovarian cyst excision (Figs. 35-22 and 35-23 reprinted with permission from Semm[4]).

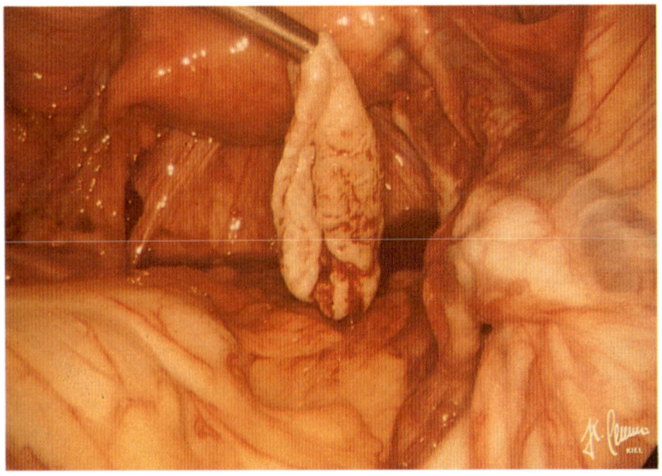

Fig. 35-22

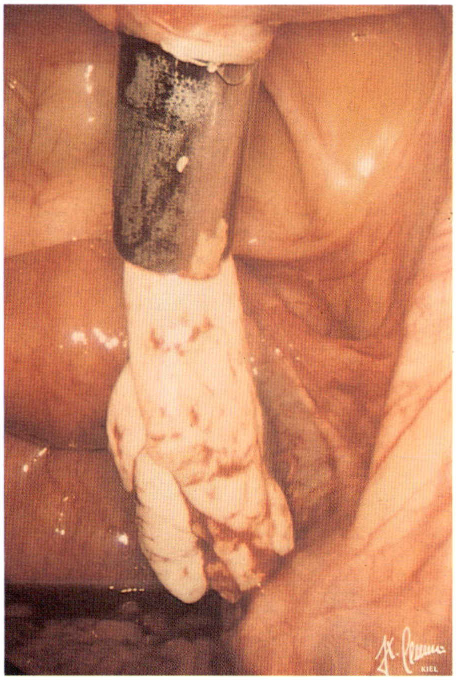

Fig. 35-23

Ovarian cyst removal by laparoscopy evacuator.

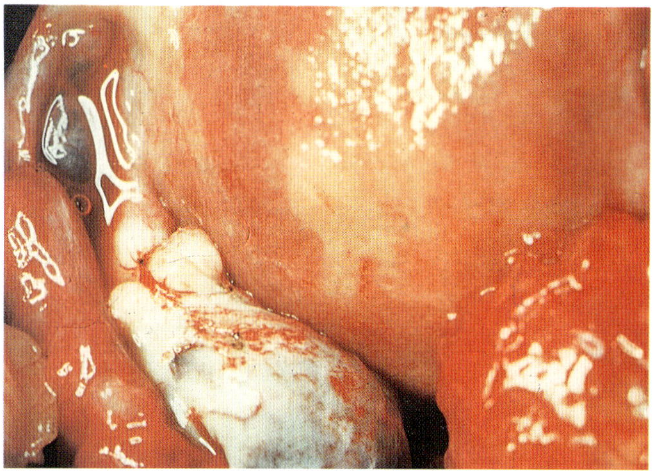

Fig. 35-24

Tubal anastomosis after endometriosis therapy.

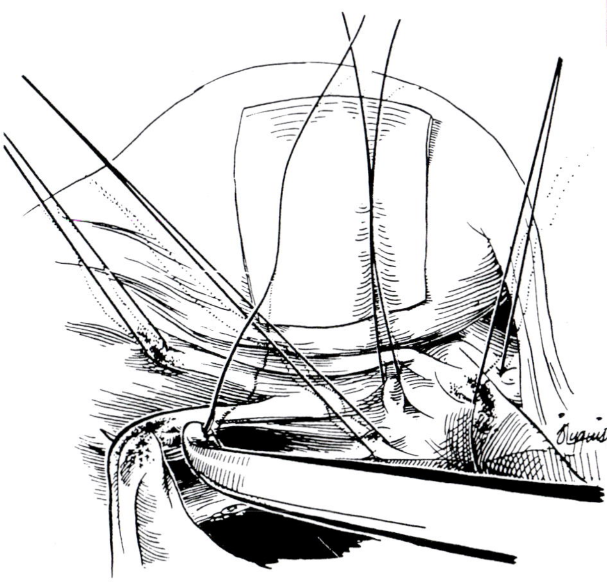

Fig. 35-25

Isolation of pelvic endometriotic lesions, marked with sutures (Figs. 35-24 through 35-29 reprinted with permission from Hunt[5]).

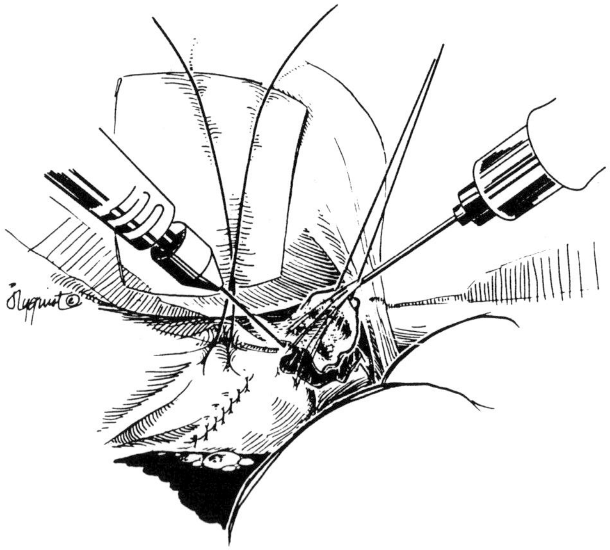

Fig. 35-26

Deep nodule removed by cautery, cul-de-sac closed.

Peritoneal wound closure no longer correct, leave open.

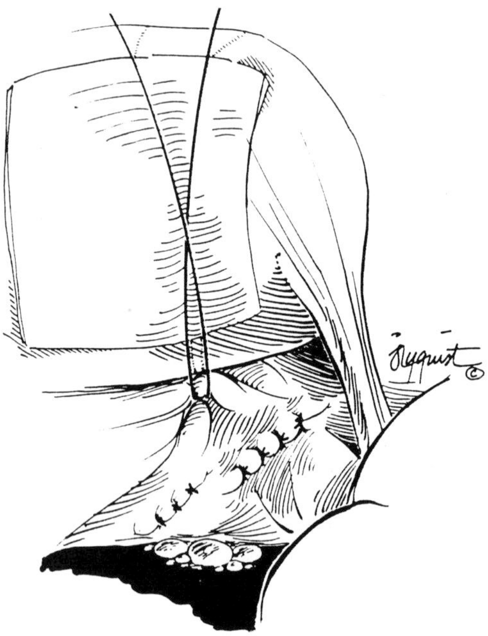

Fig. 35-27

Removal of endometriotic lesion leaves clean wound, do not close.

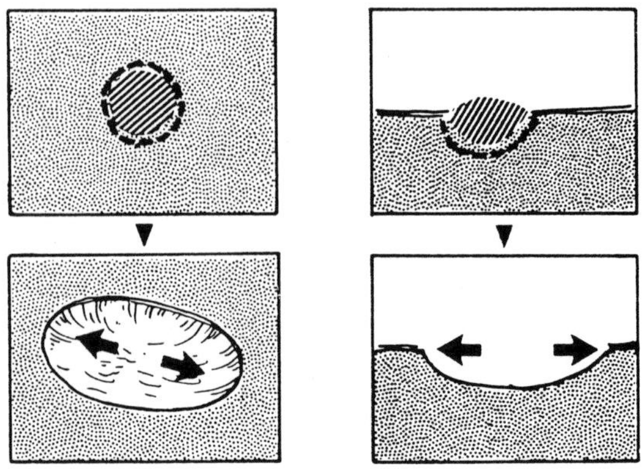

Fig. 35-28

Repaired ovaries and cul-de-sac patch.

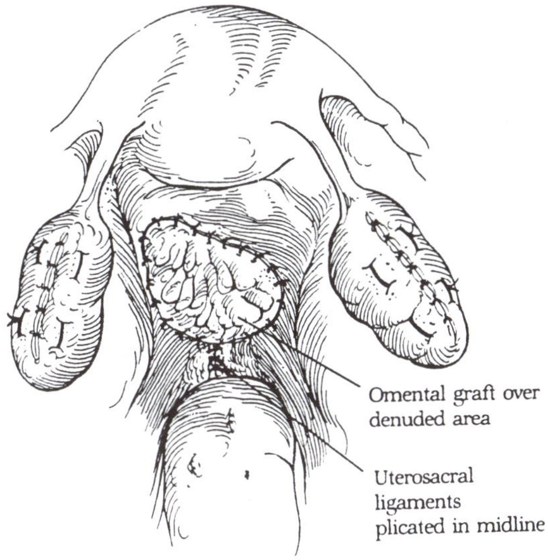

Fig. 35-29

Fine, easily lysed postoperative adhesions (Reprinted with permission from Phillips[1]).

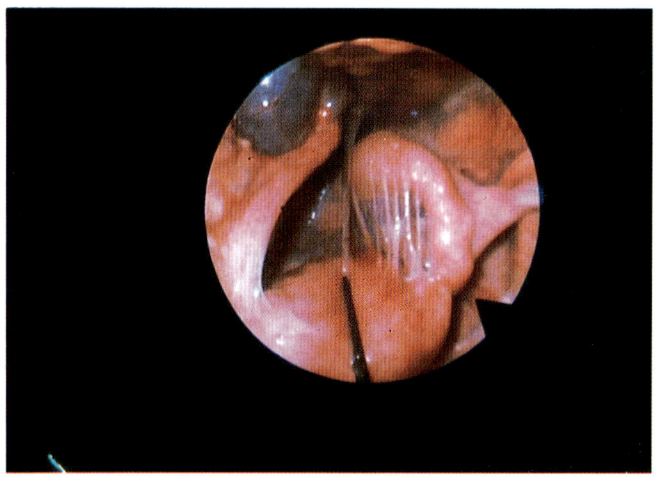

Fig. 35-30

Multiple lesions of severe endometriosis require multiple modes of treatment.

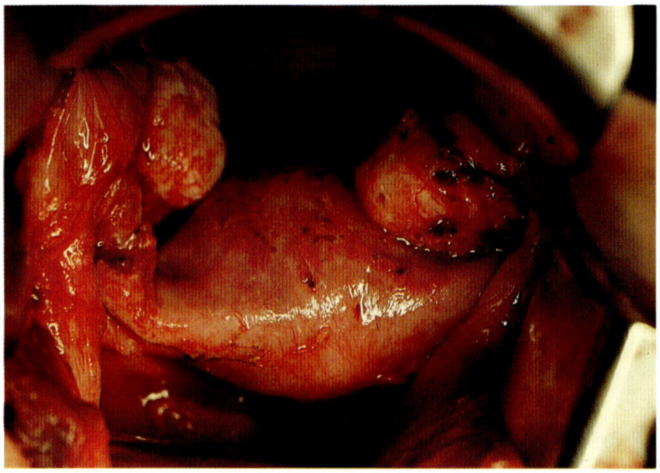

Fig. 35-31

Salpingectomy for severe endometriosis.

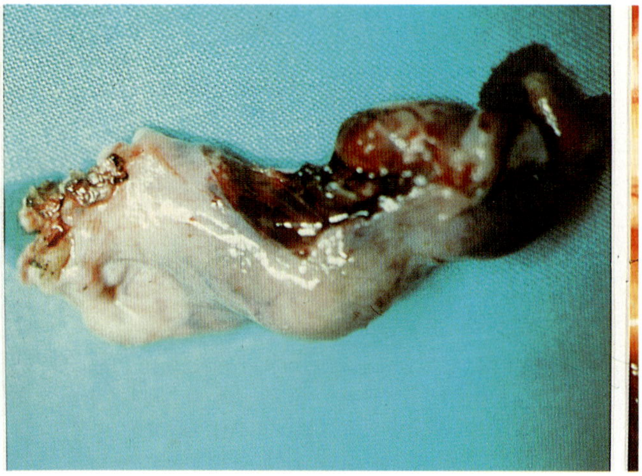

Fig. 35-32

References

1. Phillips J. Instructional slides from: *Endoscopy in Gynecology*. Published by A.A.G.L., Downey, Calif; 1985.
2. Patton G, Kistner R. *Atlas of Infertility Surgery*. 2nd ed. Boston, Mass: Little, Brown and Company; 1984.
3. McLaughlin J. *Lasers in Gynecology*. Philadelphia, Penn: JB Lippincott Co; 1992. Adapted by O.L.R., Medical Illustration Division, University of California, San Diego, Calif.
4. Semm K. *Atlas of Gynecology and Hysteroscopy, Slide-Atlas*. Philadelphia, Penn: WB Saunders Company; 1980.
5. Hunt R. *Atlas of Female Infertility Surgery*. Chicago, Ill: Year Book Publishers; 1986.

Chapter 36

Early and Late Postoperative Complications And Ectopic Pregnancy

Raphael B. Durfee, MD

Intraoperative complications and postoperative problems, both early and late, are encountered, fortunately, infrequently. These depicted here were not all repairable and many were referrals. One of these was a postoperative PID referral that proved to be inoperable. The management of tubal pregnancies has improved greatly with the development of reliable early pregnancy tests, laparoscopy, and microtubal surgical repair. Some of these very early pregnancies with minimal tubal damage can be corrected by laparoscopy alone; some can be repaired at a later date by laparotomy; and still others can be repaired at the time of diagnosis, frequently through a minilaparotomy incision. Cornual or interstitial ectopic pregnancy can be fatal if it ruptures late, fourteen weeks or more, and requires considerable surgical repair. It may be best to defer treatment until later when the patient is in better condition and one can survey the damage to the cornual area much better; if the opposite side is nonfunctional, tubouterine implantation may be considered.

Adhesion formation may be a late complication that can occasionally be managed through the laparoscope and lends itself readily to combination with the laser. Microsurgical reoperation requires skill and experience and is usually never as successful as the first attempt. High molecular weight dextran solution may be helpful when placed intraperitoneal at the time of closure of the abdominal wound. No potential for adhesion formation should remain intact.

An ability to diagnose early ectopic pregnancy by the use of accurate tests and an increased awareness of the early symptoms of impending tubal rupture have greatly improved the management of these problems. More importantly, this clinical acumen has reduced the mortality rate. Conservative treatment of tubal pregnancy either by laparoscope or minilaparotomy with preservation of the tubal tissue is the main treatment of extrauterine pregnancy.

Contemporary medical management of early ectopic pregnancy with reversible Methotrexate or Actinomycin-D and other modalities has proved to be possible. The effectiveness of this kind of therapy is evidenced by sequential refined measurement of the decrease or even disappearance of chorionic hormone.

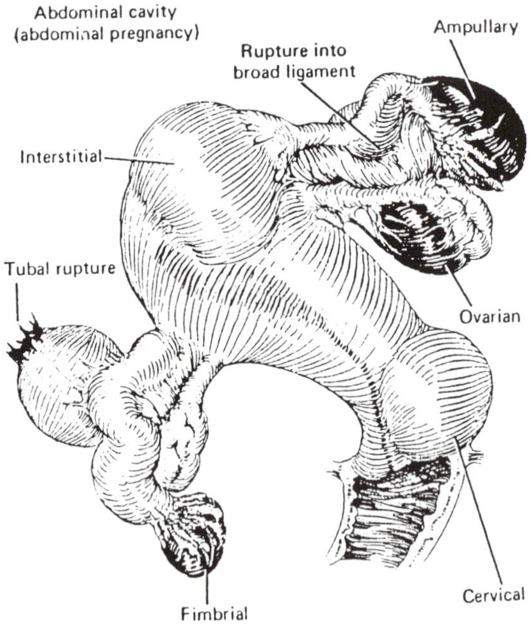

Fig. 36-1

Ectopic pregnancy sites (Reprinted with permission from Pernoll[1]).

Early fimbrial ectopic pregnancy.

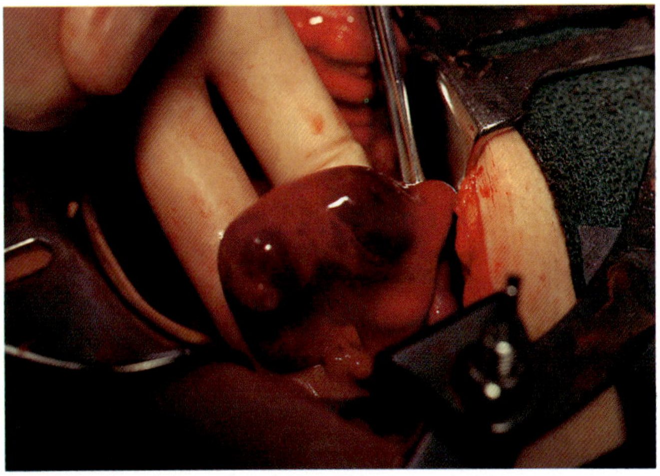

Fig. 36-2

Extrusion by gentle, careful pressure.

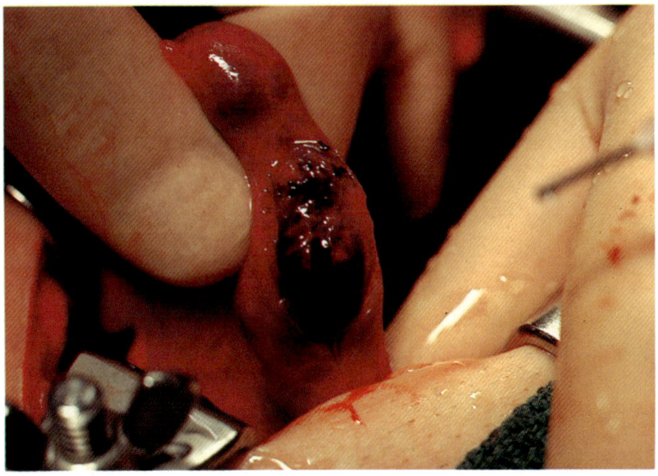

Fig. 36-3

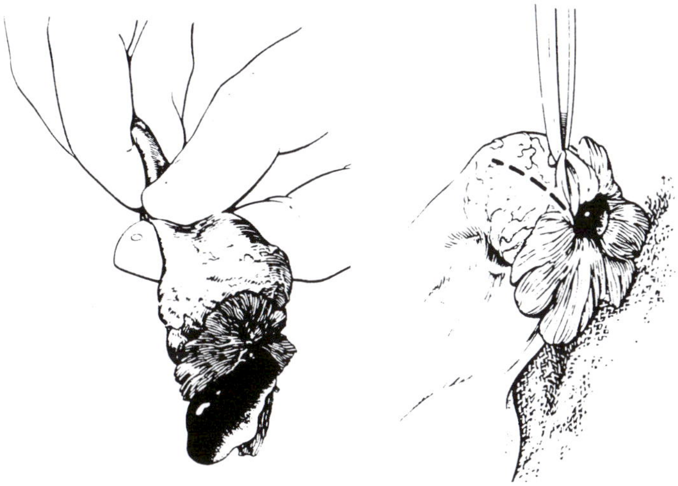

Fig. 36-4

Tube can be opened by superior incision if necessary (Reprinted with permission from Patton[2]).

Early and late postoperative complications

These complications all happened prior to the conclusion of surgery or within the first three to eight months. Not all were repairable. Some were referrals.

Immediate postanastomotic hematoma, repaired at once.

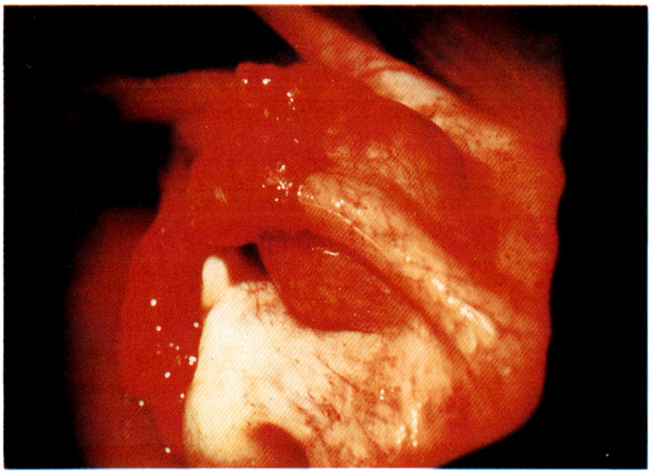

Fig. 36-5

Developing hydrosalpinx, reanastomosed at once.

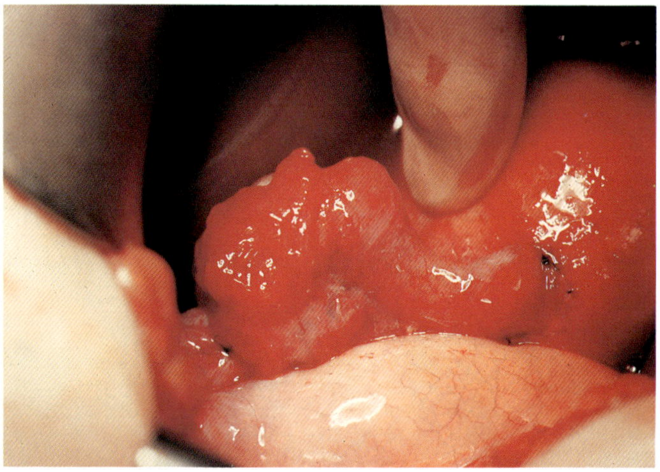

Fig. 36-6

Nonrepairable fimbrial release.

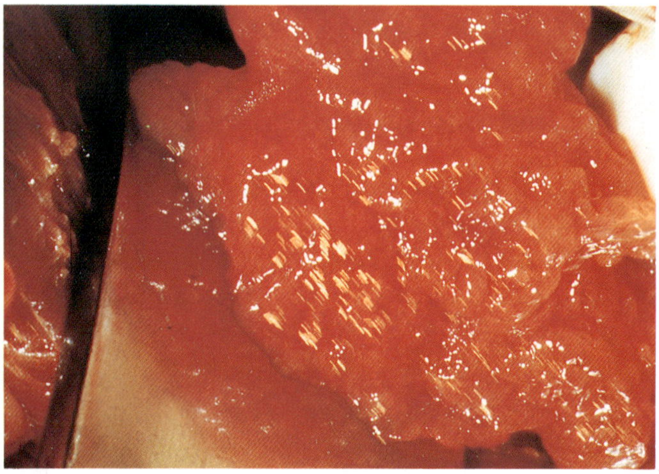

Fig. 36-7

Anatomic malpositioned fimbria, not replaceable.

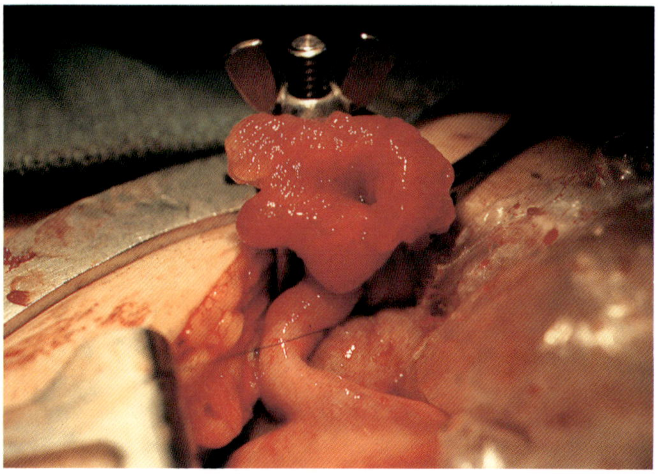

Fig. 36-8

Anastomotic separation, late.

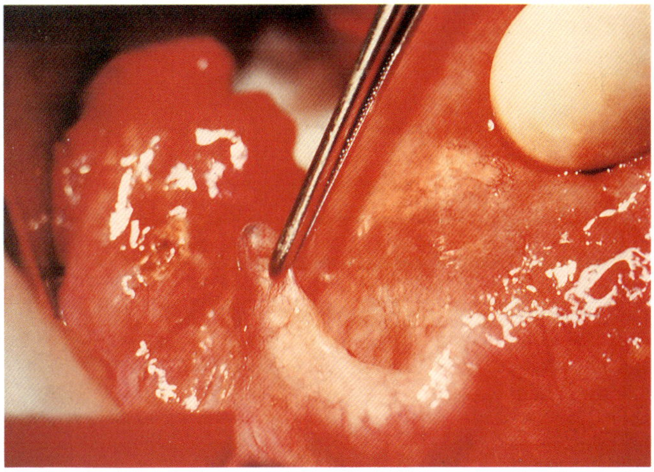

Fig. 36-9

Anastomotic separation, early.

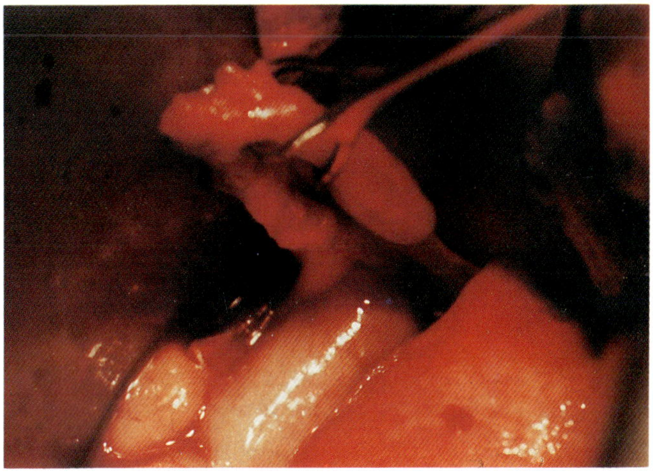

Fig. 36-10

Fimbrial-ovarian adhesions.

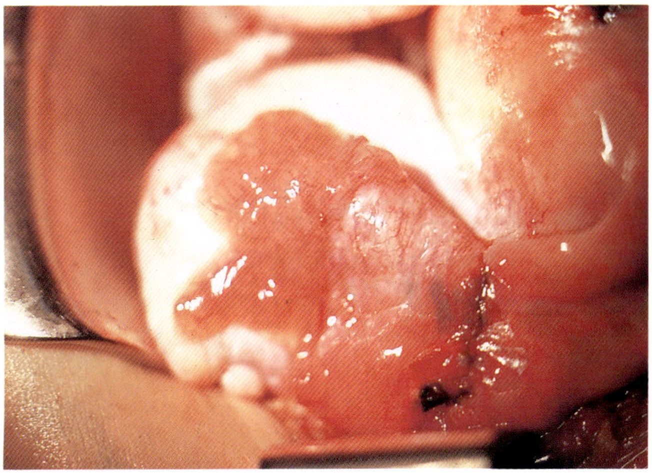

Fig. 36-11

Normal fimbrial-ovarian contact.

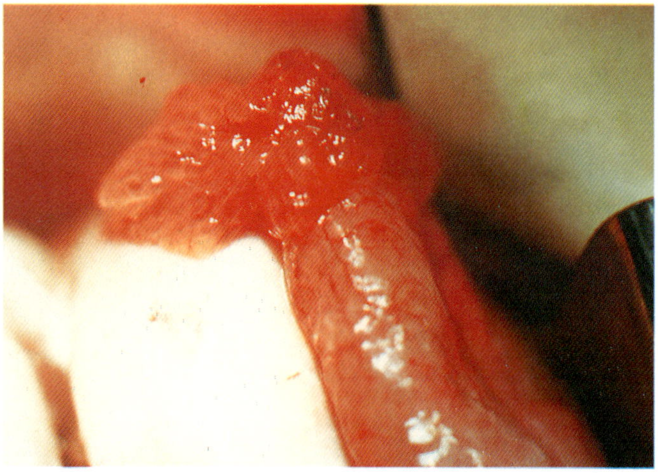

Fig. 36-12

Early postoperative adhesions.

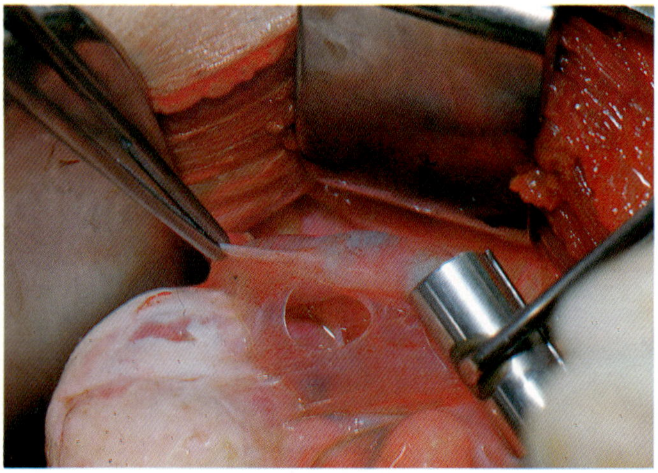

Fig. 36-13

Late postoperative adhesions.

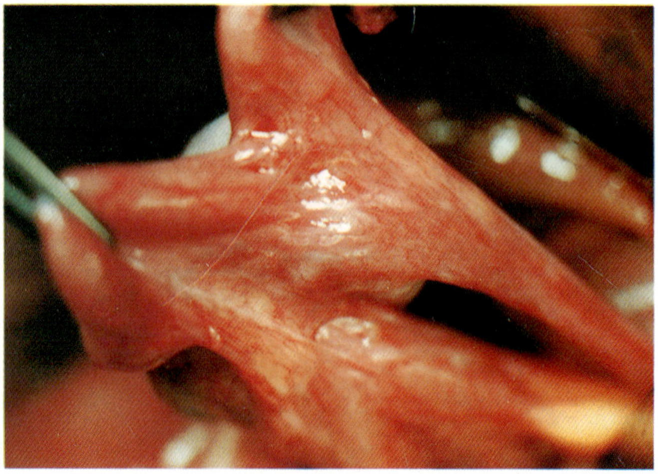

Fig. 36-14

Postoperative agglutination fimbria, hydrosalpinx.

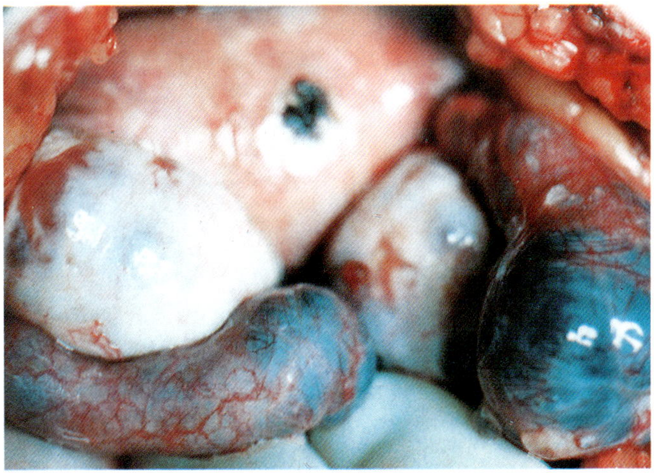

Fig. 36-15

Ligation adhesion, after Pomeroy procedure.

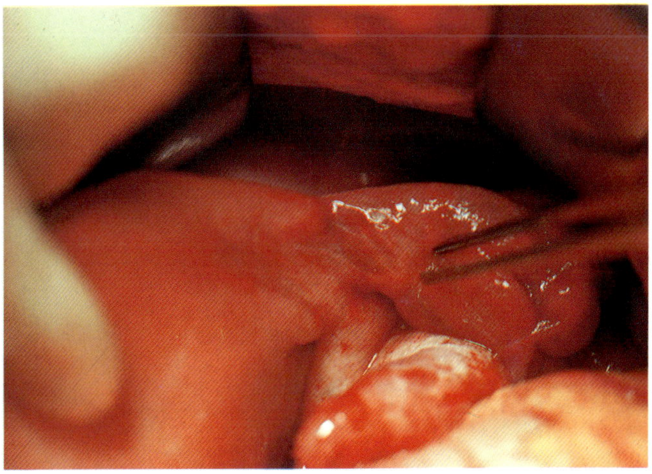

Fig. 36-16

Isthmic ectopic pregnancy removed with tubal preservation.

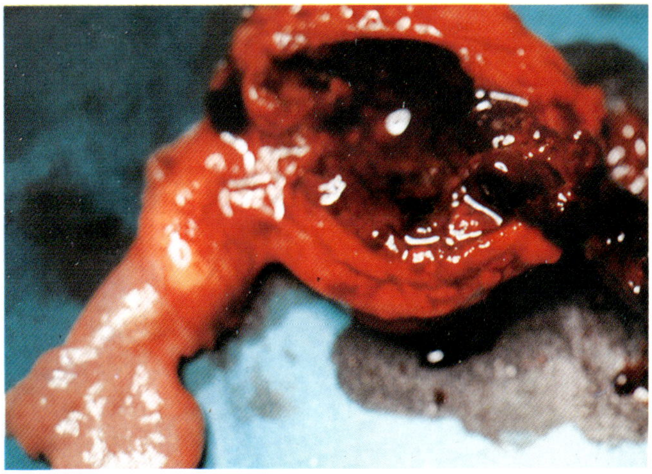

Fig. 36-17

Hemostasis in tissue bed by cautery. Tube closed by fine suture (Reprinted with permission from Patton[2]).

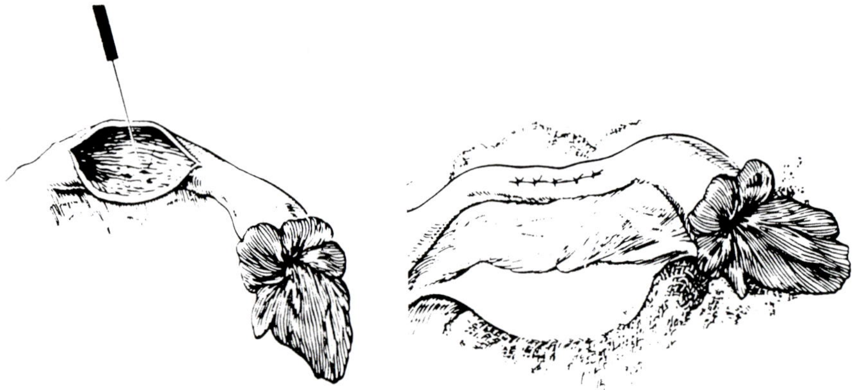

Fig. 36-18

Tubal suture closure. May be left open.

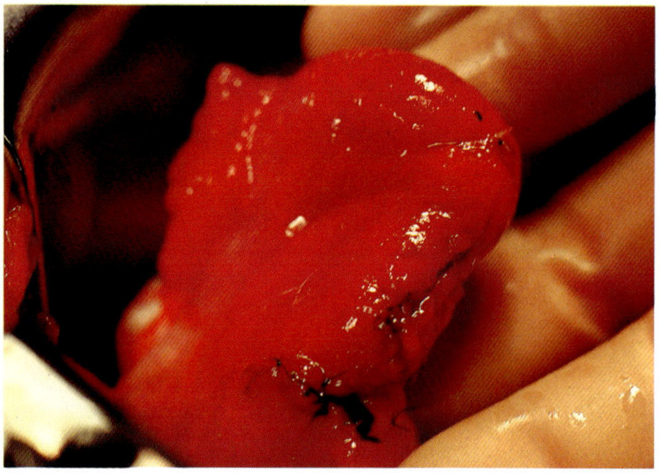

Fig. 36-19

Tube cut across, tissues removed, anastomosed if possible, ligated if not (Figs. 36-20 through 36-23 reprinted with permission from Patton[2]).

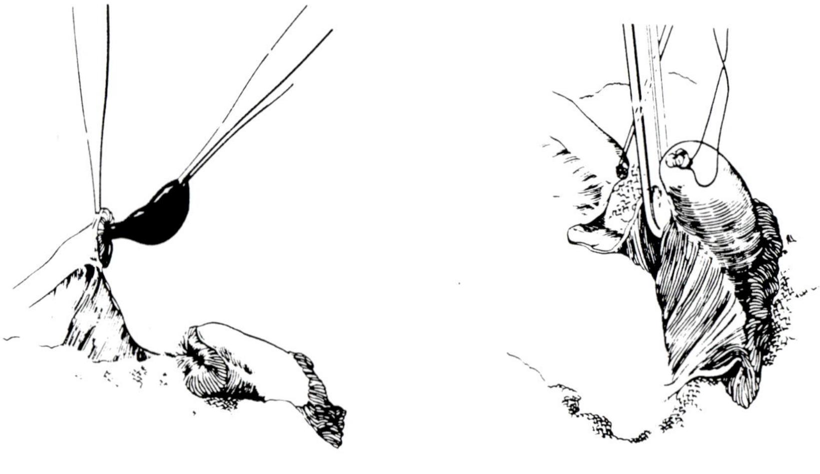

Fig. 36-20

If anastomosed, serosa is closed.

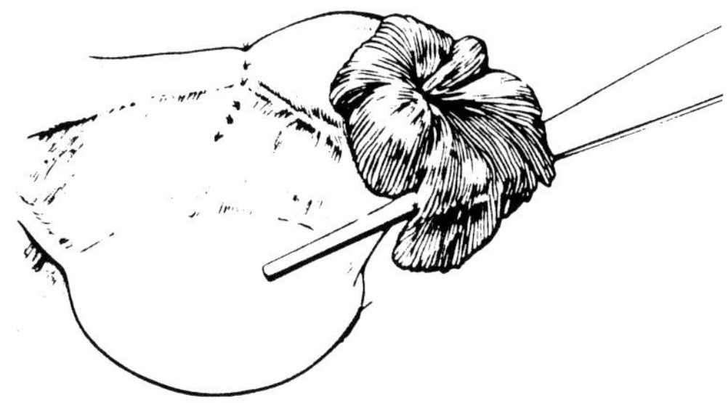

Fig. 36-21

Ampullary ectopic pregnancy, treated the same.

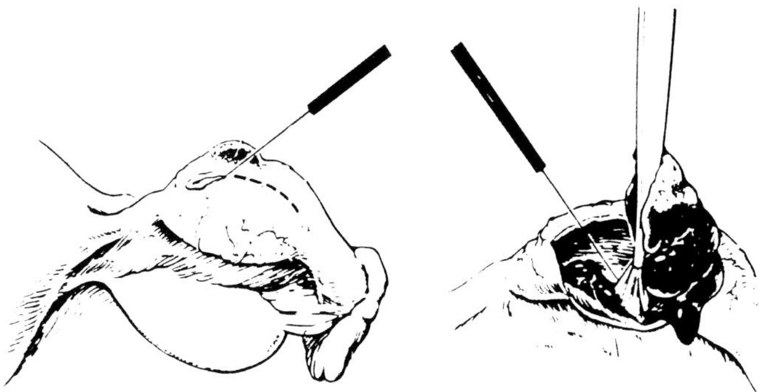

Fig. 36-22

Clots and tissues removed, hemostasis obtained.

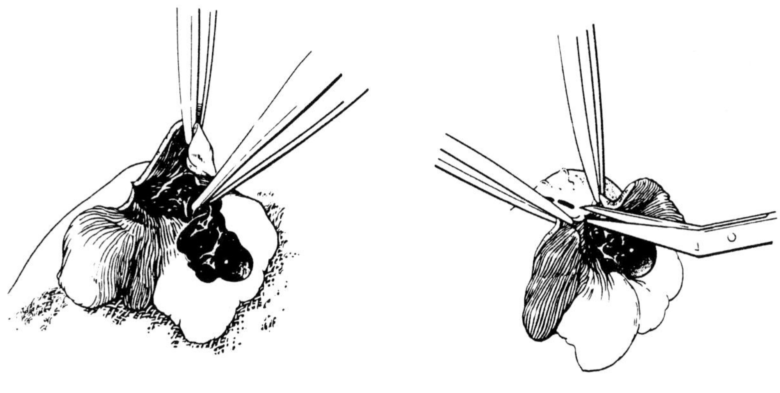

Fig. 36-23

Similar appearance, same condition.

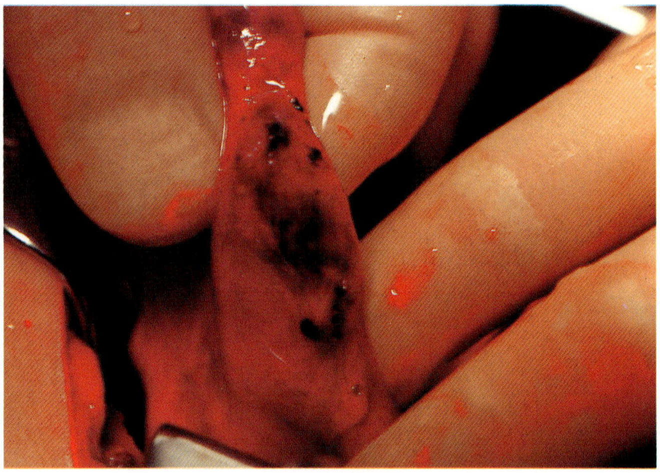

Fig. 36-24

Tube closed by fine suture (Reprinted with permission from Patton[2]).

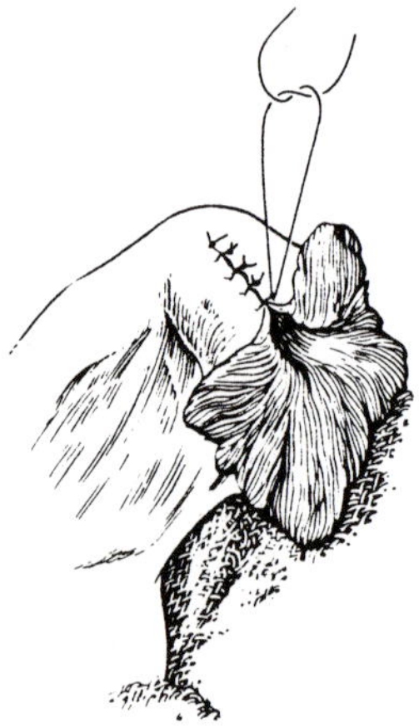

Fig. 36-25

Tube may be left open.

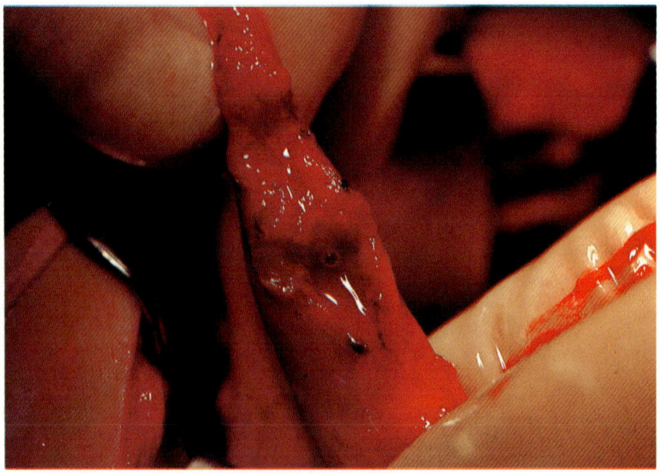

Fig. 36-26

Isthmic ectopic pregnancy.

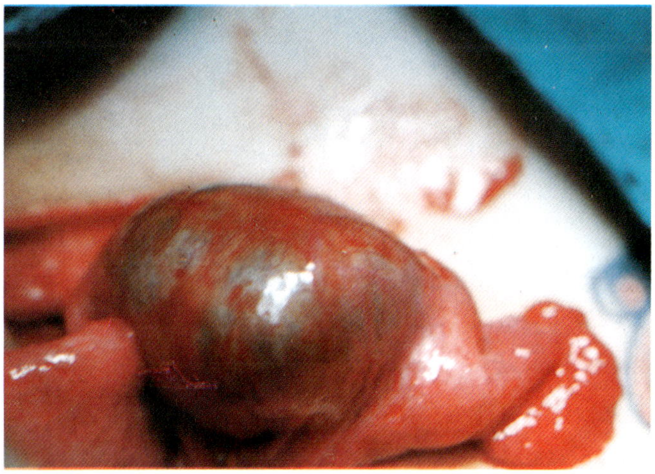

Fig. 36-27

Tissues removed from isthmus by coagulation and dissection, superior incision (Reprinted with permission from Patton[2]).

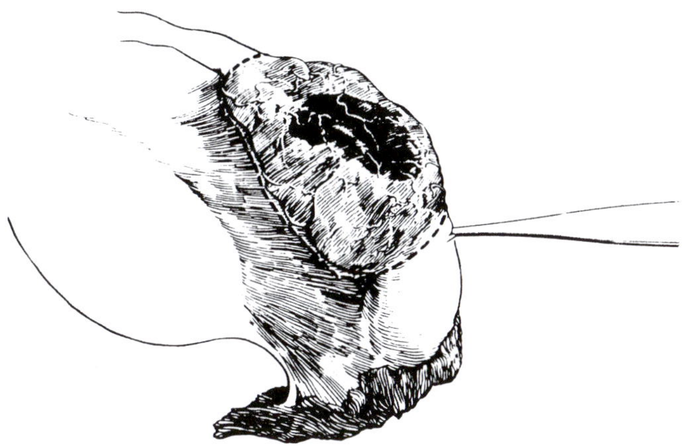

Fig. 36-28

Lateral view of interstitial pregnancy after cornual-tubal anastomosis.

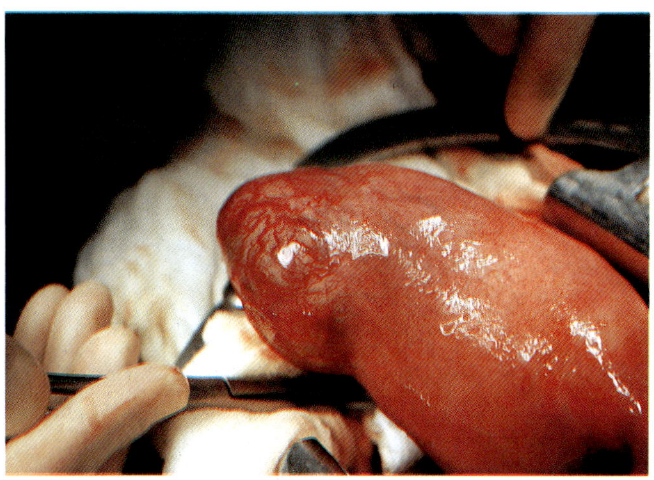

Fig. 36-29

End-on view of same. Treated by excision and plastic uterine repair.

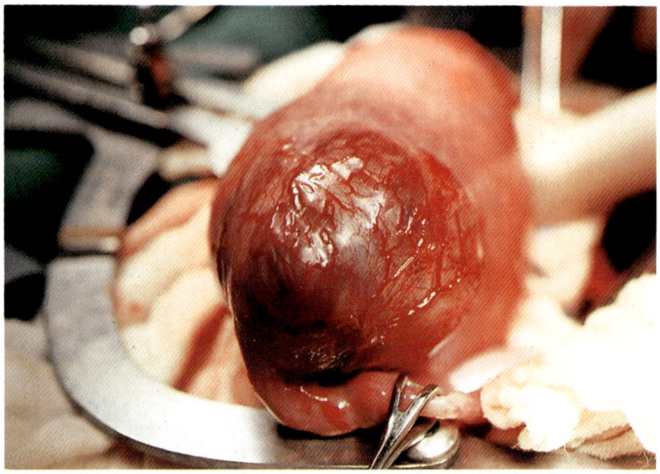

Fig. 36-30

Abdominal pregnancy.

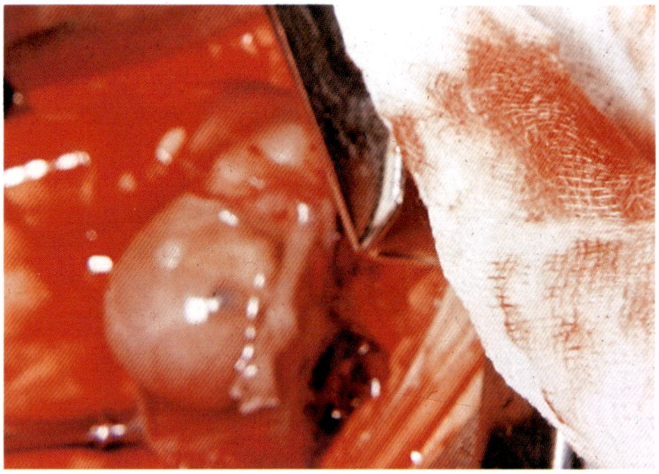

Fig. 36-31

References

1. Pernoll M, Benson R. *Current Obstetric and Gynecologic Diagnosis and Treatment*. 6th ed. East Norwalk, Ct: Appleton-Lange; 1989.
2. Patton G, Kistner R. *Atlas of Infertility Surgery*. 2nd ed. Boston, Mass: Little, Brown and Company; 1984.

Chapter 37

Points of Interest in Gynecologic Microsurgery

Raphael B. Durfee, MD

A summary of some of the details of pathology and procedures in the course of using microsurgery and the laser in Gynecology will complete this review. The value of new methods of examination, even though invasive, is that information on the condition of the pelvic organs is now available. The "blind eye" of the surgeon's index finger has been replaced by direct vision. The application of therapeutic manipulation by many and various means has improved the outcome of therapy in Gynecology.

CO_2 dispensing and monitoring device for endoscopy (Eder).

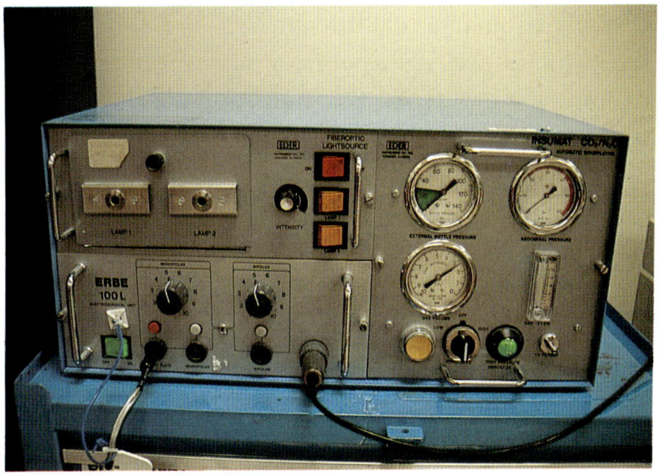

Fig. 37-1

Ancillary instruments together.

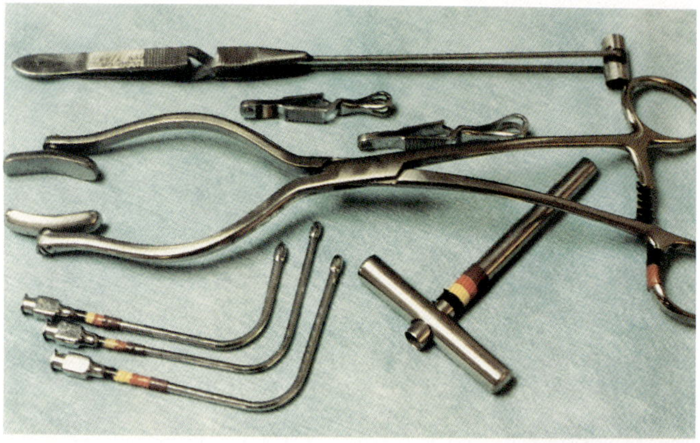

Fig. 37-2

Note exchange of instruments between scrub nurse and the operator. This reduces eye movement from the field, preventing fatigue.

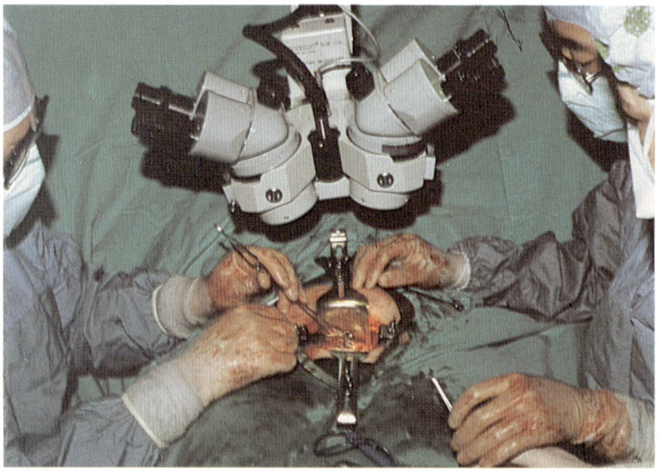

Fig. 37-3

Long handle tube holder facilitates tubal manipulation.

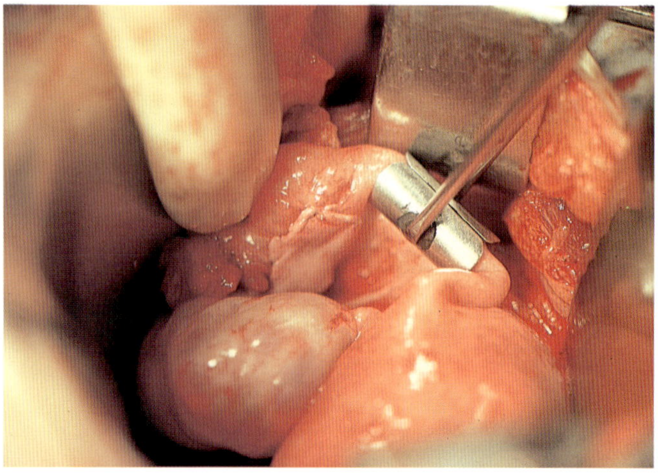

Fig. 37-4

Custom-made loupes may be used instead of a microscope.

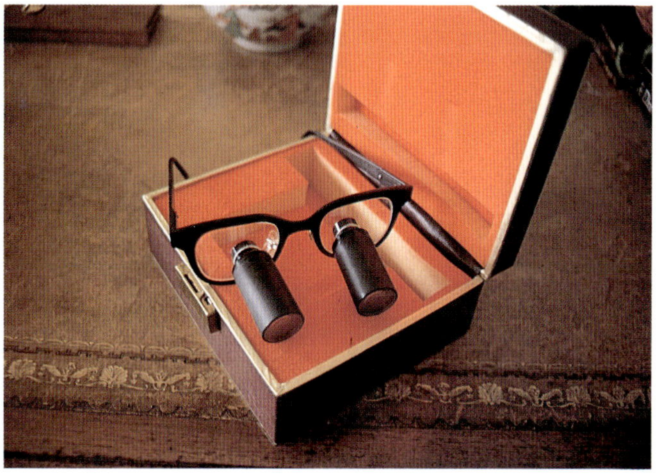

Fig. 37-5

Loupes may be made in individual magnification.

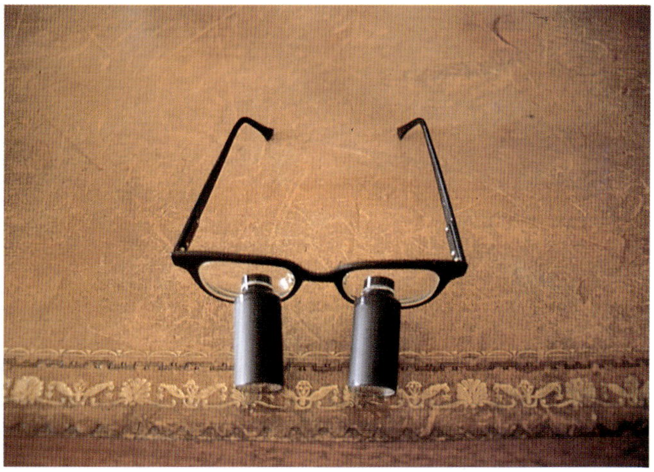

Fig. 37-6

Loupes have an advantage of being more adaptable to situations in which it is necessary to move back and forth from macro to micro surgery. Loupes also allow movement of the surgeon's head to vary the field that is observed. One problem is to be able to hold the head steady for a long time without tiring. Some people have too much of a tremor in the muscles of the neck to use loupes efficiently.

Number 18 intracath for dye injection through the uterine cavity.

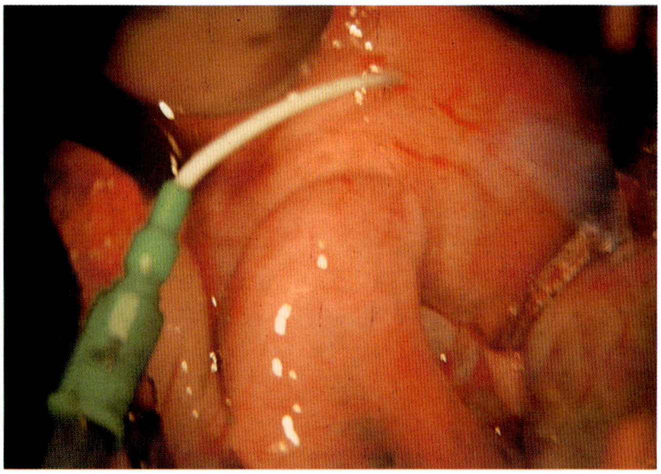

Fig. 37-7

A bulldog clamp to atraumatically occlude the tube as needed.

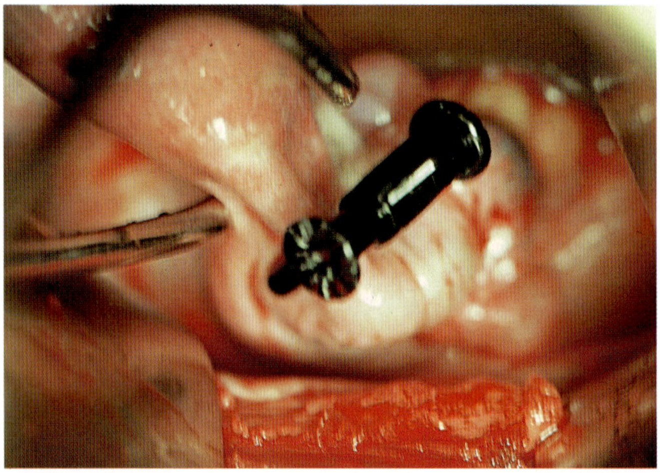

Fig. 37-8

Subcuticular wound closure with collodian seal and suprapubic catheter.

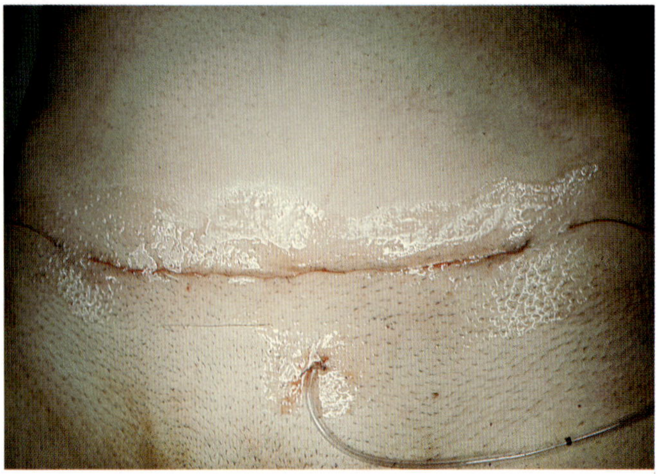

Fig. 37-9

Lachrymal probe used to test for patency, most effective for interstitial cornual lumens.

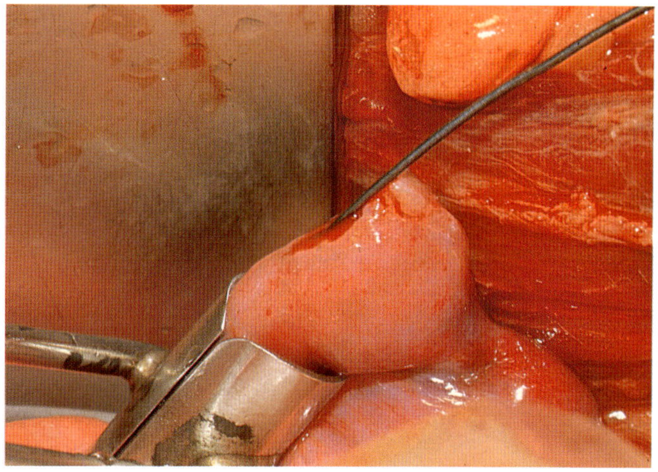

Fig. 37-10

The use of stents with tubal anastomosis is controversial. The advantages are stabilization of the movable tube to facilitate suture placement, and to maintain a lumen without constriction. The disadvantage is the probable trauma to the fragile cellular components of the tubal mucosa. Stents are essential in tubal implantation.

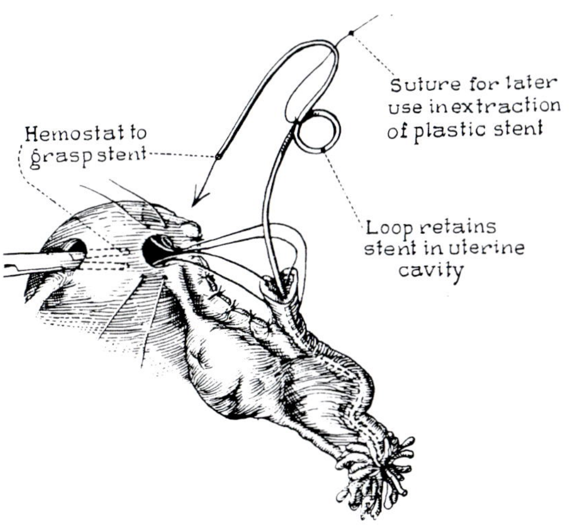

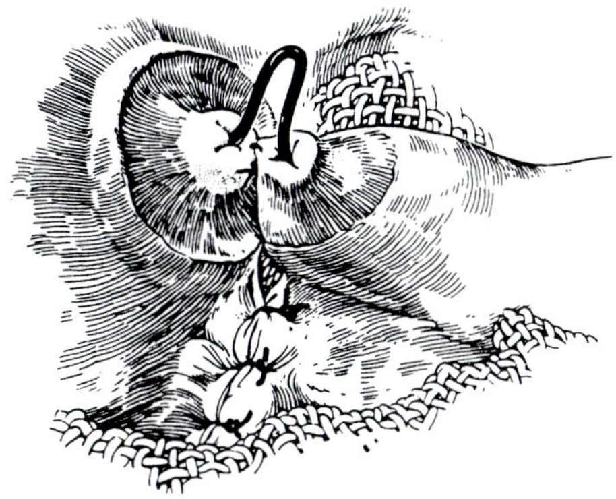

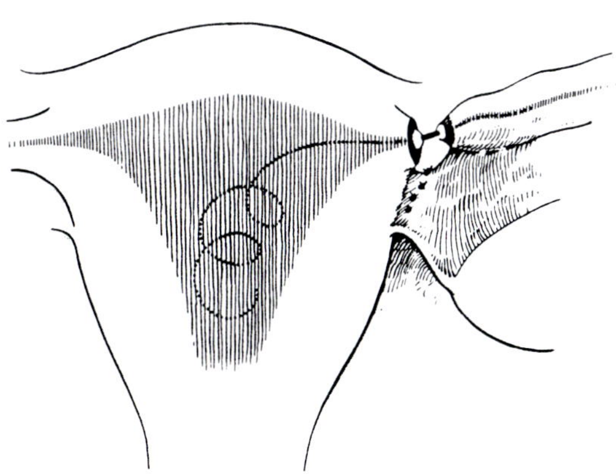

Fig. 37-11 Various uses of stents (Reprinted with permission from Jones[1] and Patton[2]).

Short reinforced instrument for tying.

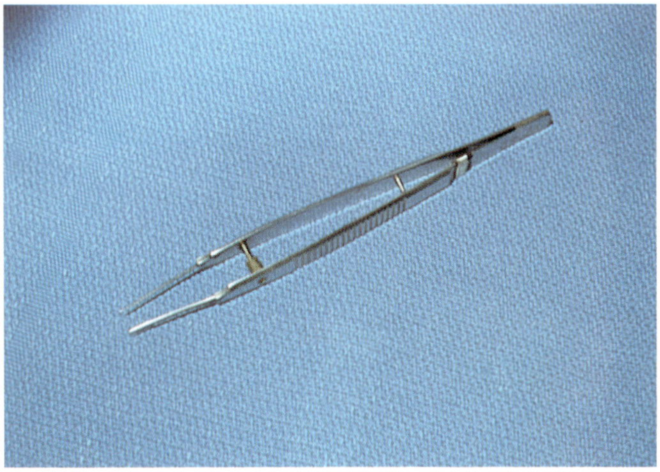

Fig. 37-12

Long handle tissue forceps.

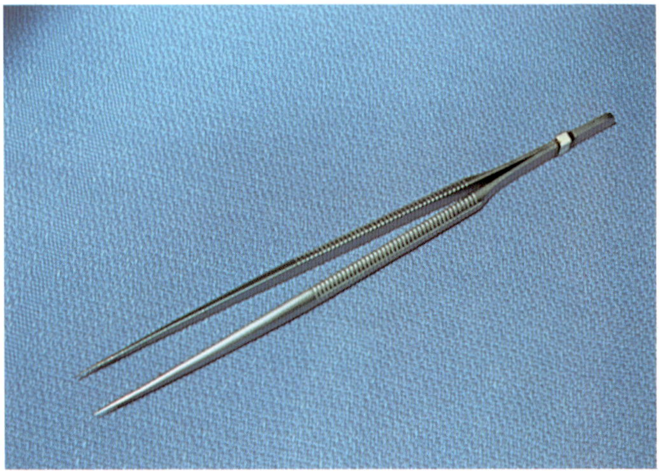

Fig. 37-13

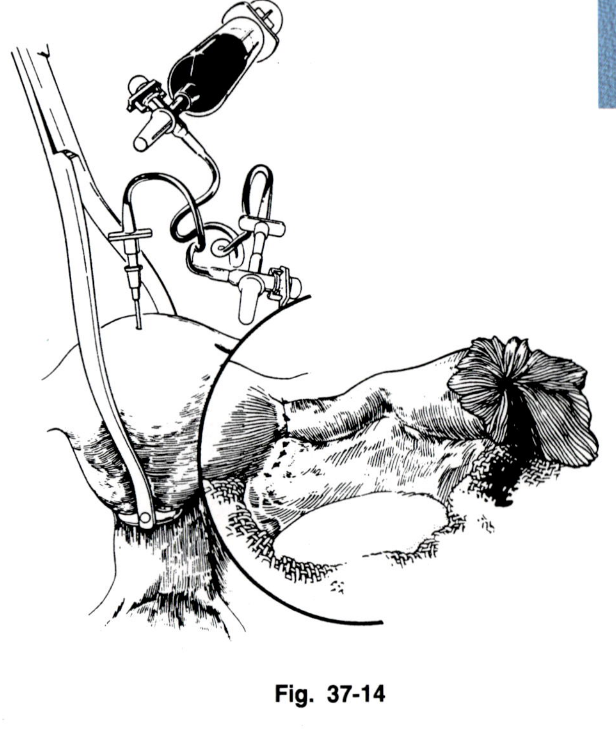

Fig. 37-14

Transuterine dye injection using Buxton clamp obstruction (Reprinted with permission from Patton[2]).

Serosal surface with reaction to drying causes adhesions.

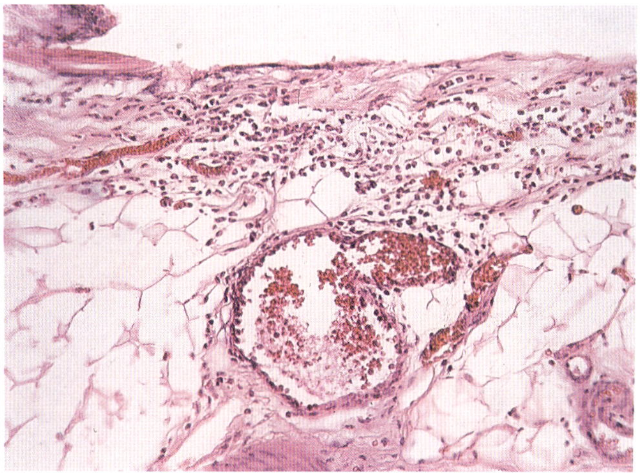

Fig. 37-15

Fine cautery tip for dissection.

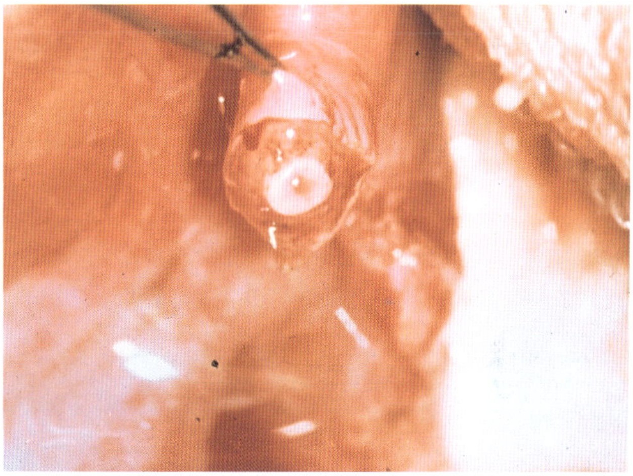

Fig. 37-16

Fine cautery tip for hemostasis.

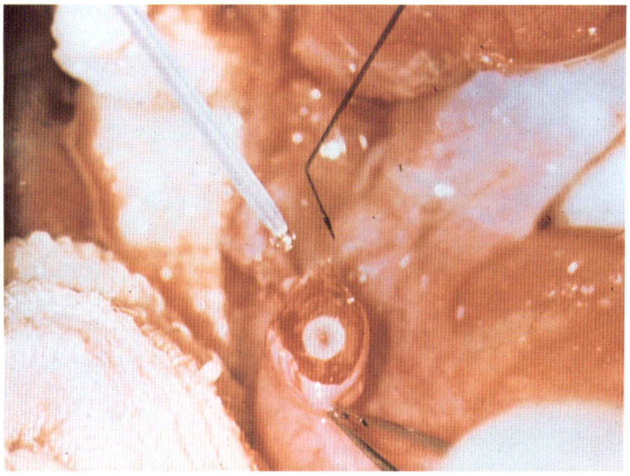

Fig. 37-17

Torsion of the Fallopian tube.

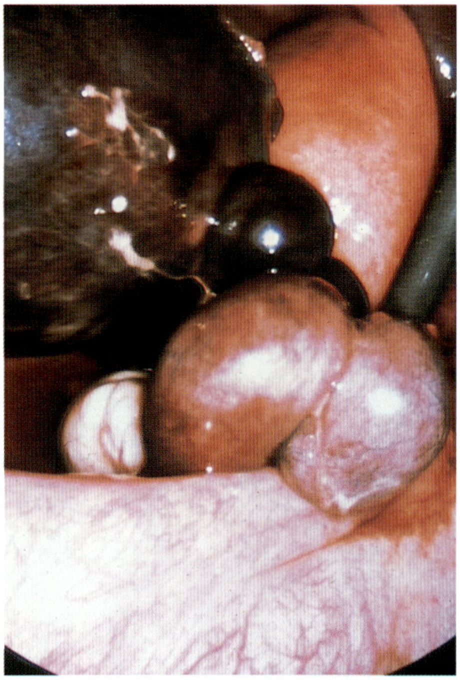

Fig. 37-18

Right hemiuterus (Reprinted with permission from Phillips[3]).

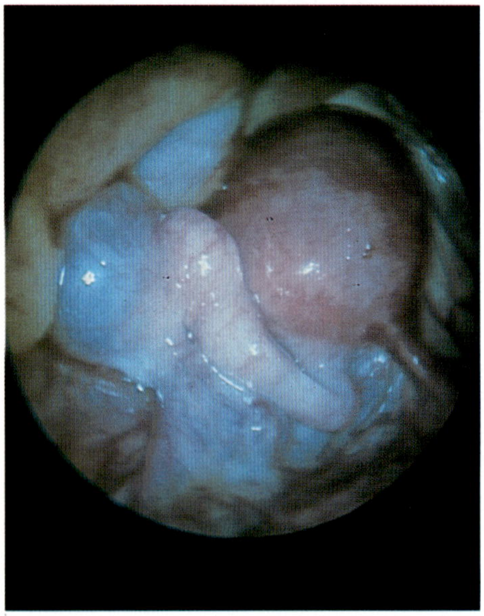

Fig. 37-19

Dilated ampulla.

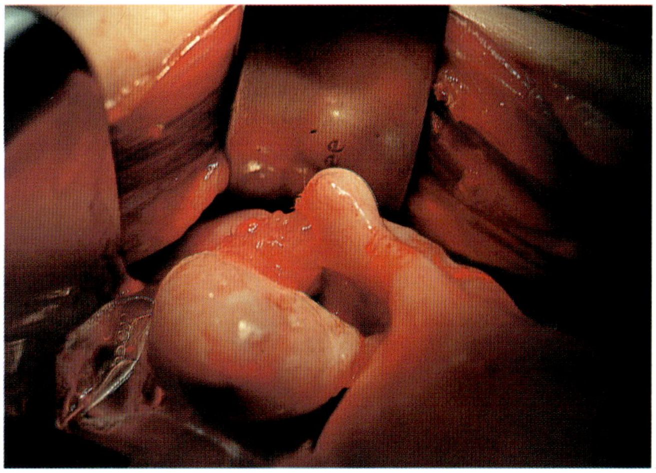

Fig. 37-20

Buried Fallope ring.

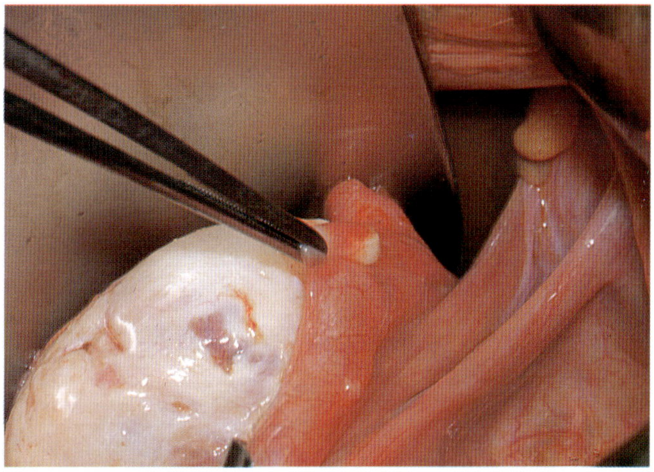

Fig. 37-21

Tubal transplant donor tissue (Figs. 37-23 through 37-29 reprinted with permission from Silber[5]).

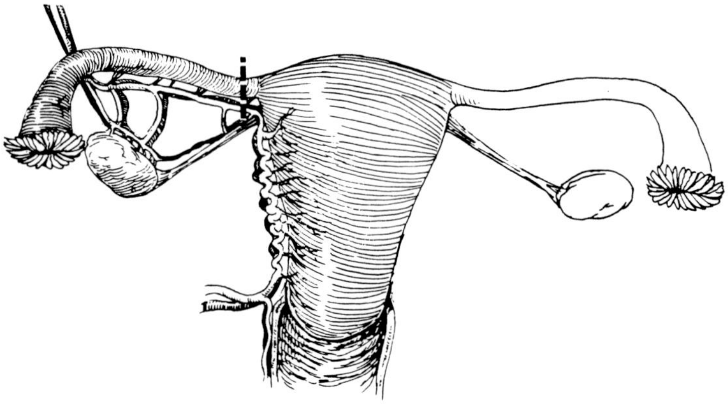

Fig. 37-22

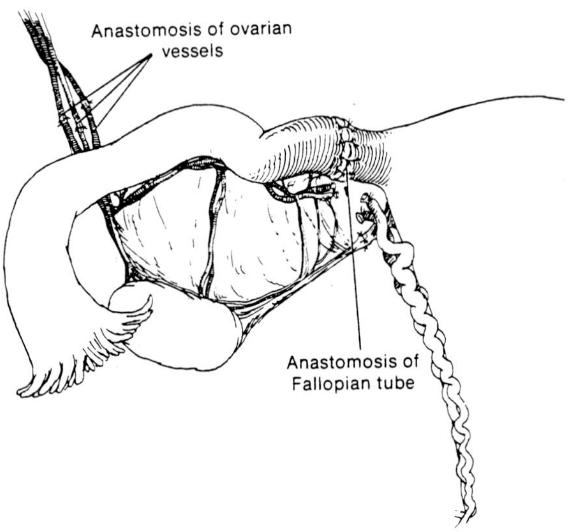

Fig. 37-23

Recipient, using anastomosed ovarian circulation and isthmic tubal anastomosis.

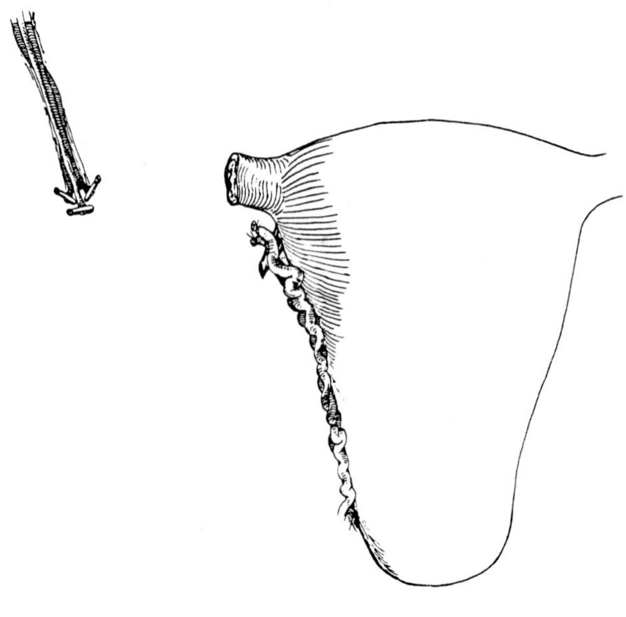

Fig. 37-24

Tube and ovary are removed from donor site.

Recipient, using ovarian artery and vein.

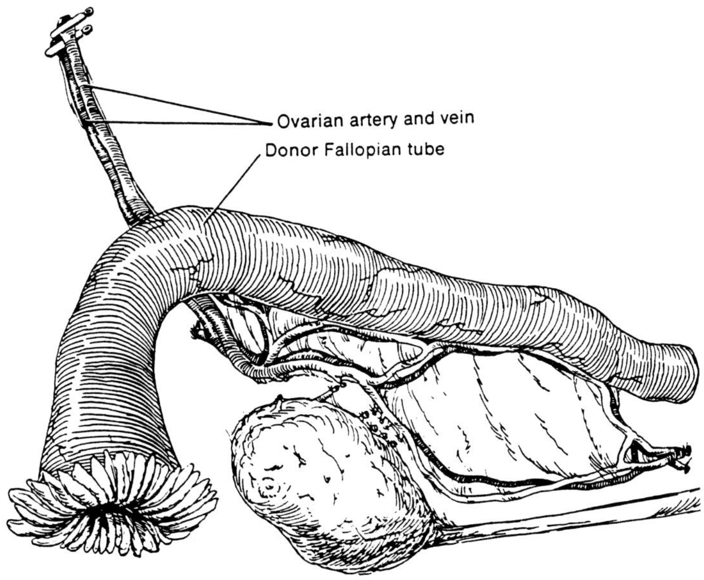

Fig. 37-25

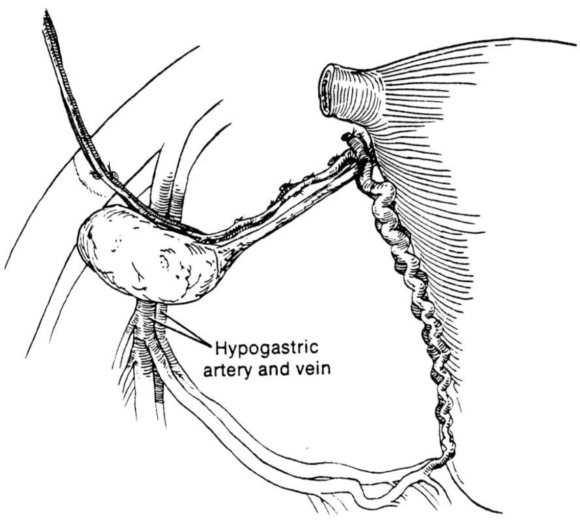

Fig. 37-26

Donor site, leaving ovary in place.

Recipient, ovarian vessels anastomosed to hypogastric vessels.

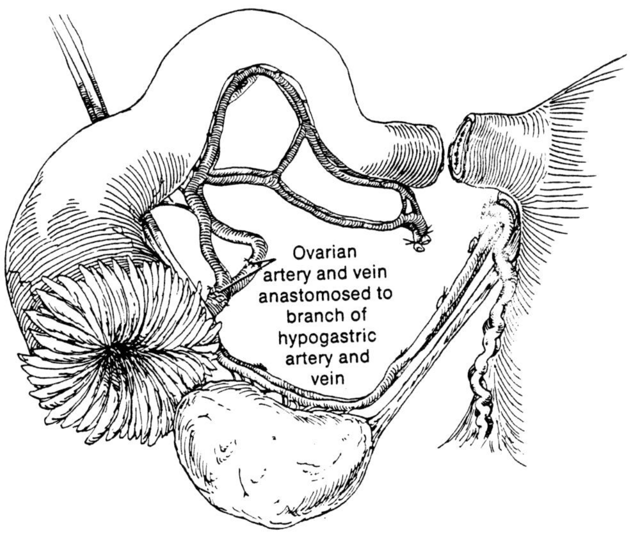

Fig. 37-27

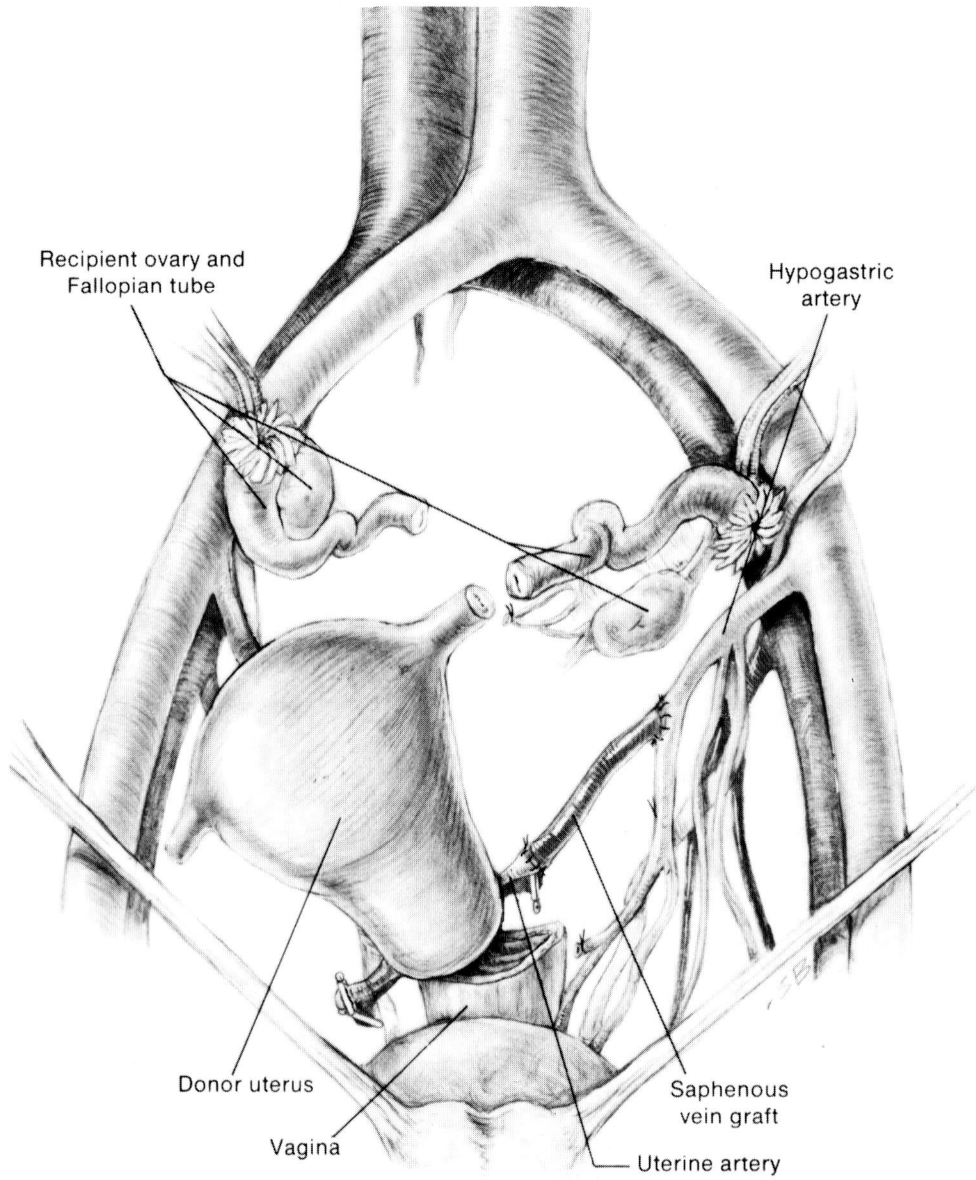

Fig. 37-28 Hypothetical uterine transplant.

Autogenous tubal and ovarian transplants have been successful. They utilize the opposite organs for the donor site and require meticulous, very fine microsutures: 10-0, 11-0, 12-0. Each vessel anastomosis must be fluid tight and without tension. The tubal anastomosis should be isthmic-isthmic for best results. All sutured areas must be examined under the microscope before closure of the abdomen. Tubal patency must be proven as well.

Heterologous transplants, especially uterine, have given way to IVF, since with the possible exception of the ovary, there are no markers to measure tissue rejection in the tube or uterus at the present time.

References

1. Jones H, Rock J. *Reparative and Constructive Surgery of the Female Generative Tract*. Baltimore, Md: Williams and Wilkins; 1983.
2. Patton G, Kistner R. *Atlas of Infertility Surgery*. 2nd ed. Boston, Mass: Little, Brown and Company; 1984.
3. Phillips J. Instructional slides from: *Endoscopy in Gynecology*. Published by A.A.G.L., Downey, Calif; 1985.
4. Gomel V. *Microsurgery in Female Infertility*. Boston, Mass: Little, Brown and Company; 1983.
5. Silber P. *Reproductive Infertility Microsurgery in Males and Females*. Baltimore, Md: Williams and Wilkins; 1986.

Chapter 38

Clinical Cases

Raphael B. Durfee, MD

Case #1. Isthmus-Fimbria Tubal Anastomosis

The patient had had bilateral laparoscopic tubal ligation with unipolar coagulation. Severe left-sided pain several weeks postoperative. She wanted ligation reversal following the death of two children.

General appearance of pelvic organs.

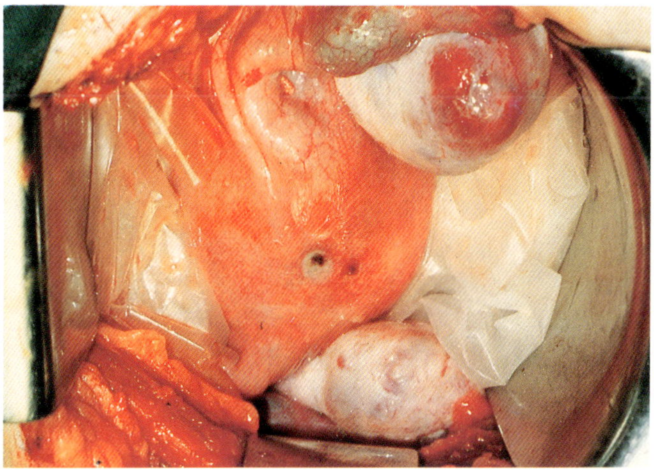

Fig. 38-1

Distal obstruction, hydrosalpinx, left.

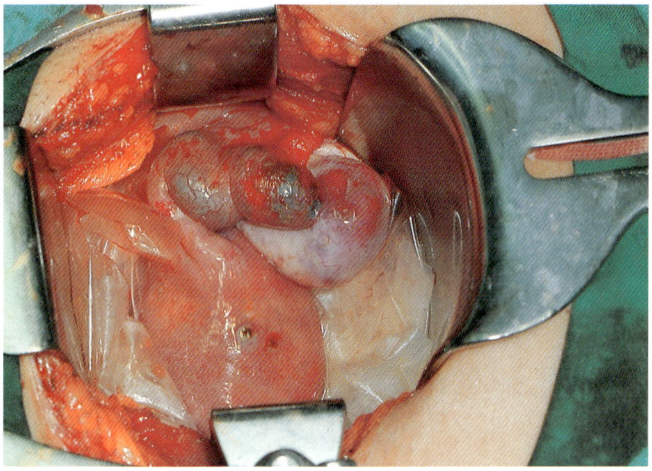

Fig. 38-2

Extensive isthmical damage, right.

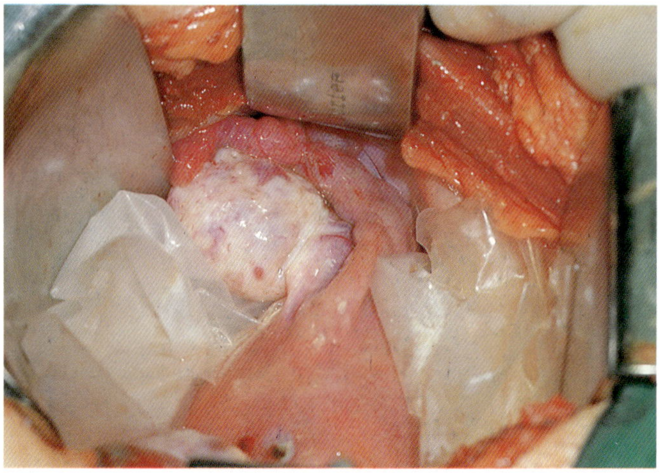

Fig. 38-3

Intact fimbria and some ampulla.

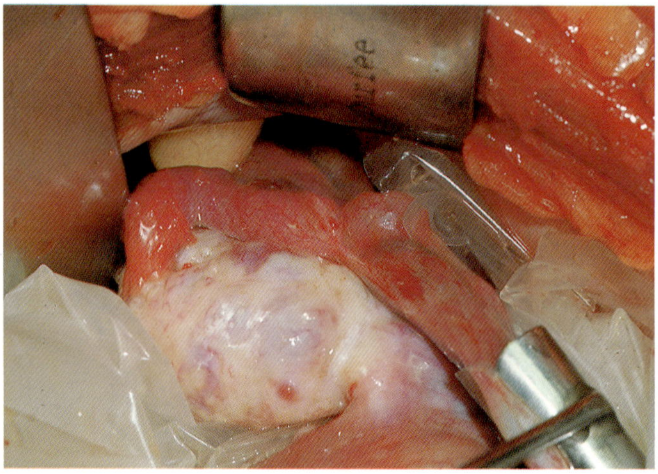

Fig. 38-4

Mobilization, proximal tube.

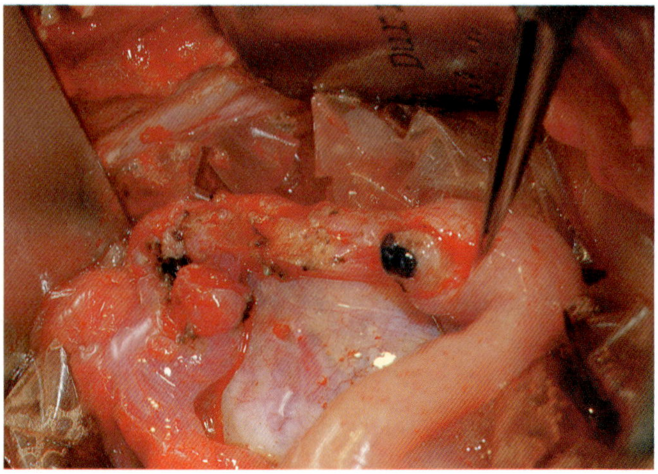

Fig. 38-5

First suture, isthmus-ampulla.

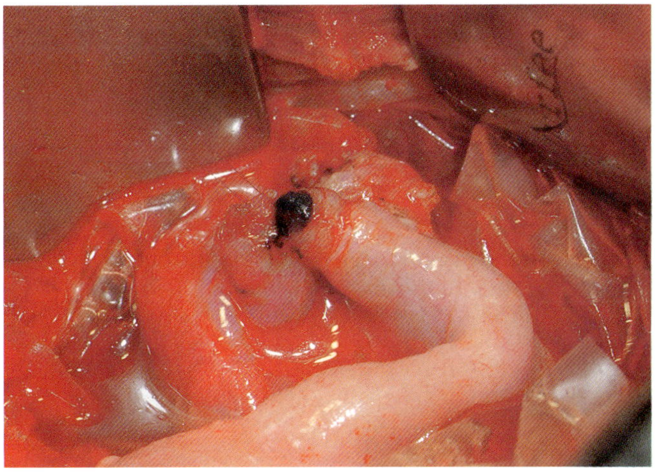

Fig. 38-6

Second suture, isthmus-ampulla.

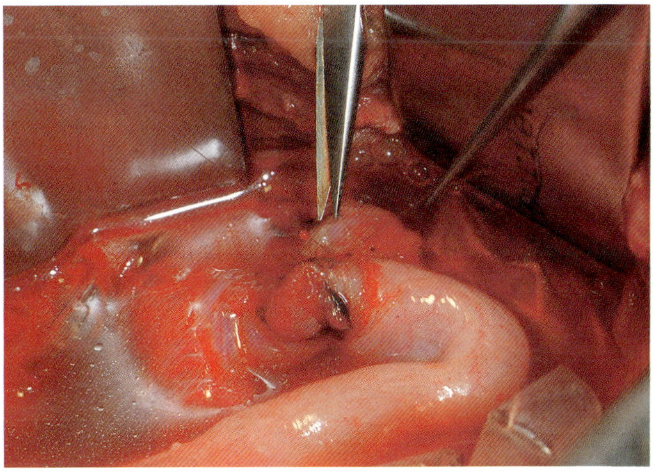

Fig. 38-7

Third suture, same.

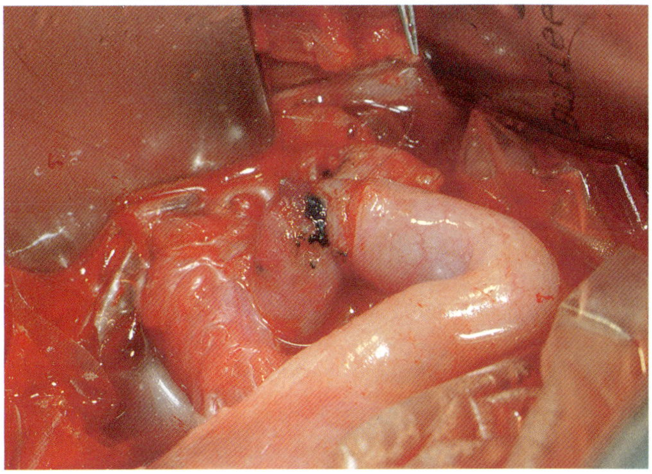

Fig. 38-8

Anastomosis completed, isthmus-ampulla.

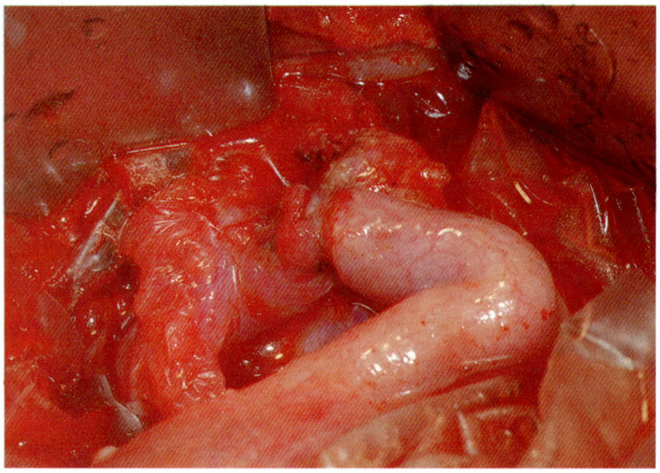

Fig. 38-9

Serosal closure, final appearance, patent.

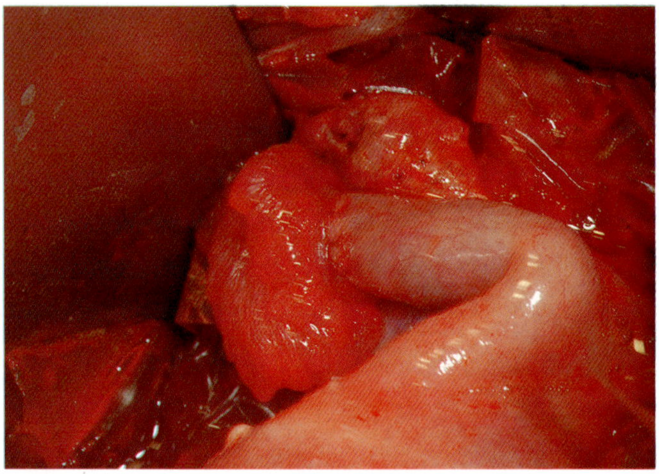

Fig. 38-10

Patient has since conceived twice, aborted both times. One year following the last abortion a live child was delivered prematurely.

Case #2.
Isthmic Neosalpingostomy

Patient had bilateral fimbriectomy sterilization (the California operation; Kroener). She had proven fertility and wanted restoration for more children.

Bilateral patency, good length.

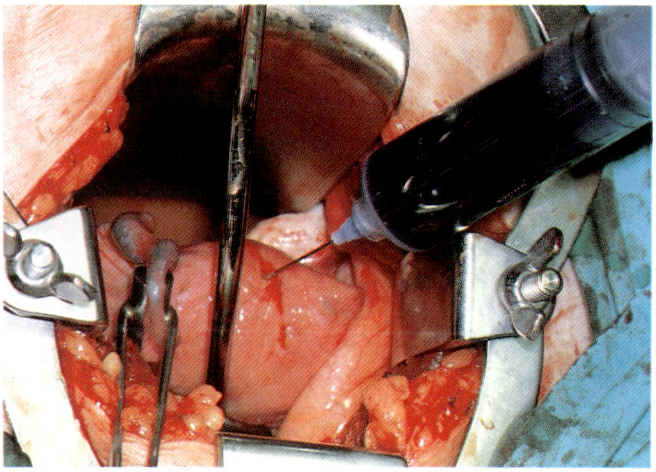

Fig. 38-11

Distal end of tube.

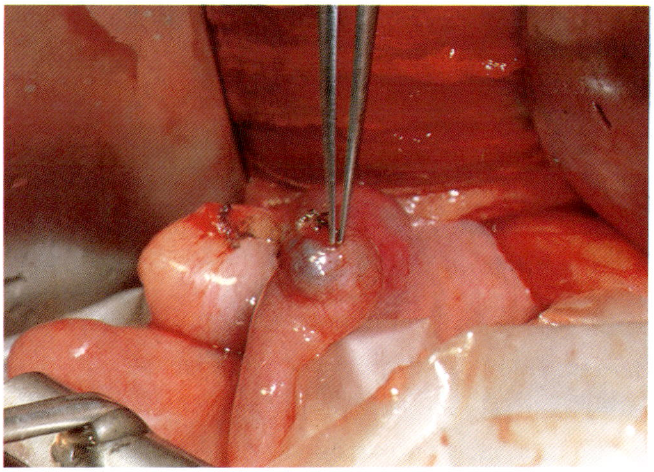

Fig. 38-12

Distal tube open for incision.

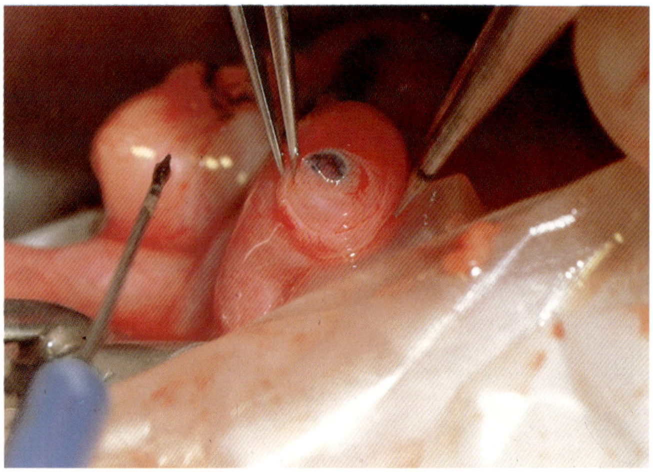

Fig. 38-13

Superior incision.

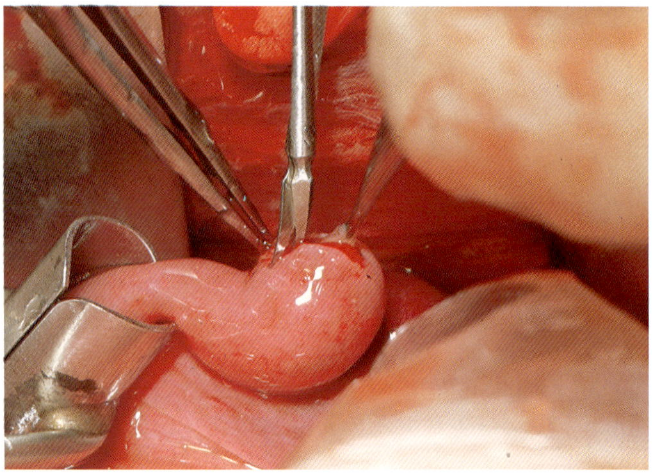

Fig. 38-14

Superior incision extended.

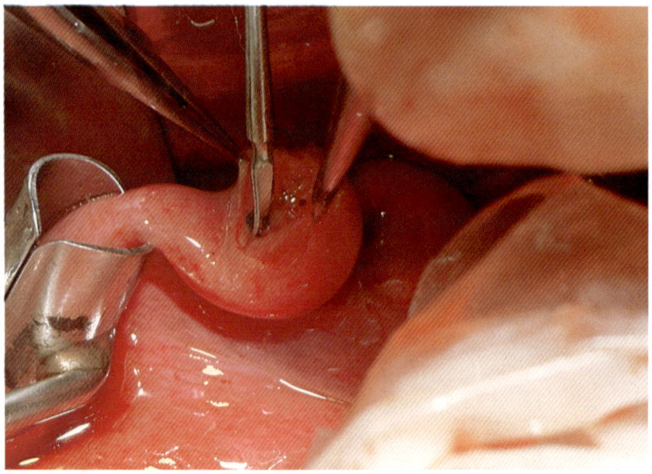

Fig. 38-15

First suture, mucosa to serosa.

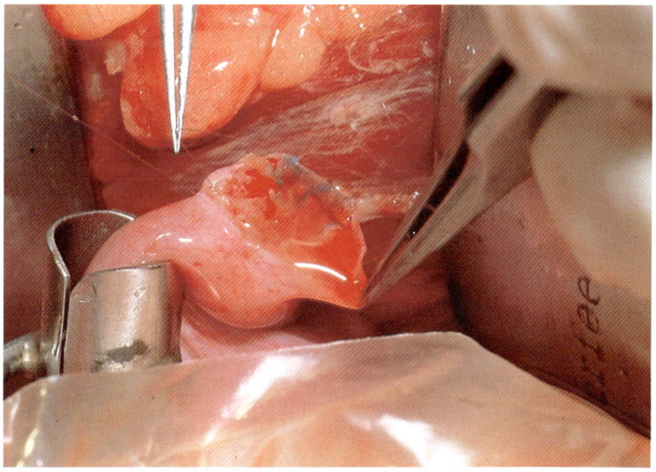

Fig. 38-16

Third suture, 7-0 Vicryl.

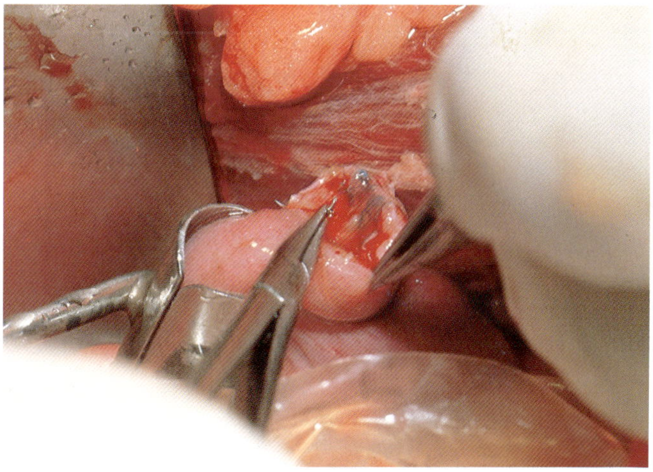

Fig. 38-17

Final appearance, cup-like.

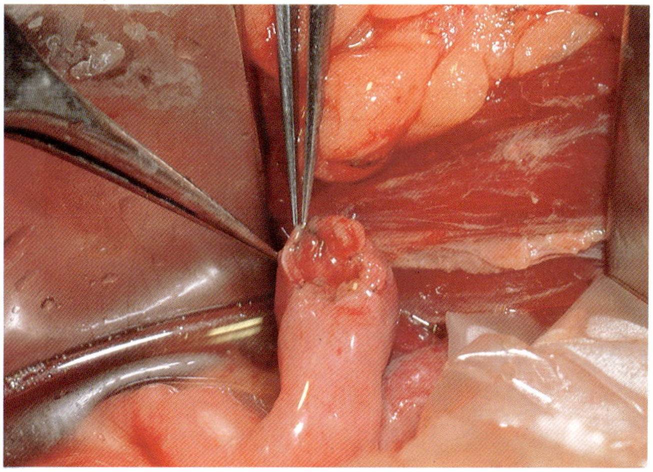

Fig. 38-18

Demonstrating patency.

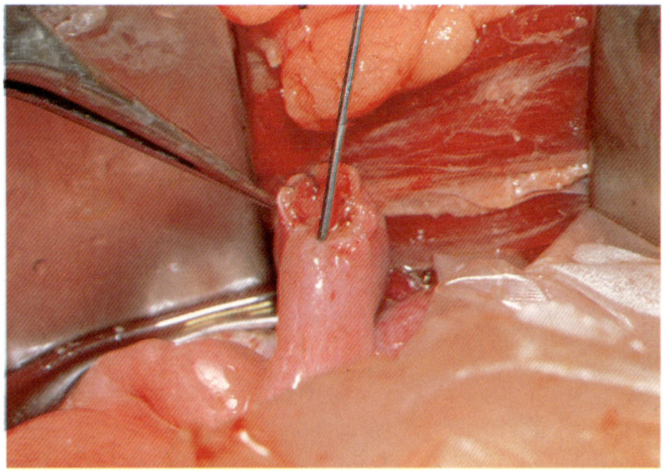

Fig. 38-19

First suture, other side. Mucosa to serosa, 7-0 Vicryl.

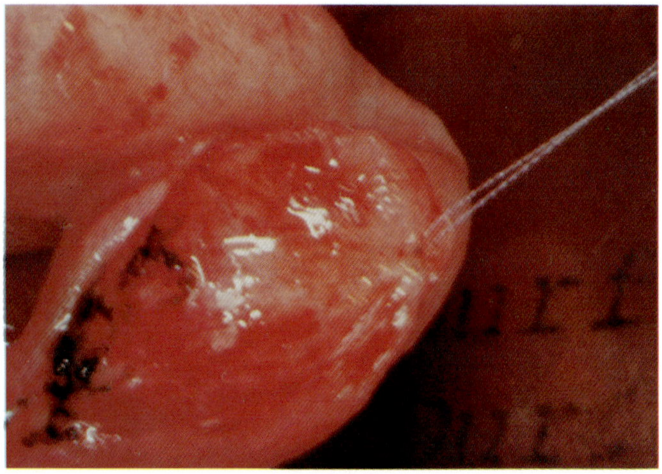

Fig. 38-20

Next-to-last suture.

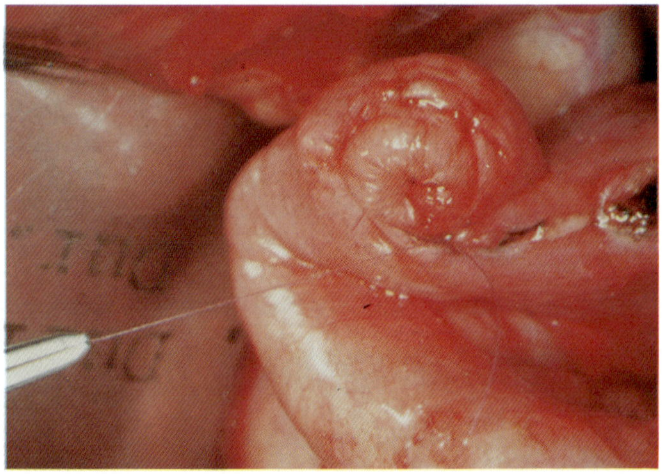

Fig. 38-21

Final suture, note umbilical-like appearance.

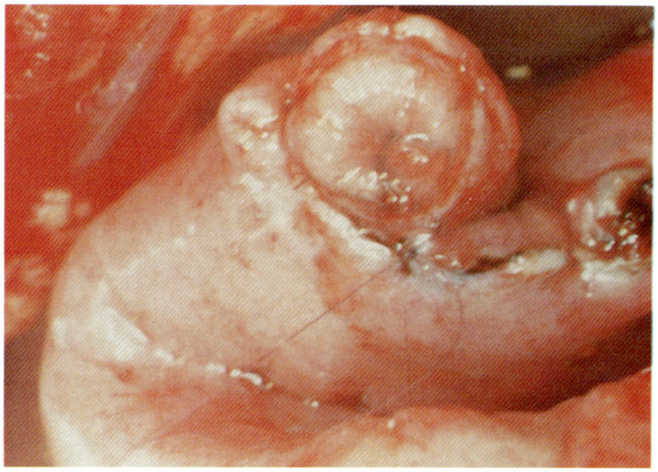

Fig. 38-22

Patient was patent bilaterally by X-ray at four months postoperative. Pregnant approximately eight months later; aborted spontaneously at three months. Term pregnancy one year later.

Case #3.
Ampulla-Cornua Tubal Anastomosis

The patient had Hulka clip ligation by colpotomy, severe postsurgical peritonitis treated with antibiotics, and a five-day hospital stay. HSG showed an obstruction at the cornua; laparoscopy showed marked fibrinous reaction, absent isthmus, clips free in cul-de-sac with adhesions. The patient wanted reversal. Ampulla-cornua anastomosis was attempted. Extensive laser removal of the serosal fibrin was accomplished, uneventful postoperative course.

Sharp adhesion lysis, note the bilateral ovarian enlargement.

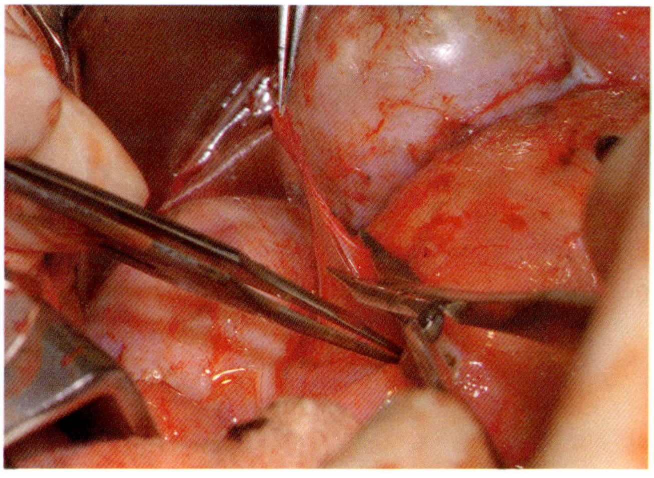

Fig. 38-23

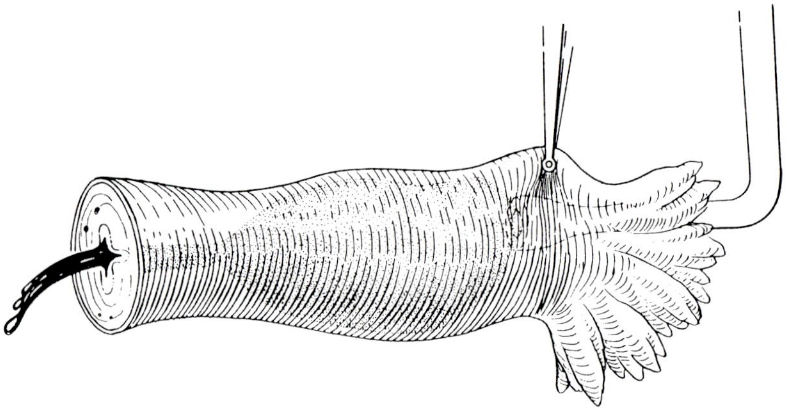

Fig. 38-24

Distal tube patency test, Stangel tubes (Figs. 38-24 and 38-25 reprinted with permission from Hunt[1]).

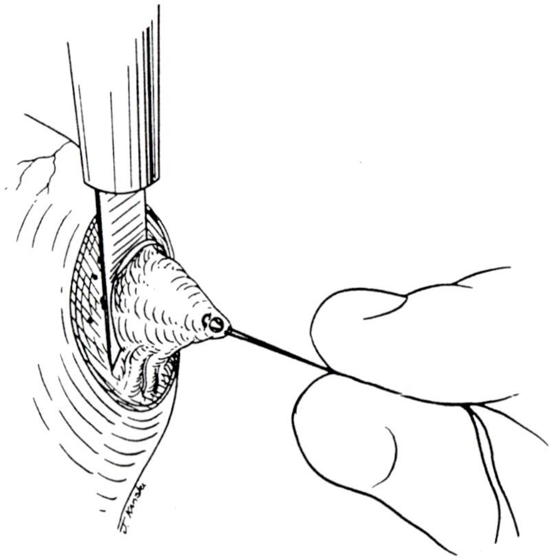

Fig. 38-25

Method of cornual dissection to patent interstitial lumen.

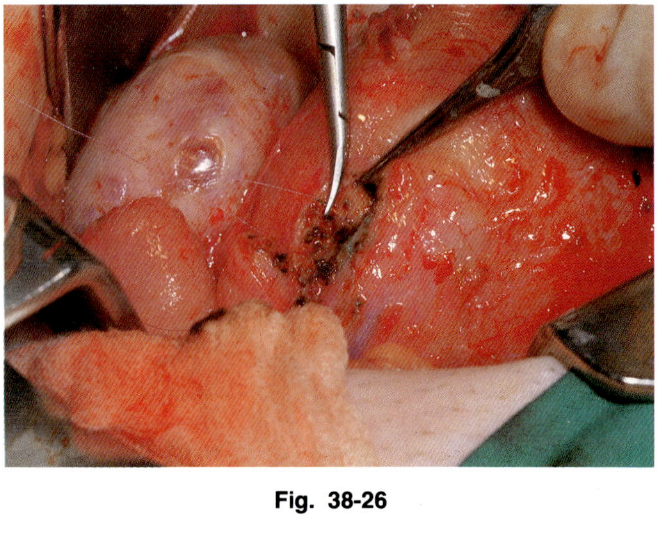

Fig. 38-26

First anastomosis suture, mesosalpinx has been sutured to the uterine wall.

A note about technique. This is a complicated anastomosis and a complicated case. On the next page are two ways of reducing the size of the ampullary lumen (Hunt). A #2-00 polyglycolic suture should be placed through the uterine wall about 1.5 cm deep, just below the round ligament, to reduce the blood supply to the cornua. The mesosalpinx should be secured to the uterine wall with several sutures of permanent suture material. The previously placed #2-00 suture is removed at the end of the bilateral anastomosis.

Ampulla lumen reduction (Figs. 38-27 and 38-28 reprinted with permission from Hunt[1]).

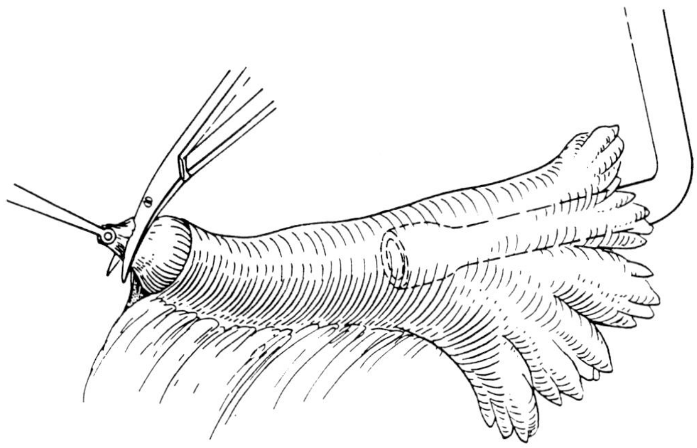

Fig. 38-27

#8-0 or #9-0 direct, same.

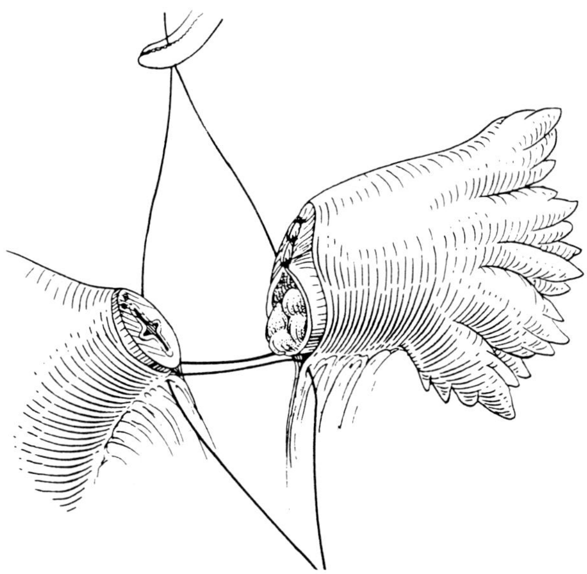

Fig. 38-28

Second suture, anastomosis.

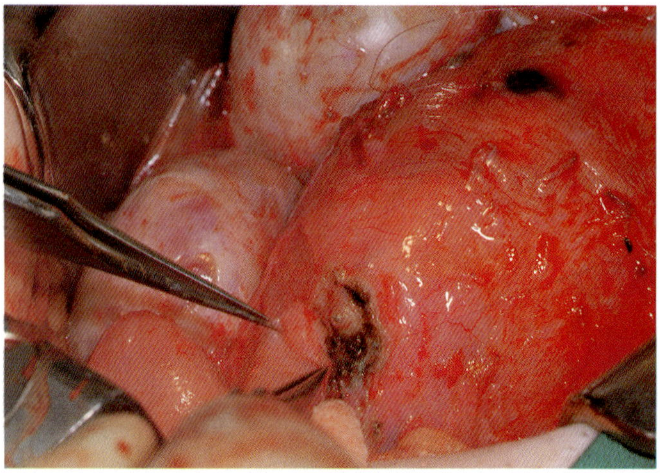

Fig. 38-29

Third suture, same.

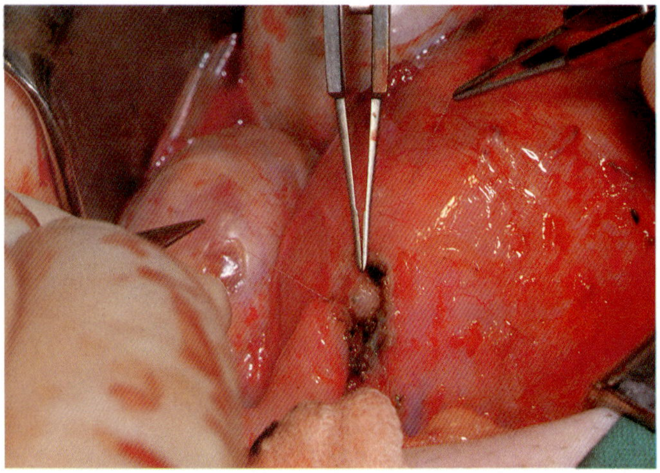

Fig. 38-30

Fourth suture, same.

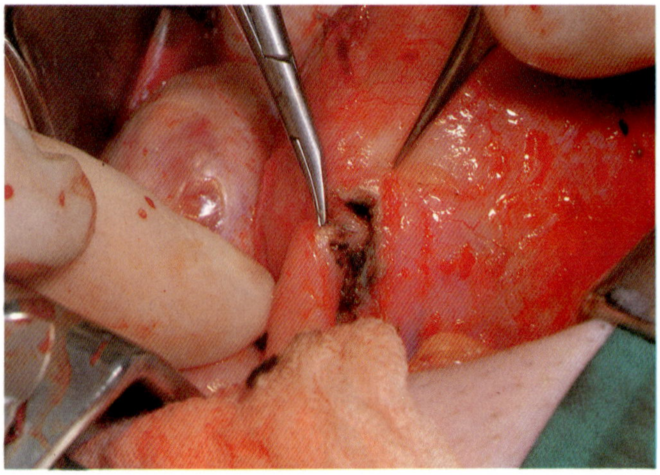

Fig. 38-31

Fifth suture, same.

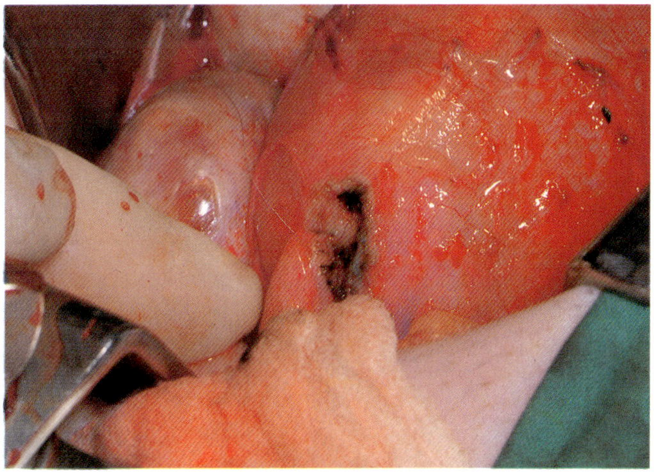

Fig. 38-32

Sixth suture secures ampulla to cornua.

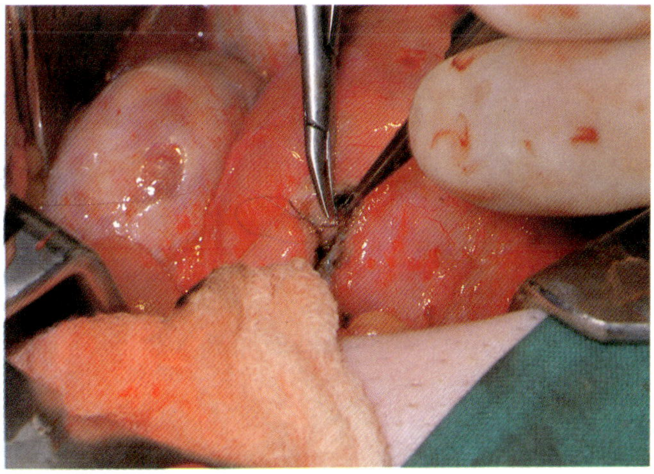

Fig. 38-33

Partial serosal closure.

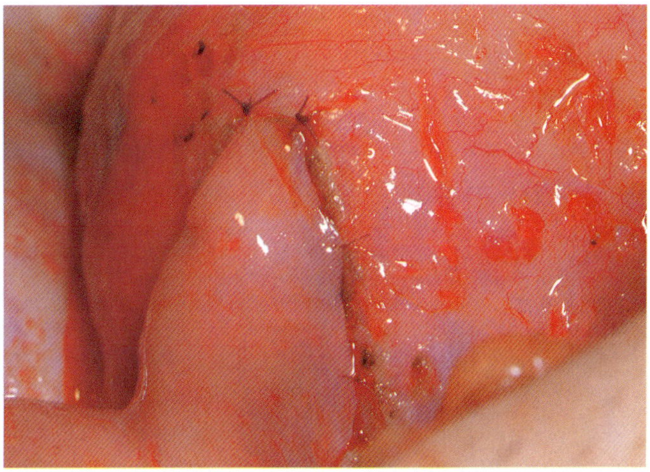

Fig. 38-34

One or two more sutures will complete the anastomosis.

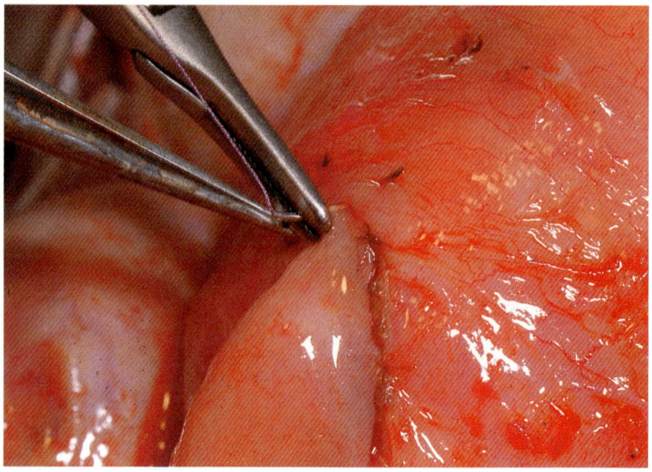

Fig. 38-35

Ovarian repair and mobilization of the other tube.

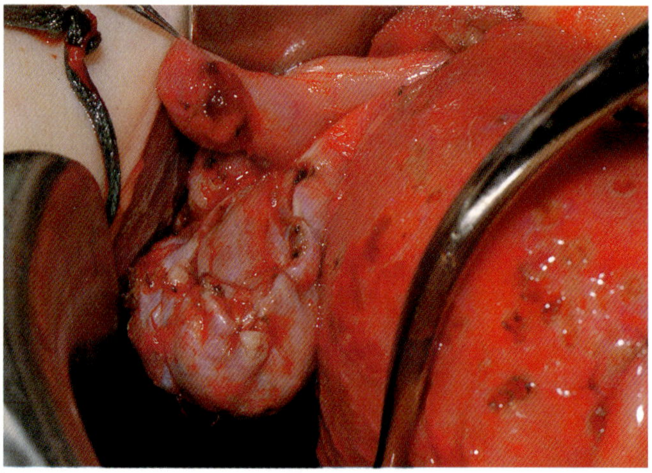

Fig. 38-36

This anastomosis was facilitated by the thickened wall of the ampulla (which is usually not the case). High magnification of the serosa in figure 38-34 shows the fibrin collection on the uterine fundal surface. All of this was readily removed by unfocused laser. Unfortunately, this patient was lost to follow-up so that there is no record of success or failure.

Case #4.
Isthmus-Ampulla Anastomosis with Fimbrial Release

Patient had had an Irving procedure following a complicated first pregnancy. She wanted restoration of fertility.

Proximal tube buried subserosal.

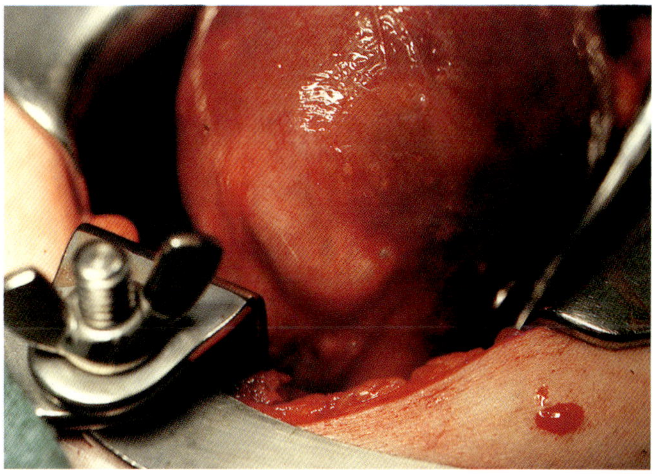

Fig. 38-37

Tube subserosal, other side.

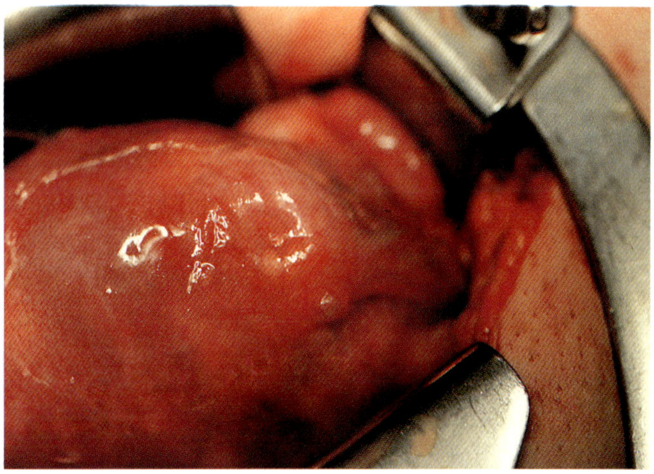

Fig. 38-38

Distal tube, endometriotic cyst.

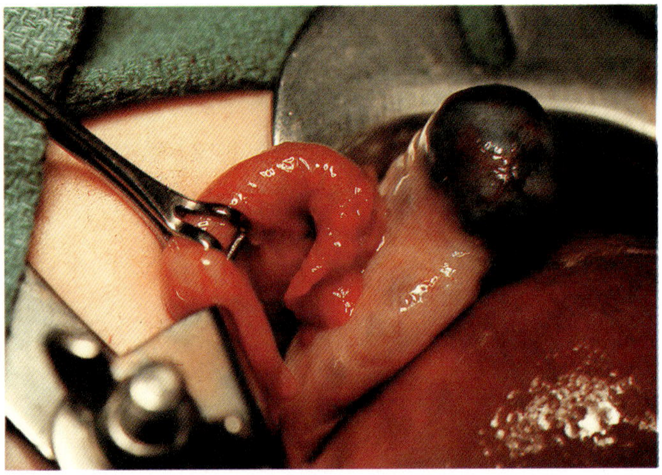

Fig. 38-39

Distal obstruction of tube, right side.

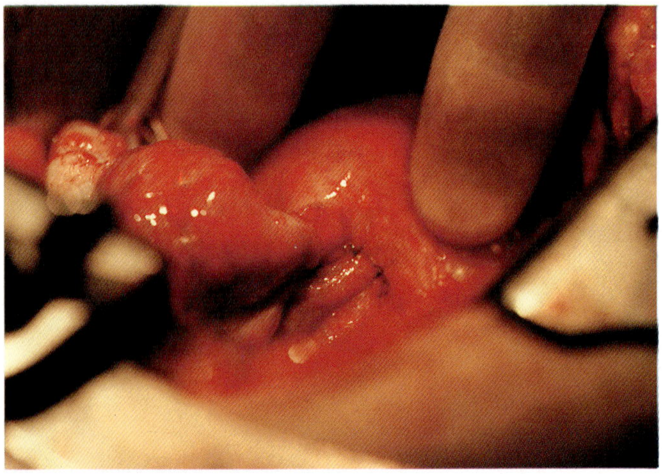

Fig. 38-40

Umbilicated obstruction, right side.

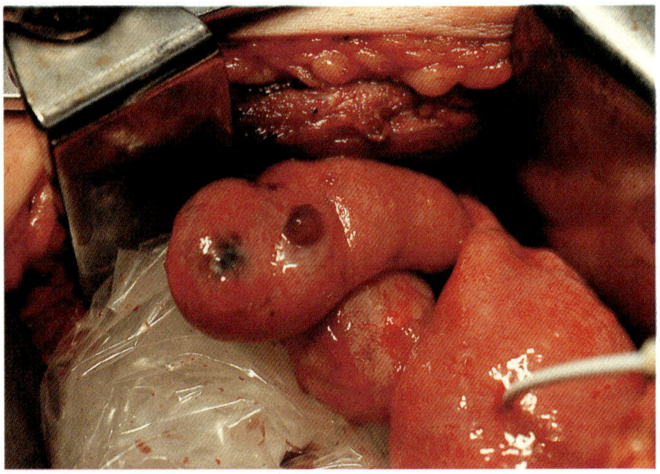

Fig. 38-41

Fimbrial release, right side.

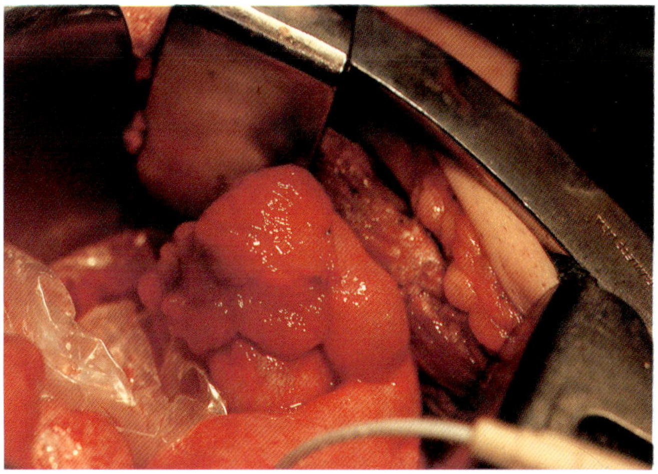

Fig. 38-42

Anastomosis complete, one side.

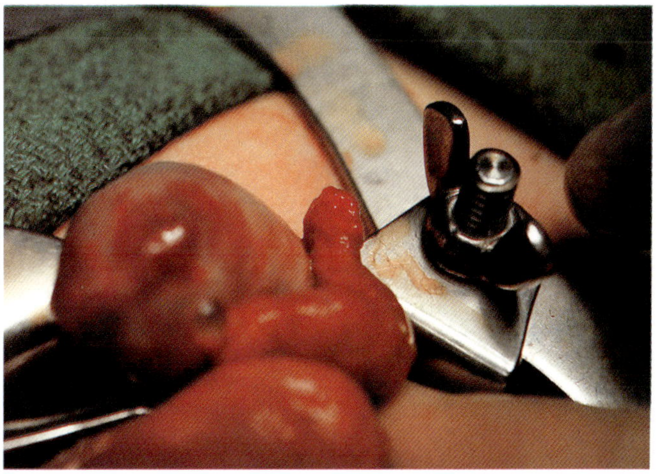

Fig. 38-43

Anastomosis, other side.

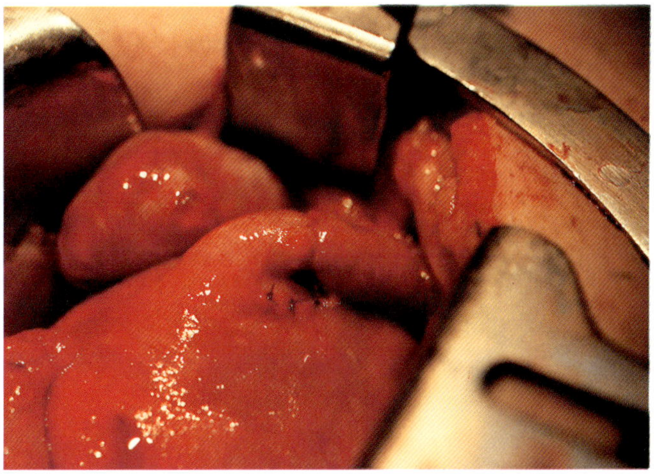

Fig. 38-44

Patency, one side.

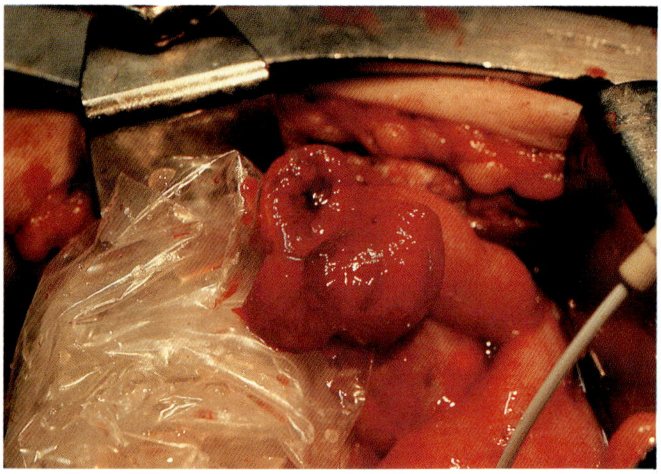

Fig. 38-45

Patency, other side.

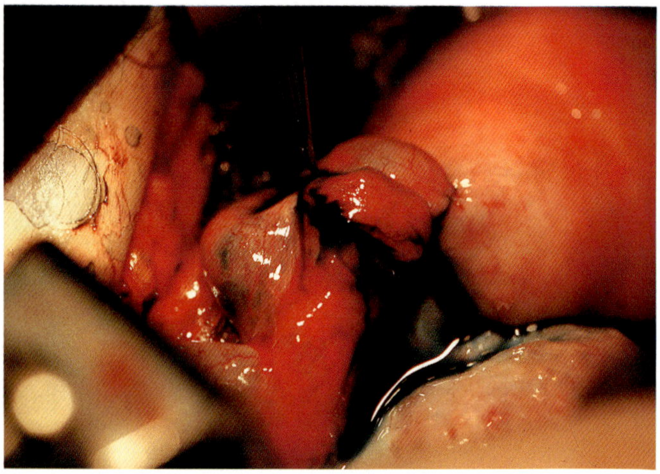

Fig. 38-46

Completed procedure.

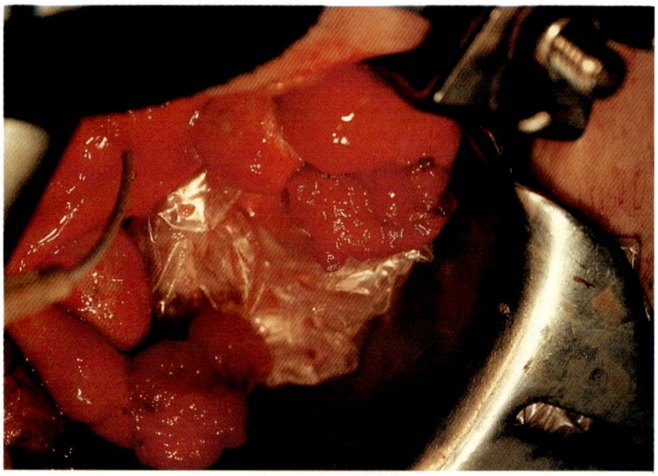

Fig. 38-47

Case #5.
Isthmus-Cornua Tubal Anastomosis

The patient had bilateral cornual block confirmed by HSG, proved to be isthmica nodosa at laparoscopy; excision and anastomosis.

Excision of pathology.

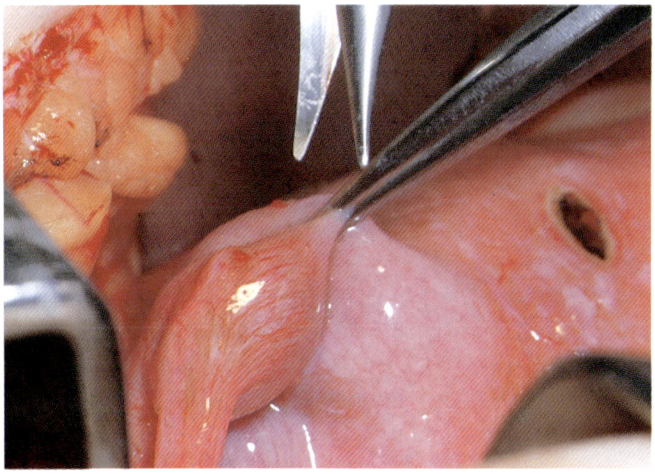

Fig. 38-48

External cornual involvement.

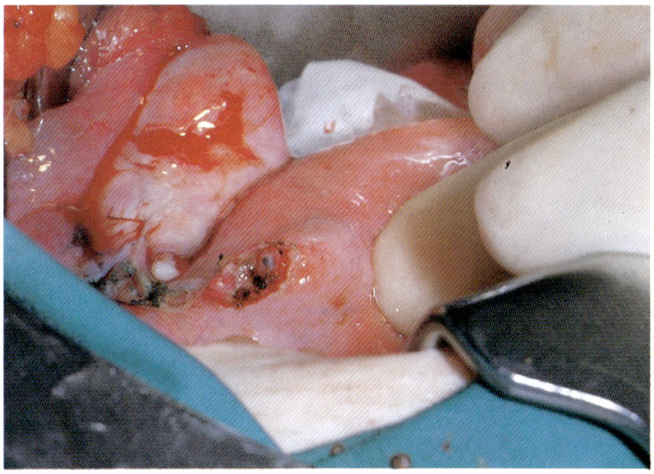

Fig. 38-49

Defined patent interstitial lumen.

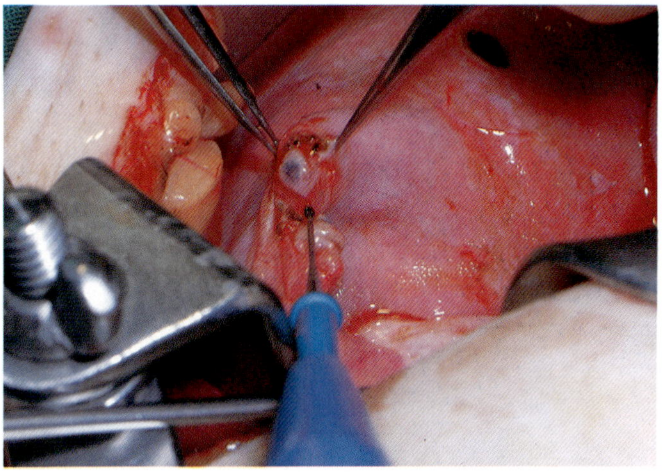

Fig. 38-50

Distal tube testing.

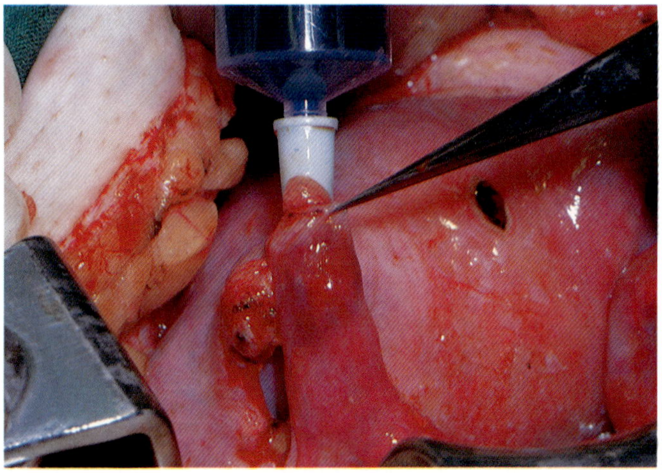

Fig. 38-51

Mobilizing distal tube.

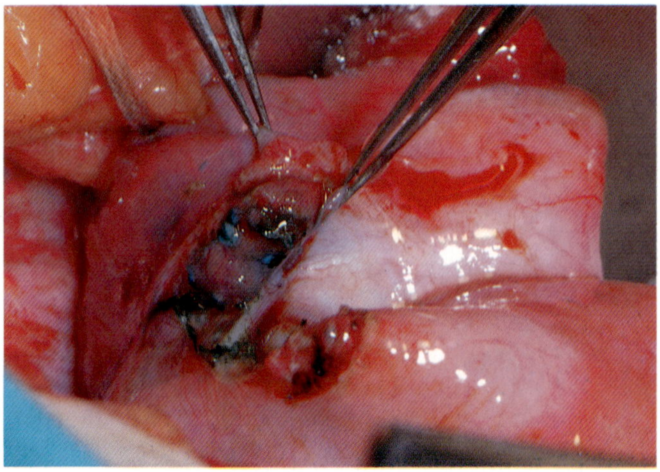

Fig. 38-52

Second tubal suture.

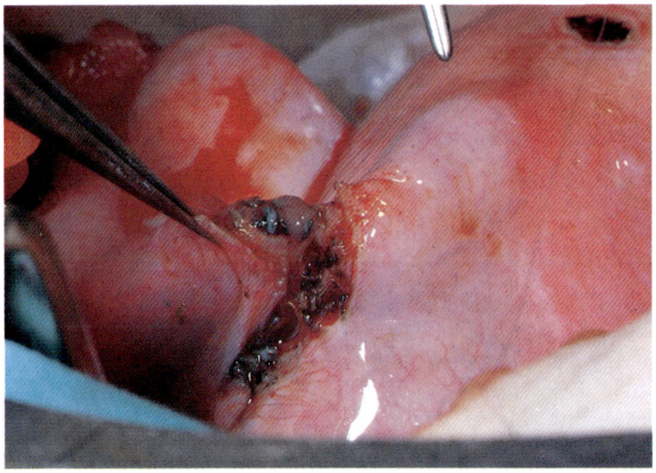

Fig. 38-53

Third tubal suture.

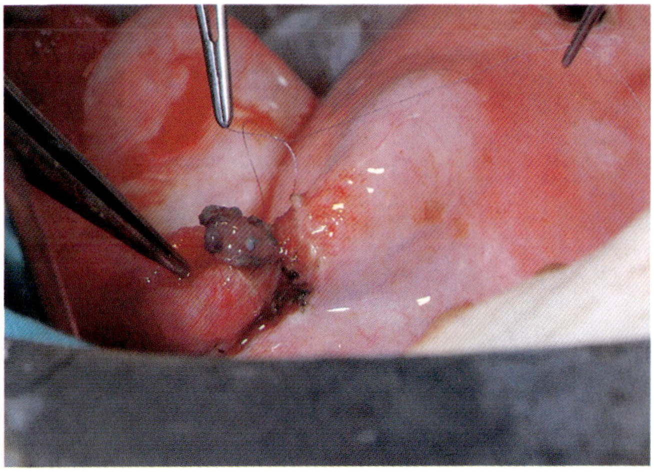

Fig. 38-54

Fourth tubal suture.

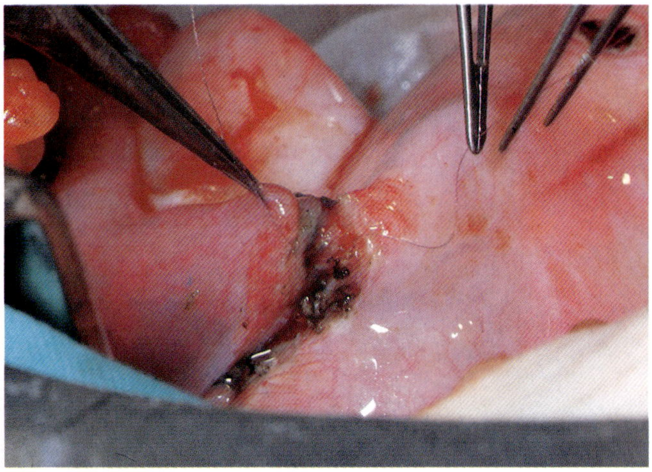

Fig. 38-55

Anastomosis complete.

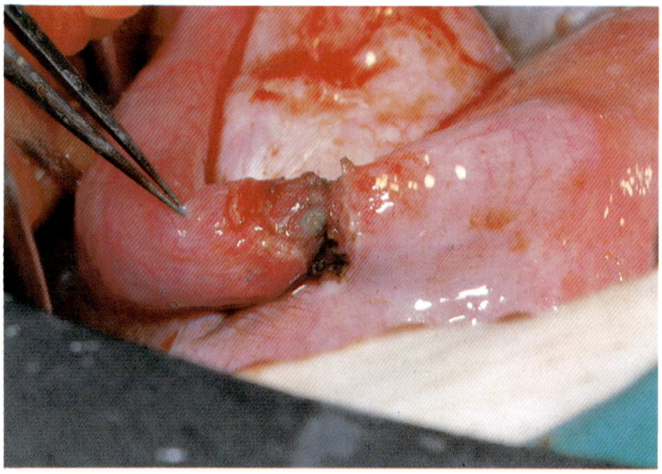

Fig. 38-56

Beginning serosa closure.

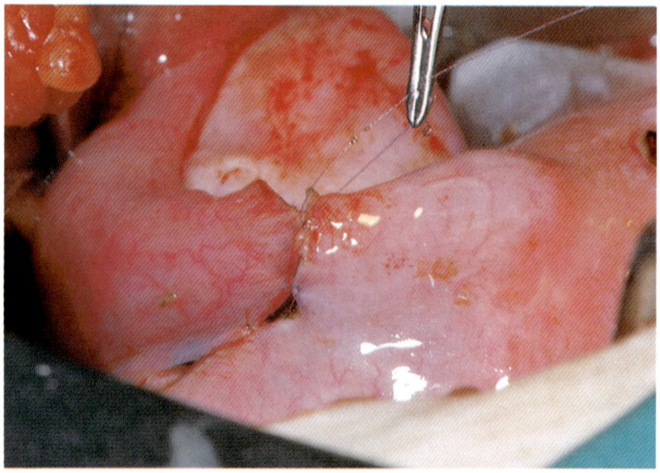

Fig. 38-57

The patient did not conceive for more than eighteen months. She had bilateral patent tubes confirmed by HSG. Pregnancy followed intra-tubal lavage, normal child at thirty-seven weeks.

Case #6.
Isthmus-Isthmus Anastomosis

The patient had Fallope ring sterilization by laparoscopy after two children. She had a moderate febrile postoperative course. She wanted reversal three years later. Observe the marked serosal reaction.

Fallope ring in situ.

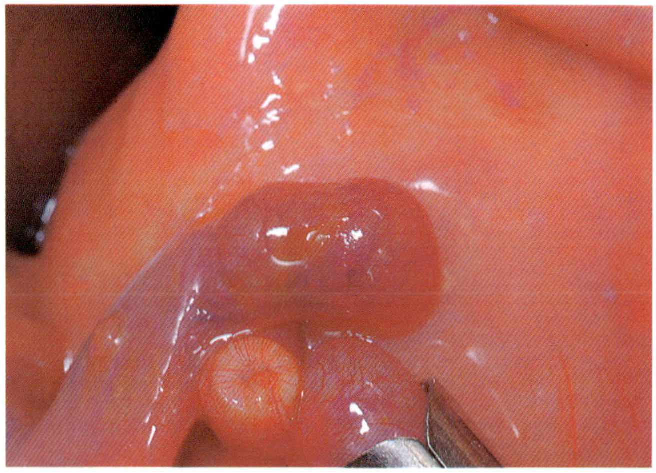

Fig. 38-58

Generalized pelvic reaction.

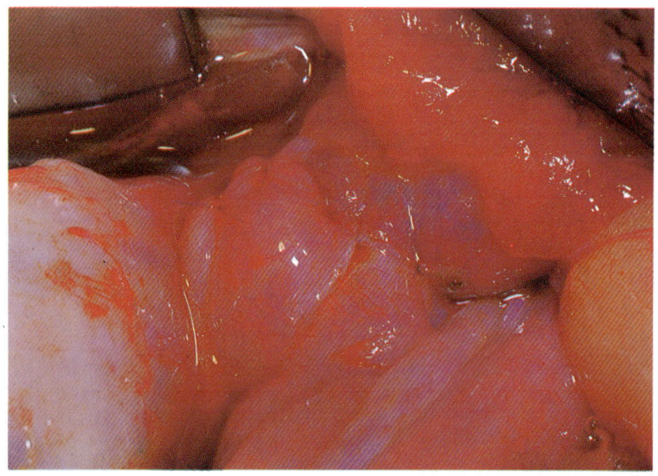

Fig. 38-59

Tube is mobilized.

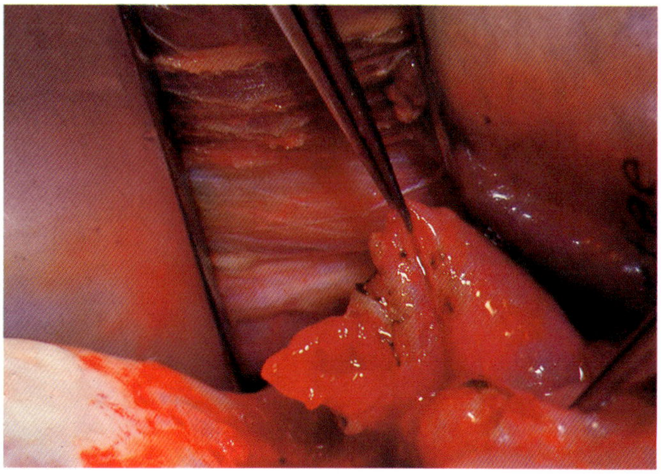

Fig. 38-60

Mesosalpinx repaired (Reprinted with permission from Reyniak[2]).

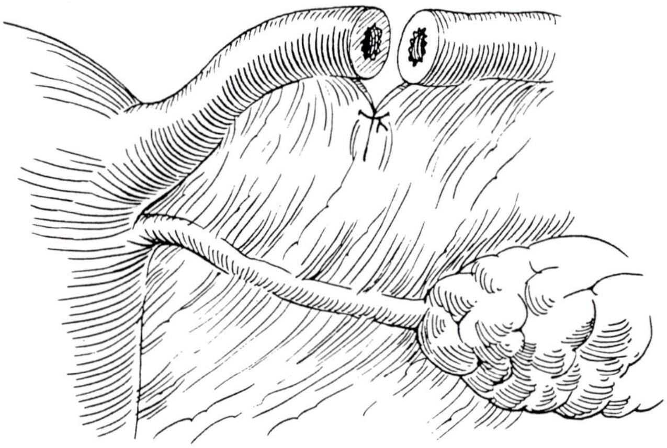

Fig. 38-61

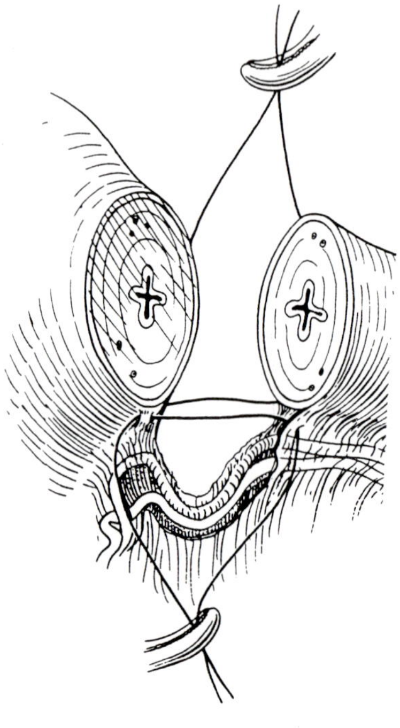

Fig. 38-62

Traction sutures (Figs. 38-62 and 38-3 reprinted with permission from Hunt[1]).

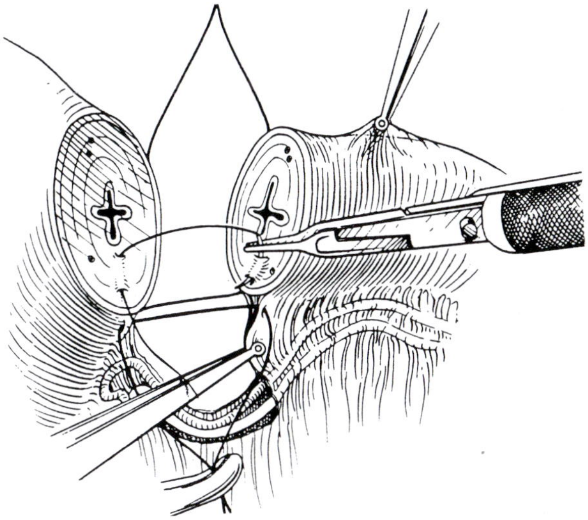

Fig. 38-63

Suture placed at 6 o'clock, traction sutures tied.

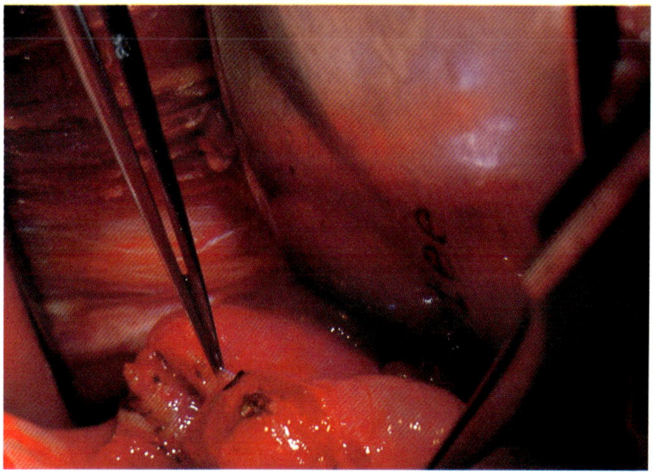

Fig. 38-64

Suture placed at 6 o'clock.

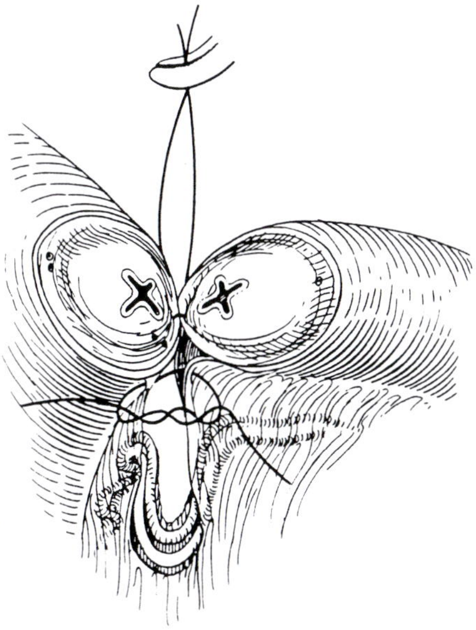

Fig. 38-65

Traction sutures tied, suture at 6 o'clock (Reprinted with permission from Hunt[1]).

First lateral suture.

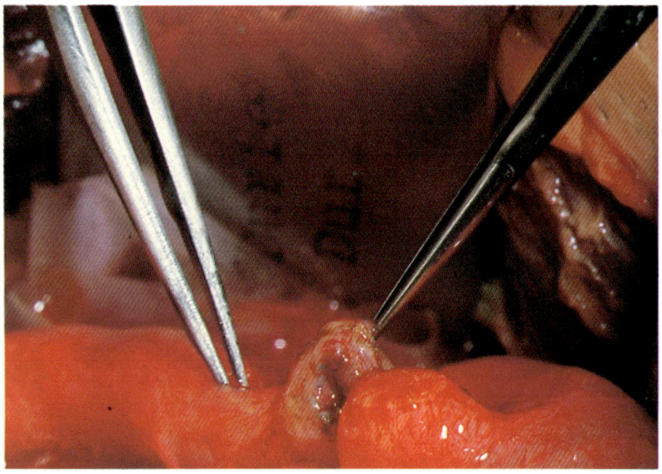

Fig. 38-66

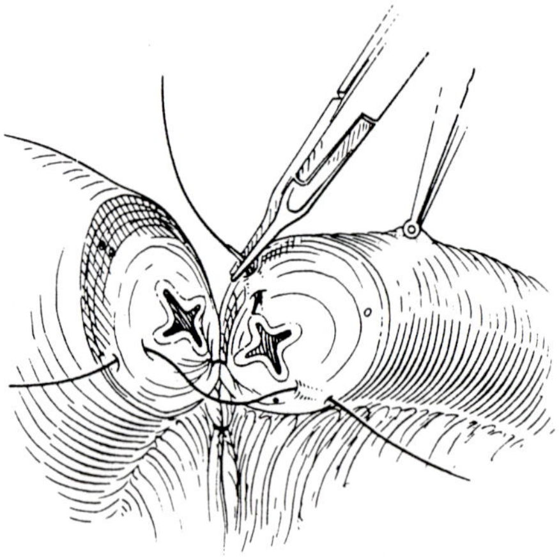

Fig. 38-67

Lateral suture in, second being placed (Reprinted with permission from Hunt[1]).

Superior suture placed.

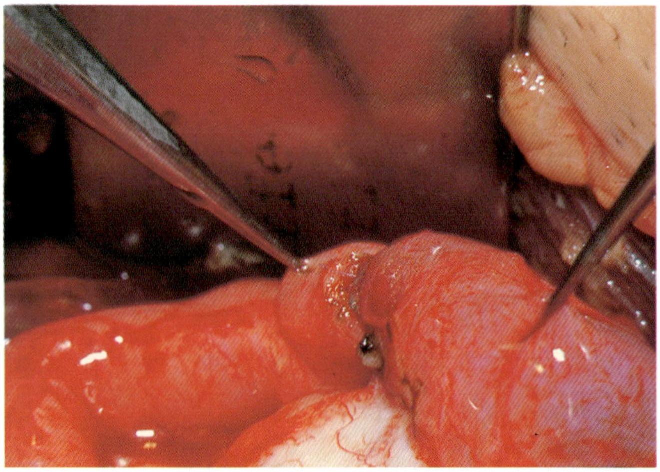

Fig. 38-68

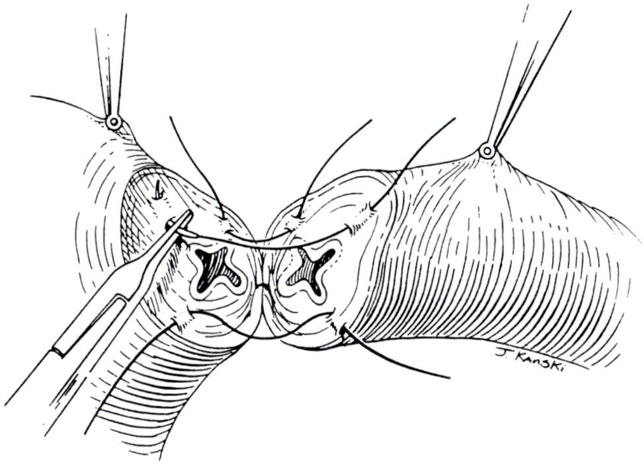

Fig. 38-69

Same, see Fig. 38-68 (Reprinted with permission from Hunt[1]).

Top, fourth suture tied.

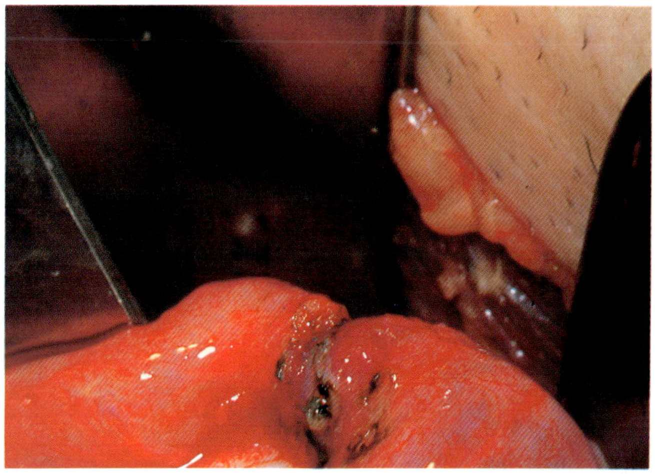

Fig. 38-70

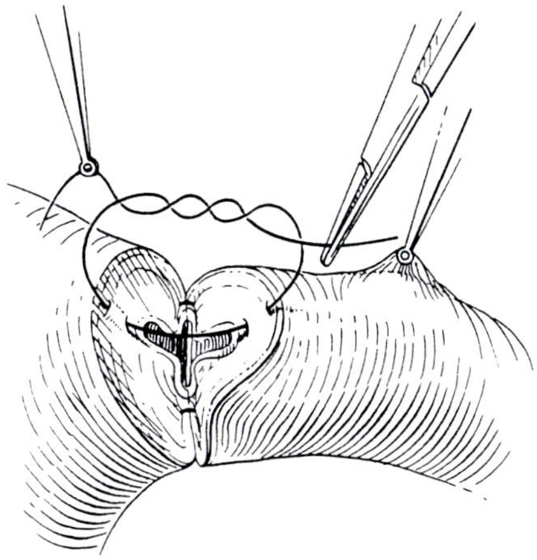

Fig. 38-71

Same, see Fig. 38-70 (Figs. 38-71 and 38-72 reprinted with permission from Hunt[1]).

Final serosal closure, running closure also used.

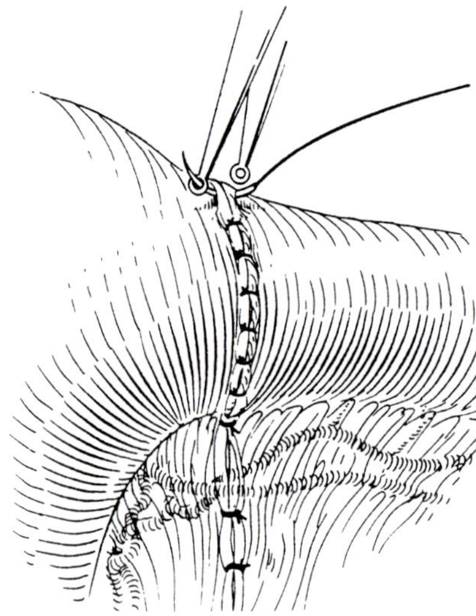

Fig. 38-72

Final appearance.

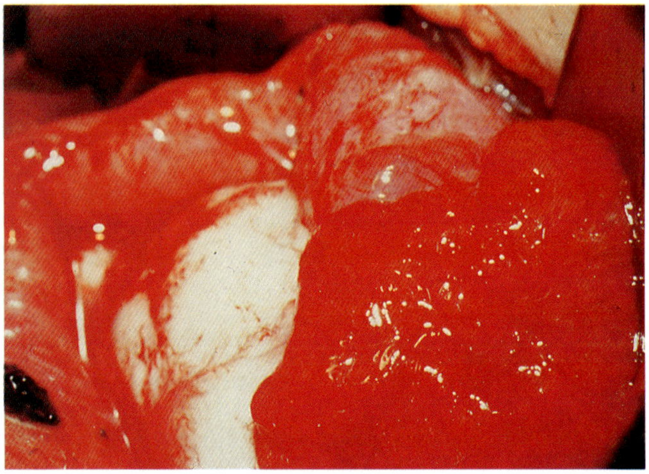

Fig. 38-73

The etiology of the intense serosal reaction is unknown. The postoperative recovery was uneventful. At closure, 400 ml 70% Dextran was placed intraperitoneally. The patient became pregnant within four months and a normal full-term child was delivered.

All black-and-white line art is from Hunt. The details of the operation are clarified by these pictures. The superficial fibrinous reaction was removed by unfocused laser as much as possible.

Case #7.
Fimbria-Cornua Anastomosis

The patient had three children. Bilateral tubal ligation by electrocoagulation had been performed. She divorced, remarried, and wanted fertility restored. Very little tissue was available, but because of urgency, the operation was done.

Distal fimbria and ovary, Corpus Luteum.

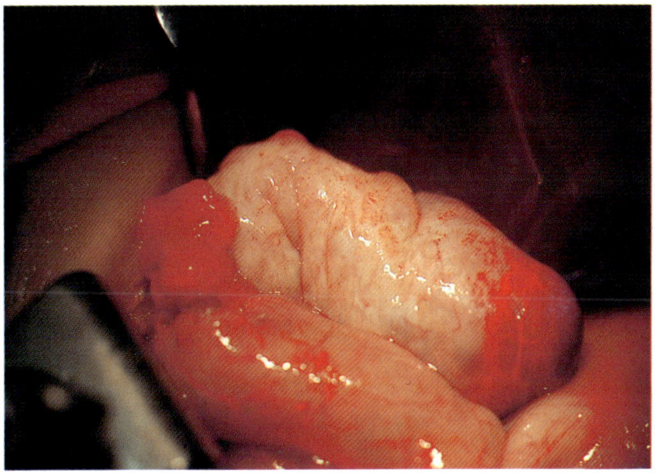

Fig. 38-74

Anastomosis using stent.

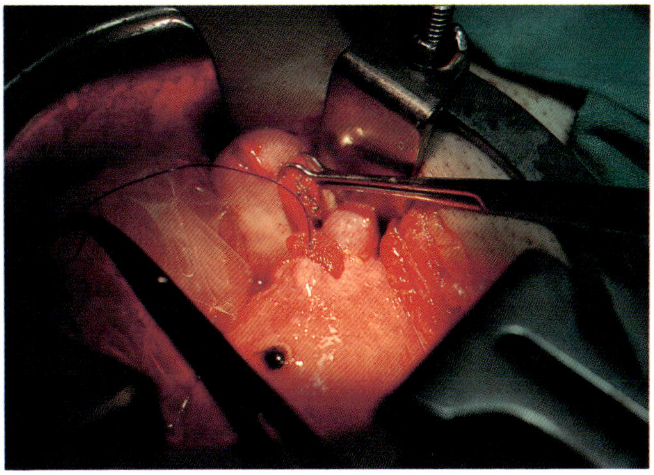

Fig. 38-75

Final suture, 8-0 Vicryl.

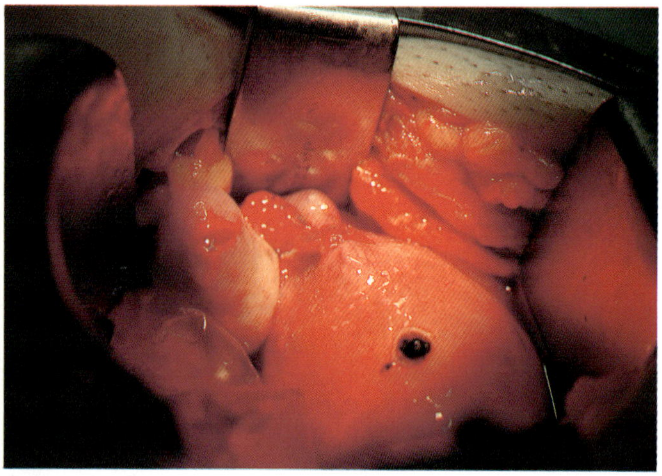

Fig. 38-76

Result one side, patent.

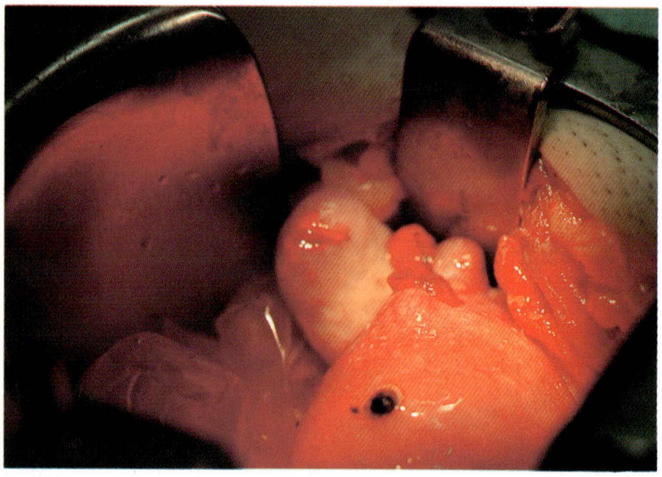

Fig. 38-77

Result other side, more tissue; also patent.

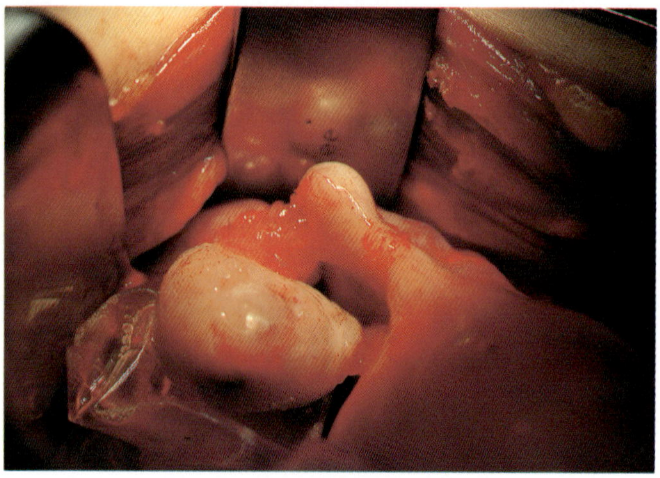

Fig. 38-78

Lateral appearance.

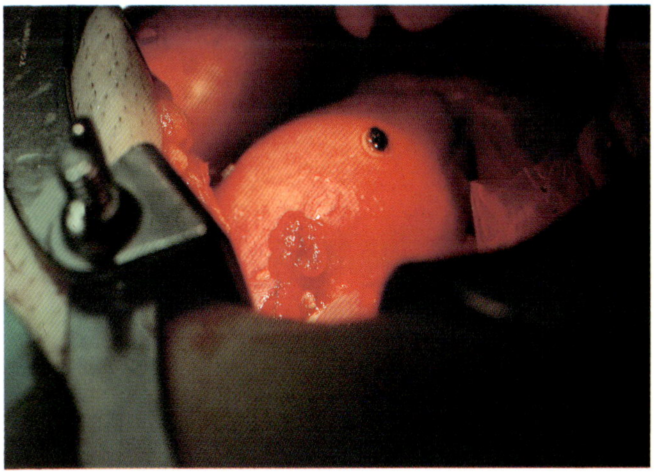

Fig. 38-79

Normal-appearing anastomosed fimbria, bilateral.

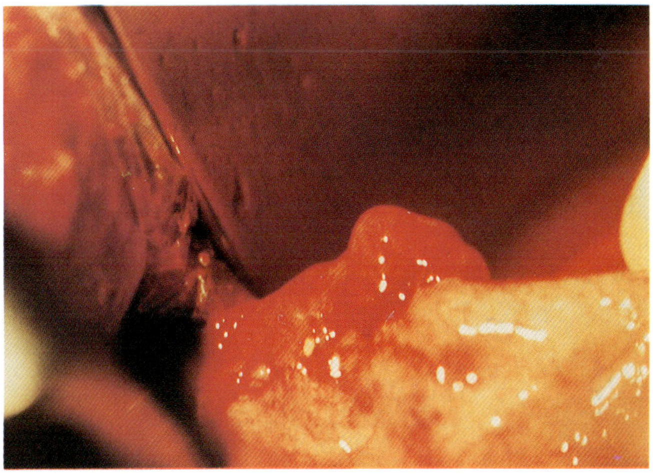

Fig. 38-80

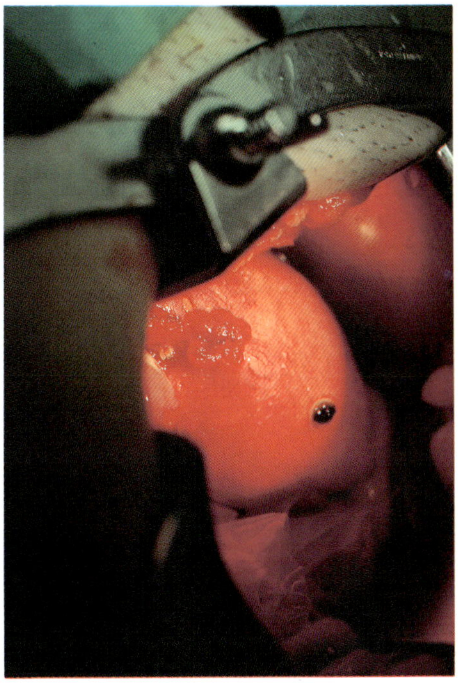

Fig. 38-81

Normal-appearing anastomosed fimbria, bilateral.

The patient became pregnant in six months, delivered a normal child at term. Longest tissue on one side, 3 cm.

Case #8.
External Adhesion Lysis, Fimbrial Release

The patient had had a ruptured appendiceal abscess, age 18; severe peritonitis, long hospital stay. She wanted the operation for fertility; micro and macro surgery as well as laser used: approximately six hours, minimal blood loss.

Pelvic appearance at surgery, no identifiable organs.

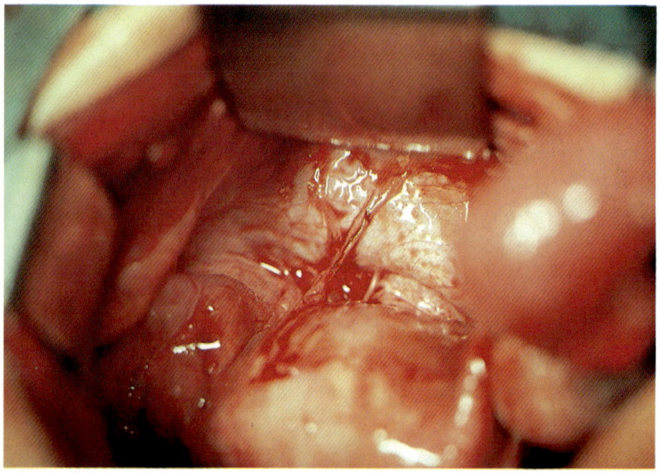

Fig. 38-82

First dissection.

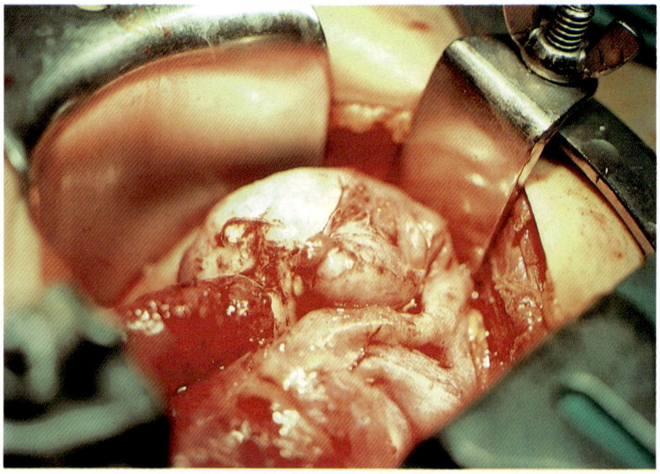

Fig. 38-83

Pelvic organs identified.

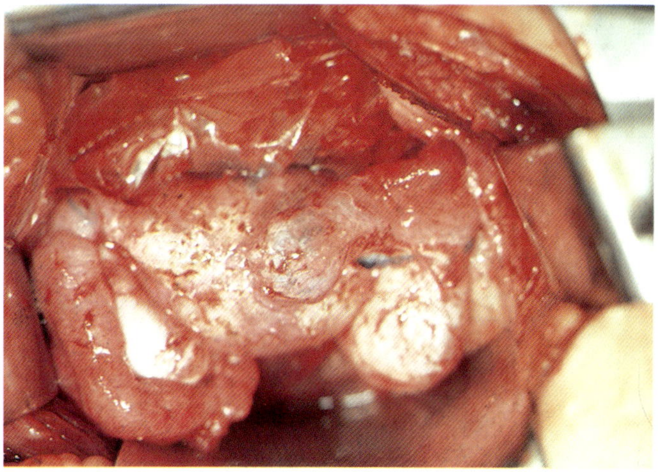

Fig. 38-84

External tubo-ovarian adhesions.

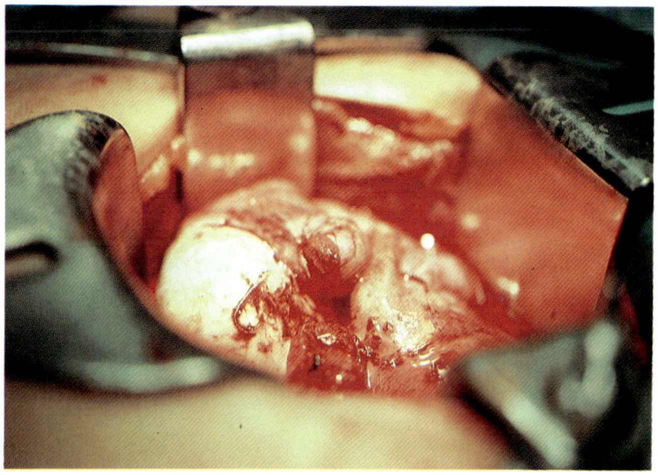

Fig. 38-85

Tubofimbrial phimosis.

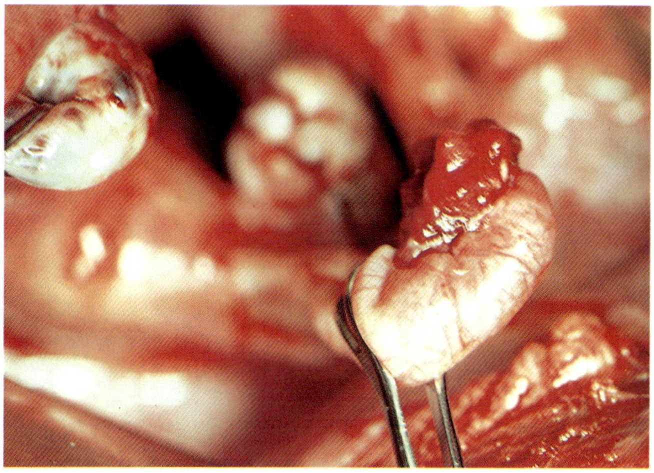

Fig. 38-86

Fimbrial release.

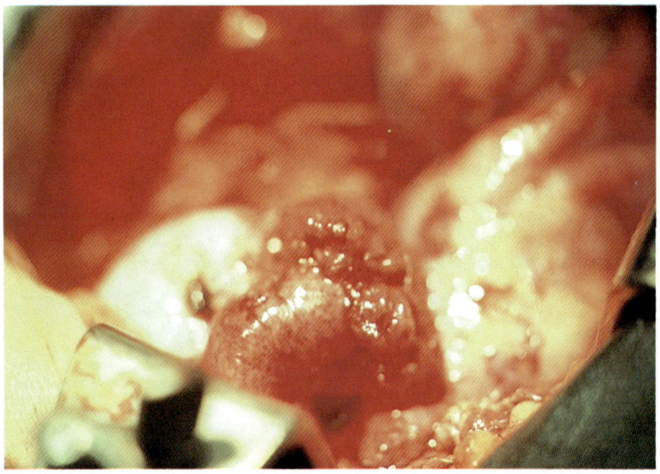

Fig. 38-87

External adhesion lysis.

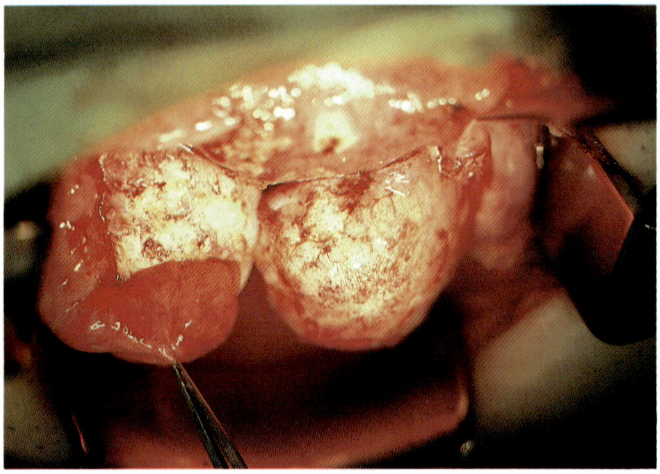

Fig. 38-88

Further adhesion lysis.

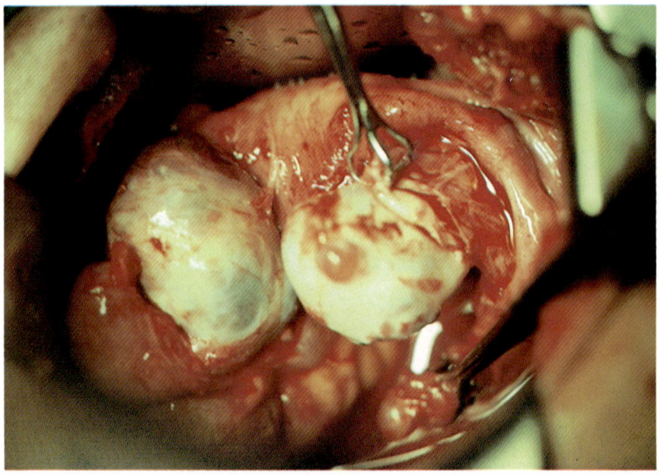

Fig. 38-89

Fimbrial release, one side.

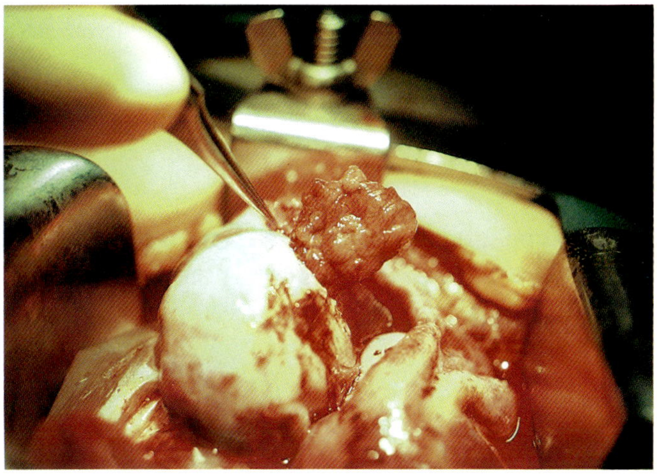

Fig. 38-90

Fimbrial release, other side.

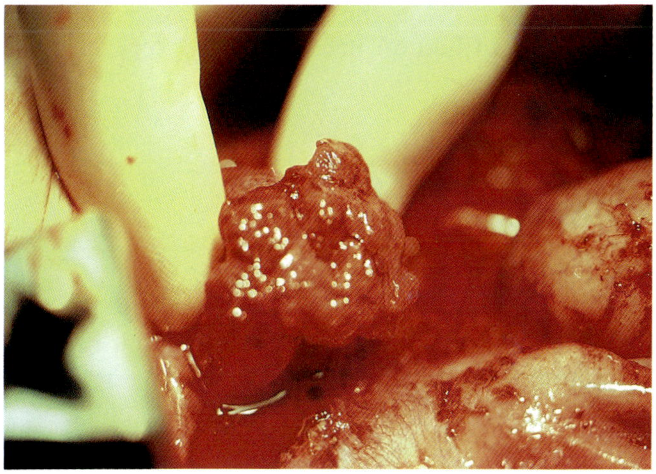

Fig. 38-91

Clearing of tube and ovary.

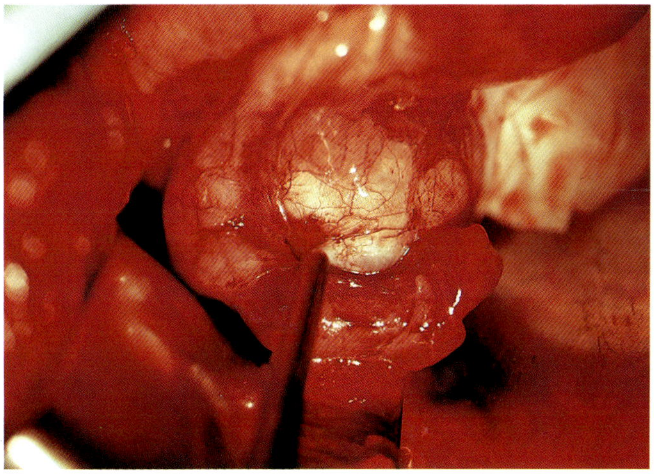

Fig. 38-92

Final appearance, good tubo-ovarian relationship.

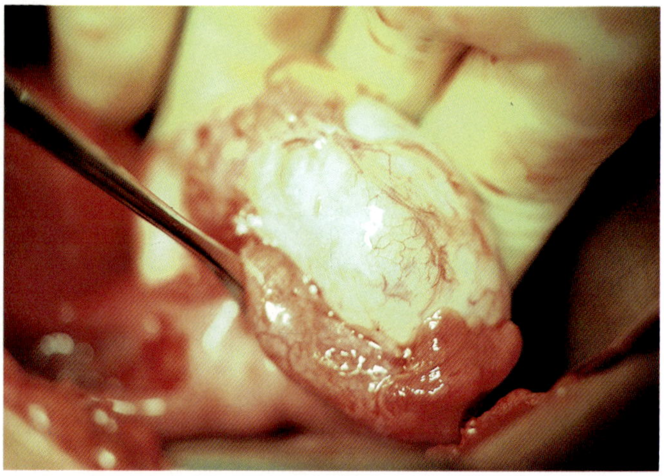

Fig. 38-93

The patient had an uneventful recovery; proven patency by HSG; had a full-term normal child within a year.

Case #9.
Uterine Unification

The patient had a diagnosis of large uterine septum with a single cervix. A Thompkins unification operation was elected. Good documentation of normal sperm—husband; obvious ovulation—patient.

HSG, septate uterus.

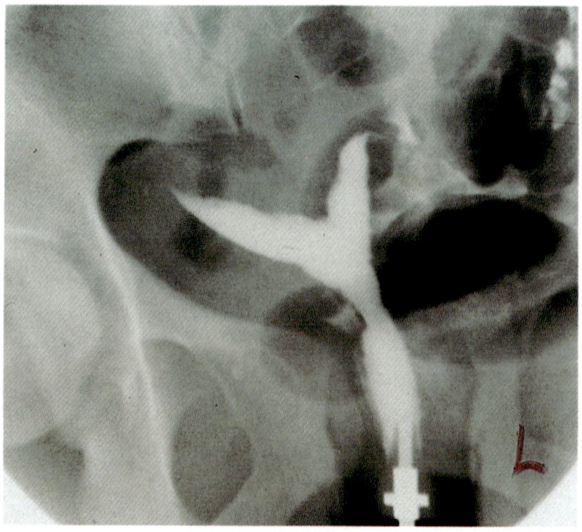

Fig. 38-94

Appearance at laparotomy.

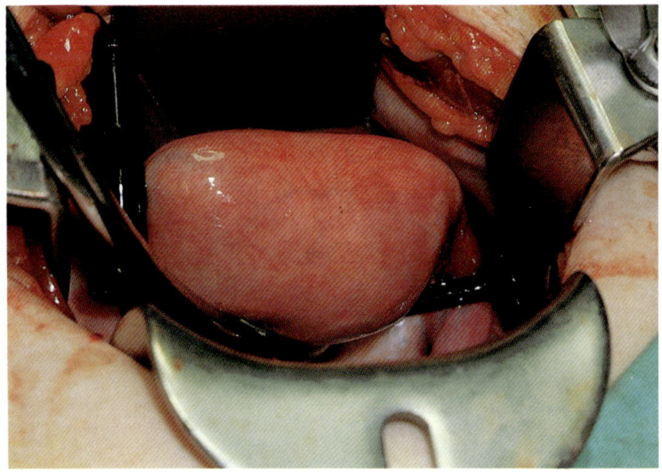

Fig. 38-95

Injection with Pitressin.

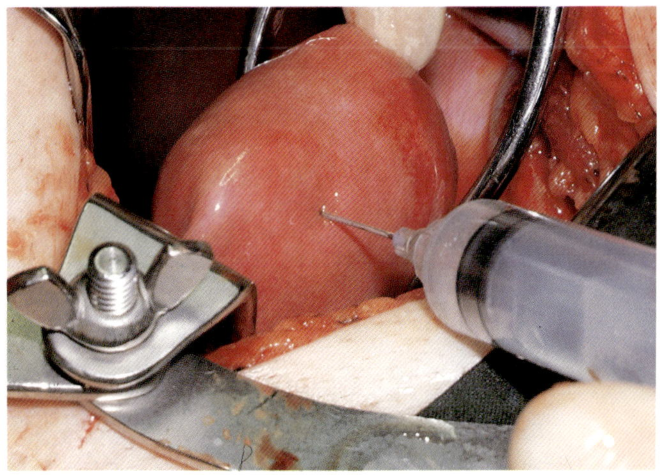

Fig. 38-96

Initial incision, note the change in color.

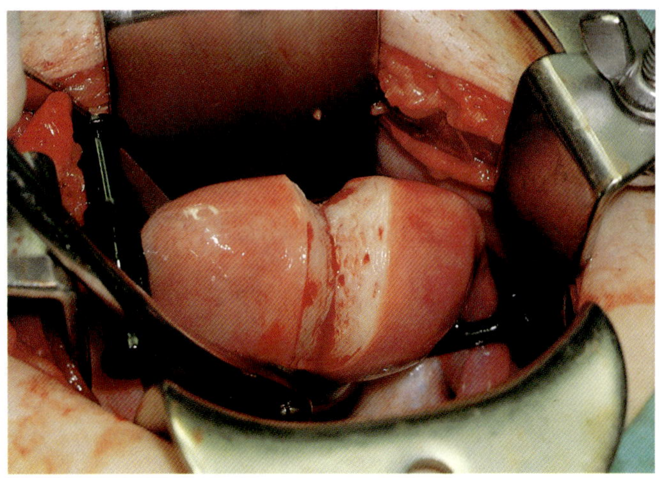

Fig. 38-97

Incision to endometrial cavity.

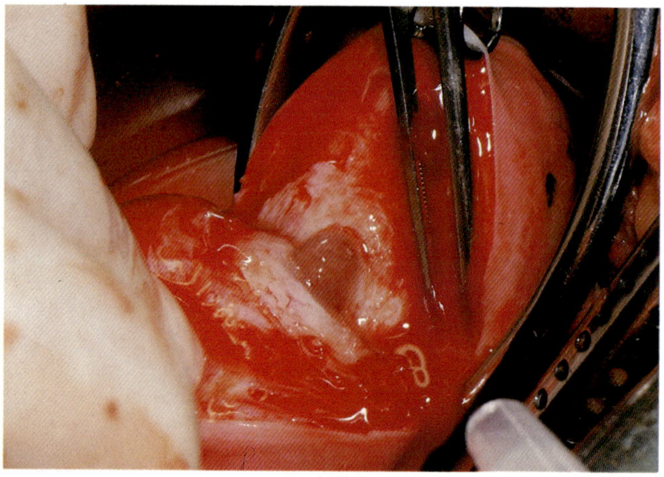

Fig. 38-98

Local hemostasis.

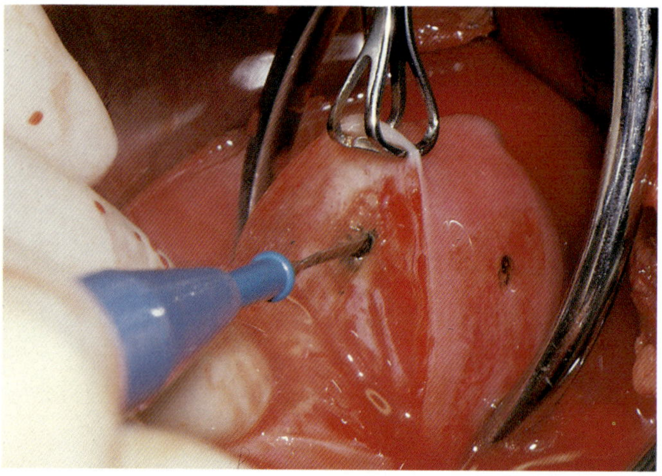

Fig. 38-99

Vertical incision into right side.

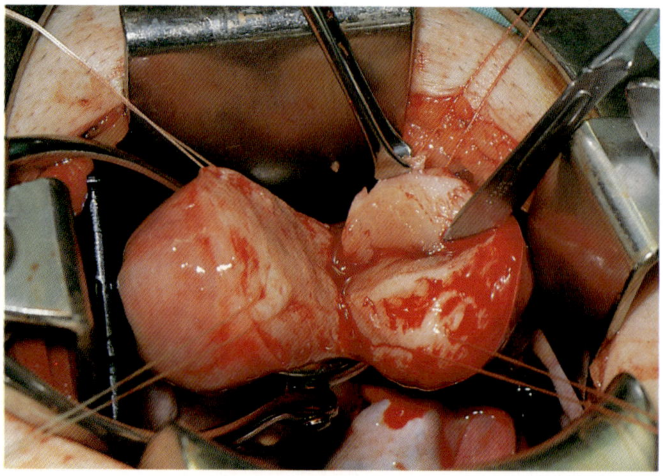

Fig. 38-100

Higher magnification, same.

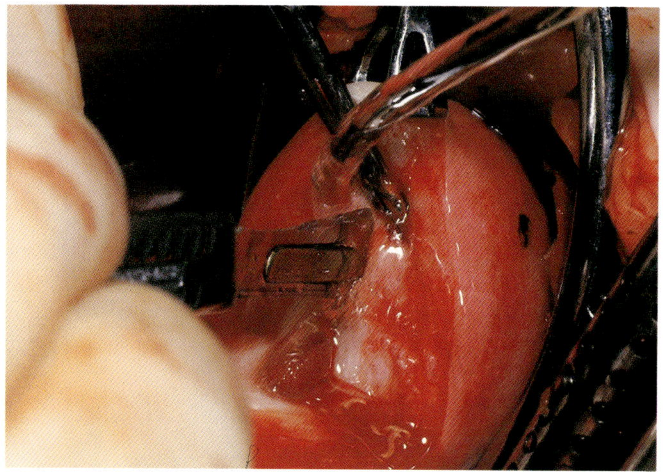

Fig. 38-101

Bilateral open endometrial cavities by vertical incisions.

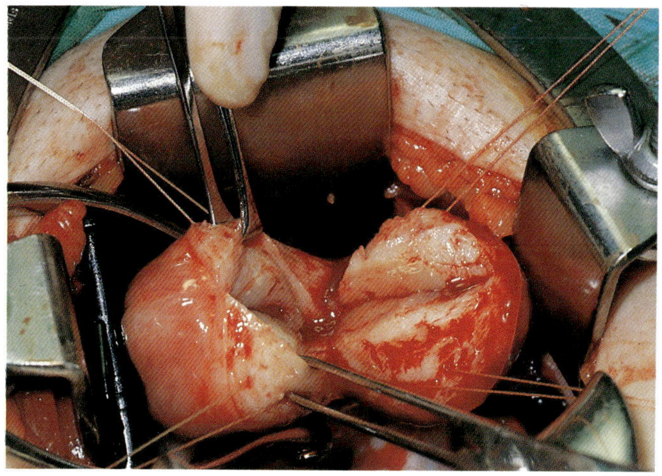

Fig. 38-102

Partial closure.

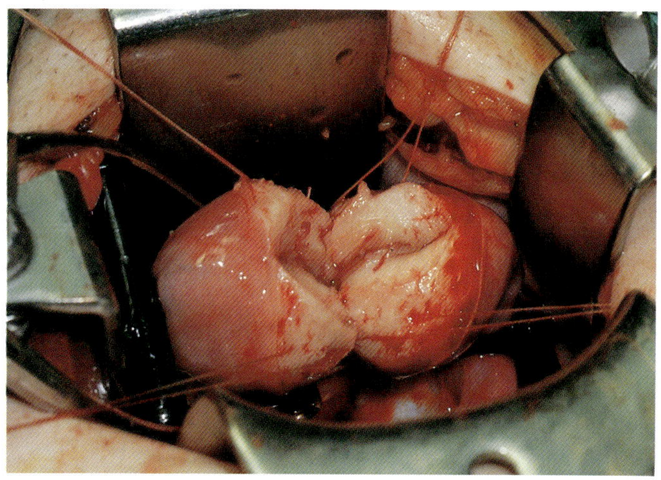

Fig. 38-103

Further closure.

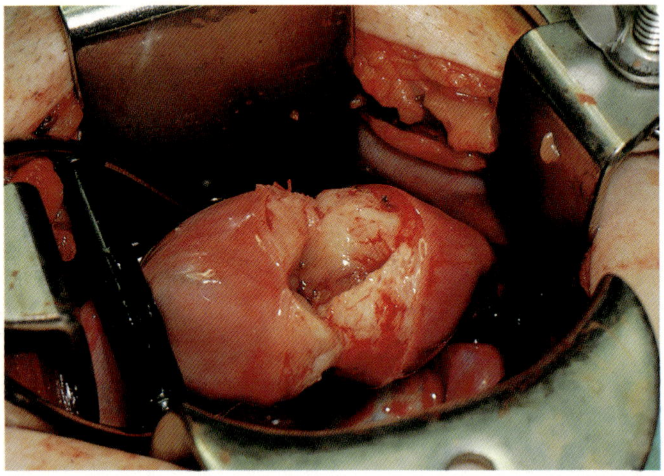

Fig. 38-104

New endometrial cavity.

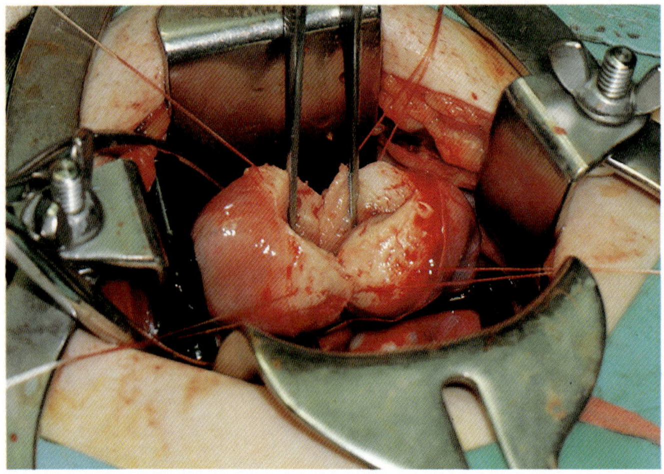

Fig. 38-105

Opening the cervix.

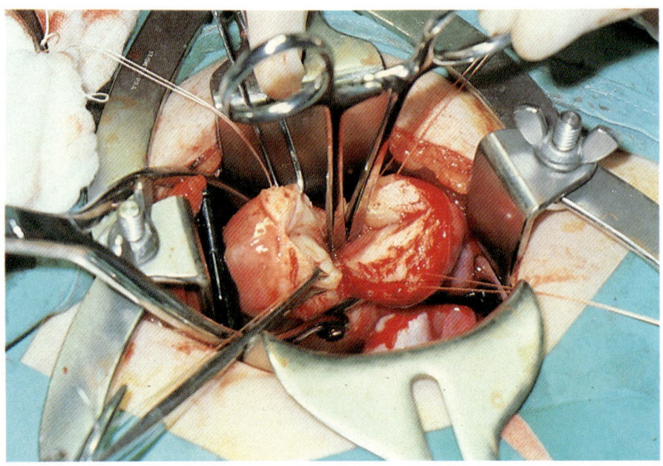

Fig. 38-106

Insertion of Lippes loop to maintain open cavity without adhesions.

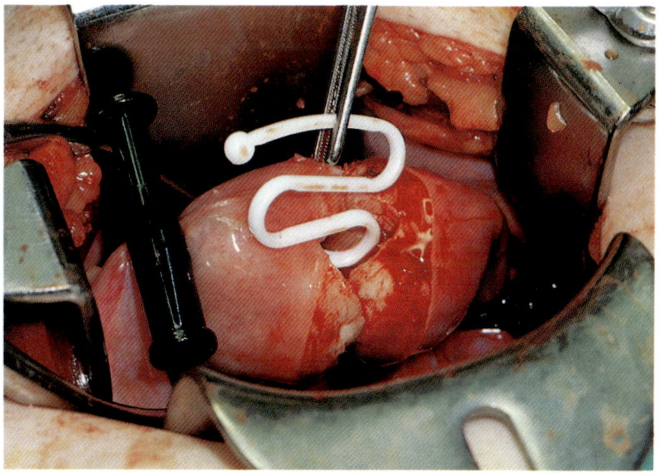

Fig. 38-107

Serosal closure with 5-0 Vicryl suture.

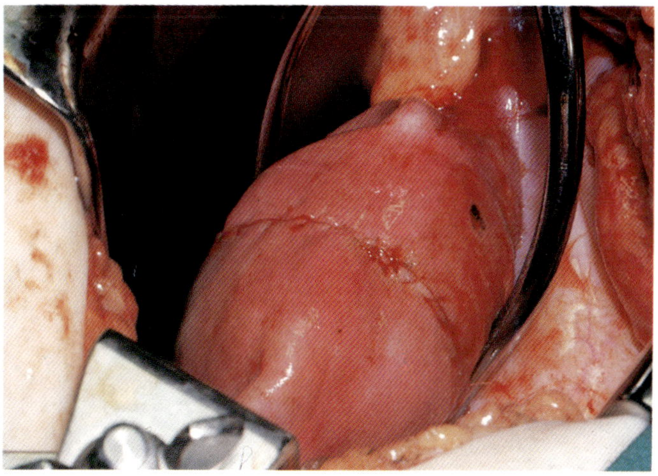

Fig. 38-108

Closure with 3-0 interrupted sutures, another case.

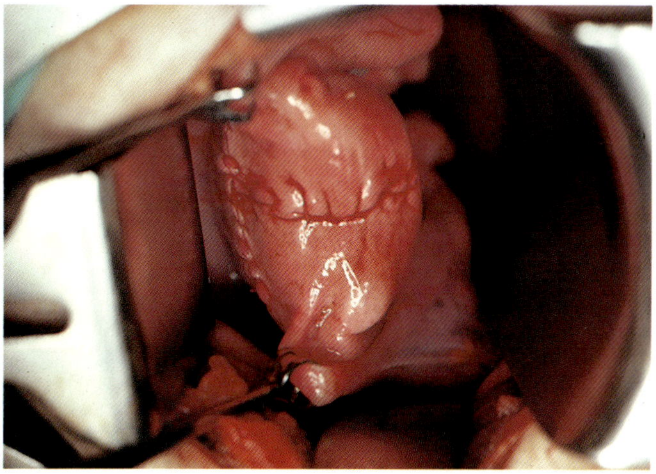

Fig. 38-109

The patient had an uneventful recovery; delivered a normal child at term by cesarean section.

References

1. Hunt R. *Atlas of Female Infertility Surgery*. Chicago, Ill: Year Book Publishers; 1986.
2. Reyniak J, Lauersen G. *Microsurgical Techniques in Infertility*. New York, NY: Plenum Medical Publishers; 1987.